# The Medical Legacy of
# Moses Maimonides

*by*

Fred Rosner, M.D.

KTAV Publishing House, Inc.
1998

Library of Congress Cataloging-in-Publication Data

Rosner, Fred.
    The medical legacy of Moses Maimonides / by Fred Rosner.
        p.    cm.
    Includes bibliographical references and index.
    ISBN 0-88125-573-4
    1. Maimonides, Moses, 1135–1204.  2. Medicine in rabbinical literature.
    3. Medicine, Medieval.   I. Title.
    R135.5.R667    1998
    610—dc21                                                                97-16874
                                                                                    CIP


                    Manufactured in the United States of America
                            KTAV Publishing House, Inc.
                        900 Jefferson St., Hoboken, NJ 07030

To my wonderful children

Mitchel and Lydia
Miriam and Motty
Aviva and Michael
Shalom and Tamar

הנה נחלת ה' בנים (תהלים קכז:ג)

Children are a blessing bestowed by the grace of God

—*Mezudat David*

# Contents

# Foreword

It may be safely asserted that no Jewish medical author of old has given rise to such a vast amount of literature as Maimonides did. I think, moreover, that I am right in maintaining that no author produced such a great number of books, monographs, translations, papers on Maimonides-the-Physician during the past thirty years as Fred Rosner did. He has certainly contributed, more than any other modern scholar, to the awareness of a wide range of readers, particularly physicians, of Maimonides' excellence as a medical author. As I remarked in the preface of a recent volume containing the Proceedings of a conference held in Jerusalem on "Moses Maimonides, Physician, Scientist, and Philosopher," both Jews and Arabs consider Maimonides among their most illustrious scholars, as an exemplary personification of the accomplished medieval scholar.

In this volume, Fred Rosner has collected some twenty essays which were (in their great majority) published in various journals, books, or collections of papers. The very fact that these sources pertain to different fields such as medicine, history, and Jewish Studies, causes difficulty of access to the wider public of readers interested in Maimonides' writings. It will be seen therefore as a welcome initiative to allow scholars and students to be able to peruse these studies more easily at leisure.

Several works of Maimonides are epitomized by Rosner in his usual clear and concise way: the Treatises on Asthma and on Poisons, and the Medical Aphorisms. I particularly value a less widely-known work of Maimonides, his Commentary on Hippocrates' Aphorisms. Rosner provides us with a translation of this work's introduction. "These are aphorisms," writes Maimonides. "which every physician, and even non-physician, should know by heart." The author announces that he will explain them briefly, and only comment on those aphorisms which require explanation. The aphorism on which he will "dwell a little longer" is the first one, indeed the most widely-cited aphorism, even in non-medical literature.

Rosner then comments on a large number of medical topics scattered throughout Maimonides' works, pertaining to cardiology, surgery, ophthalmology, geriatrics, nephrology, and dentistry (among others). Hygiene and preventive medicine follow. Here we may remark that Maimonides considered that the art of medicine should be divided into three domains, the first—and most important—being preventive medicine. He calls it "guidance of the healthy", i.e., advising how to behave in order not to lose your health. The second domain is what is called today, in a rather reductionist approach, medicine: treating the sick. The third and most original specification is in caring for those who are neither sick nor healthy, as are those who have recently been cured, while still being weak and shaky. Maimonides very cunningly includes advice to old people (i.e., gerontology) in this category.

The last chapter deals with medical notes taken from Maimonides' halakhic works, and with the Prayer which has been attributed (falsely, as Rosner well knows) to Maimonides. This lofty ethical document, unfortunately spurious, is probably the most widely-circulated text attributed to The Master of Cordoba.

In such a collection of essays, unequal in length and in scope, repetitions cannot obviously be avoided. On the other hand, the index is helpful to trace the places where a given topic can be found and diverse aspects confronted.

Let us now come back to the first aphorism of Hippocrates: "Life is short, long is the art, fleeting the occasion." It is hoped that Rosner's life will be long enough to enable him to publish, within a reasonable number of years, another volume of essays on Maimonides, who was called by the great (non-Jewish) modern medical scholar William Osler, "the prince of Physicians."

Samuel S. Kottek, M.D.
Harry Friedenwald Chair, History of Medicine
Hebrew University, Hadassah Medical School
Jerusalem

# Preface

The ten authentic medical treatises of Moses Maimonides have been published in English in seven volumes by the Maimonides Research Institute of Haifa, Israel (1984–1996). Maimonides' discussions of medical topics in his *Mishneh Torah* have been compiled in a volume entitled *Medicine in the Mishneh Torah of Maimonides* (KTAV, 1984). Statements and discussions pertaining to medicine in his *Commentary on the Mishnah* have also been published (*Koroth* 9 (1988), pp. 565–578).

*The Medical Legacy of Moses Maimonides* is a compilation of essays pertaining to the ten authentic medical books written by Maimonides, as well as essays which extract many medical discussions from his *Mishneh Torah, Guide of the Perplexed, Mishnah Commentary,* and other works. Of particular note is a responsum by Maimonides on longevity in which he proves, from medical and Jewish sources, that human lifespan is not predetermined but can be affected by our actions. Also of interest are his recommendations concerning the therapeutic efficacy of chicken soup and other fowl products. Medical aphorisms dealing with surgery, ophthalmology, urology, dentistry, geriatrics, and a host of other topics are cited. Maimonides' famous treatises on health and preventive medicine—including his depiction of the need for both physical and mental health—are presented in depth in this book.

The reader will develop a deeper insight into Maimonides the physician, his medical life, his medical thinking and his medical writings. The reader will also learn that the famous and beautiful "Physician's Prayer of Maimonides" is a fake and was not written by Maimonides but by Marcus Herz in Germany in 1783.

I am indebted to the editors of the following journals for permission to reprint several articles: *American Journal of Kidney Diseases, American Journal of Surgery, Bulletin of the History of Dentistry, Bulletin of the History of Medicine, Chest, Clio Medica, Geriatrics, Headache, Journal of Asthma, Koroth, New York State Journal of Medicine, Postgraduate Medicine.* Several of the chapters in the book have not been published elsewhere.

I am also grateful to my friend and colleague, Professor Samuel S. Kottek for his helpful advice and for writing the foreword. Finally, I thank the publisher, Mr. Bernard Scharfstein and his able staff, including editors Richard White and Sam Elowitch, for their painstaking efforts in bringing this work to the reader in an attractive and easily-read format.

Fred Rosner, M.D.
October 1997
Rosh Hashanah 5758

# Medical Writings

# The Medical
# Writings of Maimonides

Moses son of Maimon (known as Maimonides in English, and as Abu Imran Musa ibn Maimun in Arabic, and often referred to by the Hebrew acronym Rambam) was born in Cordova, Spain, on March 30, 1135 (or 1138 according to several recent essays), corresponding to Passover eve of the Hebrew year 4895. His mother died in childbirth, and consequently his father, a *dayyan* (judge), raised him. Persecution by the Almohades, a fanatical sect from North Africa, forced the Maimon family to flee Cordova in the year 1148. The family wandered through southern Spain and northern Africa for the next ten years and finally settled in Fez, Morocco.

Little is known of Maimonides' early life and medical education. There are no sources indicating that Maimonides had any formal medical education. In his *Medical Aphorisms* (see below), he mentions "the elders before whom I have read"; this is the only allusion to some semiprivate study of medicine. A few times he mentions the son of Ibn Zuhr, from whom he heard teachings of the latter's illustrious father (the great physician Abu Marwan ibn Zuhr), whom Maimonides held in great esteem.

Maimonides must have been an avid reader, since his medical

writings show a profound knowledge of ancient Greek authors in Arabic translation and of Moslem medical works. Hippocrates, Galen, and Aristotle were some of his Greek medical inspirations, and Rhazes of Persia, al-Farabi, and Ibn Zuhr, the Spanish-Arabic physician, are Moslem authors frequently quoted by Maimonides.

The Maimon family left Morocco in 1165, traveled to Palestine, landing in Acco, and from there to Egypt, where they settled in Fostat (Old Cairo). Maimonides turned to medicine as a livelihood only after the death of his father in 1166 and the death of his brother in a shipwreck shortly thereafter. Maimonides was left with his brother's wife and child to support and, after a year's illness following his brother's death, entered into the practice of medicine. He was appointed court physician to Vizier al-Fadil, regent of Egypt during the absence of the sultan, Saladin the Great, who was fighting in the Crusades in Palestine. It was at this time that Richard the Lion-Hearted, also fighting in the Crusades, is reported to have invited Maimonides to become his personal physician, an offer which Maimonides declined. His reputation as a physician grew in Egypt and neighboring countries, and his fame as a theologian and philosopher became worldwide.

In 1193, Saladin died and his eldest son, al-Afdal Nur al-Din Ali, a playboy, succeeded him. As a result, Maimonides' medical duties became even heavier, as described in the famous letter he wrote to his friend, disciple, and translator, Rabbi Samuel ibn Tibbon, in the year 1199:

> I live in Fostat and the Sultan resides in Cairo; these two places are two Sabbath limits [marked-off areas around a town within which it is permitted to move on the Sabbath; approximately one and one-half miles] distant from each other. My duties to the Sultan are very heavy. I am obliged to visit him every day, early in the morning, and when he or any of his children or concubines are indisposed, I cannot leave Cairo but must stay during most of the day in the palace. It also frequently happens that one or two of the officers fall sick and I must attend to their healing. Hence, as a rule, every day, early in the morning, I go to Cairo and, even if nothing unusual happens there, I do not return to Fostat until the afternoon. Then I am famished but I find the antechambers filled with people, both Jews and Gentiles, nobles and common people, judges and policemen, friends and enemies—a mixed multitude who await the time of my return.

I dismount from my animal, wash my hands, go forth to my patients, and entreat them to bear with me while I partake of some light refreshment, the only meal I eat in twenty-four hours. Then I go to attend to my patients and write prescriptions and directions for their ailments. Patients go in and out until nightfall, and sometimes, even as the Torah is my faith, until two hours and more into the night. I converse with them and prescribe for them even while lying down from sheer fatigue. When night falls, I am so exhausted that I can hardly speak.

In consequence of this, no Israelite can converse with me or befriend me [on religious or communal matters] except on the Sabbath. On that day, the whole congregation, or at least the majority, comes to me after the morning service, when I instruct them as to their proceedings during the whole week. We study together a little until noon, when they depart. Some of them return and read with me after the afternoon services until evening prayer. In this manner, I spend the days. I have here related to you only a part of what you would see if you were to visit me.

As this account indicates, Maimonides was also the spiritual leader of the Jewish community of Egypt. At age thirty-three, in the year 1168, shortly after settling in Fostat, he completed his first major work, the *Commentary on the Mishnah*.[1] In 1178, ten years later, his magnum opus, the *Mishneh Torah*, was finished.[2] This monumental work is a fourteen-book compilation of all biblical and talmudic law and remains a classic to this day. In 1190, Maimonides' great philosophical masterpiece, the *Guide for the Perplexed*, was completed.[3]

Maimonides died on December 13, 1204 (Tevet 20, 4965, in the Hebrew calendar), and was allegedly buried in Tiberias. Legend relates that Maimonides' body was placed upon a donkey and the animal set loose. The donkey wandered and wandered, and finally stopped in Tiberias. That is the site where the great Maimonides was buried.

---

1. See D. Kapach, *Mishneh, with the Commentary of Rabbi Moses ben Maimon.*

2. The Yale Judaica Series began publishing a translation of the entire work, entitled *The Code of Maimonides*, in 1949. Another translation of the first two volumes is M. Hyamson's, *Mishneh Torah: The Book of Knowledge by Maimonides* and *The Book of Adoration by Maimonides*. A one-volume selection of excerpts, with Hebrew and English on facing pages, is Philip Birnbaum, ed. and trans., *Maimonides' Mishneh Torah* (New York: Hebrew Publishing Co., 1967).

3. There are two English translations, that of S. Pines (Chicago: University of Chicago Press, 1963) and an earlier one by M. Friedländer (1881; reprint ed., New York: Dover Books, 1956).

Maimonides was a prolific writer. We have already mentioned his famous trilogy, the *Commentary on the Mishnah*, the *Mishneh Torah*, and the *Guide for the Perplexed*. Each of these works alone would have indelibly recorded Maimonides' name for posterity. However, in addition to these, he also wrote a *Book on Logic (Ma'amar ha-Higgayon)*,[4] a *Book of Commandments (Sefer ha-Mitzvot)*,[5] an *Epistle to Yemen (Iggeret Teman)*,[6] a *Treatise on Resurrection (Ma'amar Tehiyat ha-Metim)*,[7] commentaries on several tractates of the Talmud, and over six hundred responsa.[8] Several additional works, including the so-called Prayer of Maimonides, are attributed to him but are, in fact, spurious, the prayer having been written in 1783.[9]

Over and above all the books we have just enumerated, Maimonides also wrote ten medical works.[10] The following is a brief examination and analysis of these medical writings. The first is called *Extracts from Galen* or *The Art of Cure*. Galen's medical writings consist of over one hundred books and required two volumes just to catalogue and index them all. Maimonides therefore extracted what he considered the most important of Galen's pronouncements and compiled them verbatim in a small work intended primarily for the use of students of medicine. This work, like all of Maimonides' medical books, was originally written in Arabic. At least two Arabic manuscripts exist today, one in Hebrew letters and one in Arabic script. This work had heretofore never been published in any language, but brief excerpts in English and Hebrew appeared in a Hebrew periodical in 1955, and a complete English and Hebrew translation by Uri Barzel was published in 1992.[11]

---

4. I. Efros, *Maimonides' Treatise on Logic.*

5. C. B. Chavel, *The Book of Divine Commandments.*

6. S. Morais, "A Letter by Maimonides to the Jews of South Arabia."

7. J. Finkel, *Maimonides' Treatise on Resurrection.*

8. See below, chap. 20.

9. For a full account, see F. Rosner, "The Physician's Prayer Attributed to Maimonides," reprinted as chap. 22 of this book.

10. See F. Rosner, "Maimonides, the Physician: A Bibliography"; idem, "Maimonides the Physician: A Bibliography."

11. U. Barzel, "The Art of Cure"; idem, *Moses Maimonides' "The Art of Cure".*

The second of Maimonides' medical writings is the *Commentary on the Aphorisms of Hippocrates.* The famous *Aphorisms of Hippocrates* were translated from the Greek into Arabic by Ḥunain ibn Isḥaq in the ninth century. Maimonides wrote his commentary on this translation. Two incomplete Arabic manuscripts exist. A good medieval translation into Hebrew was made by Moses ben Samuel ibn Tibbon. In this work, Maimonides occasionally criticizes both Hippocrates and Galen where either of these Greeks differs from his own views. For example, in chapter 5, Hippocrates is quoted as having said, "A boy is born from the right ovary, a girl from the left," to which Maimonides remarks: "A man would have to be either prophet or genius to know this." The introduction to this work was edited in the original Arabic, with two Hebrew translations and one German, by Steinschneider in 1894.[12] The entire work was published by Hasida in 1935 and again in a definitive edition by Muntner in 1961.[13] Bar Sela and Hoff published Maimonides' interpretation of the first aphorism of Hippocrates.[14] This is the famous aphorism which has been called the motto or credo of the art of medicine: "Life is short, and the art long, the occasion fleeting, experience fallacious, and judgment difficult. The physician must not only be prepared to do what is right himself, but must also make the patient, the attendants, and the externals cooperate." In 1976 I published Maimonides' introduction to this work in English, and in 1987 the entire work.[15]

The third of Maimonides' medical works, the most voluminous of all, is the *Medical Aphorisms of Moses (Pirkei Moshe).* This book comprises fifteen hundred aphorisms based mainly on Greco-Persian medical writers. There are twenty-five chapters, each dealing with a different area of medicine, including anatomy, physiology,

---

12. M. Steinschneider, "Die Vorrede des Maimonides zu seinem Commentar über die Aphorismen des Hippokrates."

13. M. Z. Hasida, *Perush le-Pirkei Abukrat shel ha-Rambam*; S. Muntner, *Perush le-Pirkei Abukrat.*

14. A. Bar Sela and H. E. Hoff, "Maimonides' Interpretation of the First Aphorism of Hippocrates."

15. F. Rosner, "The Introduction of Maimonides to His *Commentary on the Aphorisms of Hippocrates.*" idem, *Moses Maimonides' Commentary on the Aphorisms of Hippocrates.*

pathology, symptomatology and diagnosis, etiology of disease and therapeutics, fevers, bloodletting, laxatives and emetics, surgery, gynecology, hygiene, exercise, bathing, diet, drugs, and medical curiosities. A complete Arabic original manuscript exists in the Gotha library in Germany. A Hebrew translation was made in the thirteenth century and published in Lemberg, Poland, in 1834 and again in Vilna in 1888.[16] The definitive Hebrew edition is that of Muntner, dated 1959.[17] Maimonides'*Aphorisms* were also translated into Latin in the thirteenth century and appeared as an incunabulum in Bologna in 1489 and again in Venice in 1497, followed by several printed Latin editions.[18] Only small fragments of this work appeared in a Western language[19] until the complete English version by myself and Muntner was published in two volumes in 1970–1.[20]

A few excerpts from this most important work will give the reader the flavor of Maimonidean medical thinking. Maimonides speaks of cerebrovascular disease:"One can prognosticate regarding a stroke, called apoplexy. If the attack is severe, he will certainly die but if it is minor, then cure is possible, though difficult. . . . the worst situation that can occur following a stroke is the complete irreversible suppression of respiration."

Maimonides explains that diabetes mellitus was seldom seen in cold Europe, whereas it was frequently encountered in warm Africa. He also reports this disease to be associated with the imbibition of suave water of the Nile (Maimonides lived in Fostat, or Old Cairo). There follows the English translation of a most important aphorism (no. 69) from the eighth chapter:

---

16. Z. Magid, *Medical Aphorisms of Maimonides (Pirkei Moshe)*.

17. S. Muntner, *Moshe ben Maimon: (Medical) Aphorisms of Moses in Twenty-five Treatises (Pirkei Moshe bi-Refuah)*.

18. See J. O. Leibowitz, "Maimonides' Aphorisms"; idem, "The Latin Translations of Maimonides' *Aphorisms*."

19. W. Steinberg and S. Muntner, "Maimonides' Views on Gynecology and Obstetrics"; F. Rosner and S. Muntner, "Moses Maimonides' Aphorisms Regarding Analysis of Urine"; idem, "The Surgical Aphorisms of Moses Maimonides"; F. Rosner, "Moses Maimonides and Diseases of the Chest."

20. F. Rosner and S. Muntner, *The Medical Aphorisms of Moses Maimonides*.

Moses says: I, too, have not seen it [diabetes] in the West [Spain, where Maimonides was born, or Morocco, where he fled from the Almoḥade persecution], nor did any of my teachers under whom I studied mention that they had seen it. However, here in Egypt, in the course of approximately ten years, I have seen more than twenty people who suffered from this illness. This leads to the conclusion that this illness occurs mostly in warm countries. Perhaps the waters of the Nile, because of their suaveness, may play a role in this.

A very accurate description of obstructive emphysema is provided during a lengthy discussion of respiratory disease: ". . . the reason [for respiratory embarrassment] is narrowing of the organs of respiration, then the breast is seen to greatly expand. This expansion produces rapid and cut off [respirations]."

Clubbing of the fingers associated with pulmonary disease, already described by Hippocrates, is beautifully depicted: "With an illness affecting the lungs called *hasal*, namely phthisis, there develops rounding of the nail as a rainbow." The signs and symptoms of pneumonia are remarkably accurately described: "The basic symptoms which occur in pneumonia and which are never lacking are as follows: acute fever, sticking [pleuritic] pain in the side, short rapid breaths, serrated pulse and cough, mostly [associated] with sputum." Hepatitis is just as beautifully described: "The signs of liver inflammation are eight in number as follows: high fever, thirst, complete anorexia, a tongue which is initially red and then turns black, biliary vomitus, initially yellow egg yolk in color which later turns dark green, pain on the right side which ascends up to the clavicle. . . . Occasionally a mild cough may occur and a sensation of heaviness which is first felt on the right side and then spreads widely."

So much for the *Medical Aphorisms of Moses.*

The fourth of Maimonides' medical writings is his *Treatise on Hemorrhoids.* This work was written for a nobleman, as Maimonides says in the introduction—probably a member of the sultan's family. There are seven chapters dealing with normal digestion, foods harmful to patients with hemorrhoids, beneficial foods, general and local therapeutic measures, such as sitz baths, oils, and fumigations. Maimonides disapproves of bloodletting or surgery for hemorrhoids except in very severe cases. Maimonides' whole approach to the problem seems to bespeak a modern medical trend. The *Treatise on Hemorrhoids* was first published by Kroner in 1911 in Arabic, Hebrew, and German.[21] A general description of the work in English appeared in 1927 by Bragman.[22] The definitive Hebrew edition is that of Muntner, dated 1965,[23] and an English translation of the entire work was published by myself and Muntner in 1969.[24] An improved, more fully annotated English translation was published in 1984.[25]

In the introduction to this work, Maimonides explains his reason for writing it:

> There was a youth, [descended] from knowledgeable, intelligent, and comprehending forebears, from a prominent and renowned family, distinguished and charitable and of great means, in whom the affliction of hemorrhoids occurred at the mouth of the rectum, who interested me in his problem and placed the task [of healing them] upon me. These irritated him on some occasions, and he treated them in the customary therapeutic manner until the pain subsided and the protruding hemorrhoids were reduced and returned to the interior of the body so that his [bodily] functions returned to normal. Because this [illness] recurred many times, he considered having them extirpated in order to uproot this malady from its source so that it would not return again. I informed him of the danger inherent in this, in that it was not clear whether these hemorrhoids were of the variety which should be excised or not, since there are people in whom they have once been [surgically] extirpated and in whom other hemorroids develop. This is because the causes which gave rise to the original ones remained, and therefore new ones developed.

Here Maimonides provides an insight into the etiology of disease in general, in that he regards operative excision of hemorrhoids with skepticism, because surgery does not remove the underlying causes that produced the hemorrhoids in the first place.

The fifth work is Maimonides' *Treatise on Cohabitation*, written for the nephew of Saladin, Sultan al-Muzaffar Umar ibn Nur Al-Din. The sultan indulged heavily in sexual activity and asked Mai-

21. H. Kroner, "Die Haemorrhoiden in der Medizin des XII und XIII Jahrhunderts."
22. L. J. Bragman, "Maimonides' Treatise on Hemorrhoids."
23. S. Muntner, *Moshe ben Maimon: On Hemorrhoids (Bi-Refuot ha-Tehorim).*
24. F. Rosner and S. Muntner, *Treatise on Hemorrhoids and Maimonides' Answers to Queries.*
25. F. Rosner, *Moses Maimonides' Treatises on Poisons, Hemorrhoids, and Cohabitation.*

monides, his physician, to aid him in increasing his sexual potency. The work consists mainly of recipes of foods and drugs which are either aphrodisiac or anti-aphrodisiac in their actions. Maimonides advises moderation in sexual intercourse and describes the physiology of sexual temperaments. There are two versions of this book, a short authentic one and a longer spurious version. Both were first edited and published by Kroner in 1906 in Hebrew and German.[26] Ten years later, Kroner published the true short version from the original Arabic manuscript in Granada.[27] An Italian edition appeared in 1906,[28] and English and Spanish translations were published in 1961.[29] The definitive Hebrew edition of both the authentic and the spurious versions of Maimonides' books on sex is that of Muntner, dated 1965.[30] A new English translation of the true work by myself was published in 1974 and subsequently reprinted.[31]

The sixth medical book of Moses Maimonides is his *Treatise on Asthma*. The patient for whom this book was written suffered from violent headaches which prevented him from wearing a turban. The patient's symptoms began with a common cold, especially in the rainy season, forcing him to gasp for air until phlegm was expelled. The patient asked whether a change of climate might be beneficial. Maimonides, in thirteen chapters, explained the rules of diet and climate in general and those rules specifically suited for asthmatics. He outlined the recipes of food and drugs and described the various climates of the Middle East. He stated that the dry Egyptian climate was efficacious for sufferers from this disease and warned against the use of very powerful remedies. The

---

26. H. Kroner, *Ein Beitrag zur Geschichte der Medizin des XII Jahrhunderts.*

27. H. Kroner, "Eine Medizinische Maimonides Handschrift aus Granada."

28. U. DeMartini, *Maimonides, Segreto dei segreti.*

29. M. Gorlin, *Maimonides' "On Sexual Intercourse" (Fi'l-Jima)*; E. Chelminski, "Notas introductorias al `Guia sobre el contacto sexual' de Maimonides."

30. S. Muntner, *Moshe ben Maimon on the Increase of Physical Vigour (Ma'amar al Ḥizzuk Ko'aḥ ha-Gavra)*; idem, "Pseudo-Maimonides on Sexual Life."

31. F. Rosner, *Sex Ethics in the Writings of Moses Maimonides*; F. Rosner, *Moses Maimonides' Treatises on Poisons, Hemorrhoids and Cohabitation.*

first critical edition of this work appeared in Hebrew in 1940, edited by Muntner.[32] Additional manuscripts became available after World War II, and a corrected, improved, and revised second Hebrew edition appeared in 1963.[33] Only three hundred copies of this edition were printed, and thus a third edition was published by Muntner in 1965.[34] An English version of Maimonides' book on asthma was published in 1963,[35] and a French translation in 1965.[36] I have commented extensively on this work elsewhere.[37]

The last chapter of this work deals with concise admonitions and aphorisms which Maimonides considered "useful to any man desirous of preserving his health and administering to the sick." The chapter begins as follows: "The first thing to consider . . . is the provision of fresh air, clean water, and a healthy diet." Fresh air is described in some detail: "City air is stagnant, turbid, and thick, the natural result of its big buildings, narrow streets, the refuse of its inhabitants. . . . one should at least choose for a residence a wide-open site. . . . living quarters are best located on an upper floor . . . and ample sunshine. . . . Toilets should be located as far as possible from living rooms. The air should be kept dry at all times by sweet scents, fumigation, and drying agents. The concern for clean air is the foremost rule in preserving the health of body and soul." Let our air-pollution-control programmers take cognizance of Maimonides' prophetic statements about eight hundred years ago.

The seventh medical work of Maimonides is his *Treatise on Poisons and Their Antidotes*. It is one of the most interesting and popular works because it is very scientific and modern in its approach and was, therefore, used as a textbook of toxicology throughout the Middle Ages. The book was written at the request of Maimonides' noble protector, the grand vizier and supreme judge al-Fadil, who asked Maimonides to write a treatise on poisons for the layman by

---

32. S. Muntner, *Moshe ben Maimon: Sefer ha-Katzeret.*
33. S. Muntner, *Rabbi Moses ben Maimon: Sefer ha-Katzeret or Sefer ha-Misadim.*
34. S. Muntner, *Moshe ben Maimon on Asthma (Sefer ha-Katzeret).*
35. S. Muntner, *The Medical Writings of Moses Maimonides: Treatise on Asthma.*
36. S. Muntner and I. Simon, "Le traité de l'asthme de Maïmonide."
37. F. Rosner, "Moses Maimonides' Treatise on Asthma." See also chap. 2 of this book.

which to be guided before the arrival of a physician. In the introduction, Maimonides praises al-Fadil and his feats in war and peace. He mentions al-Fadil's orders to import from distant lands ingredients lacking in Egypt but necessary for the preparation of two antidotes against poisoning, the "great theriac" and the "electuary of Mithridates."

The first section of the book deals with snake and dog bites and with scorpion, bee, wasp, and spider stings. The first chapter concerns the conduct of the victim in general. Thus Maimonides states as follows:

> When someone is bitten, immediate care should be taken to tie the spot above the wound as fast as possible to prevent the poison from spreading throughout the body; in the meantime, another person should make cuts with a lancet directly above the wound, suck vigorously with his mouth, and spit out. Before doing that, it is advisable to disinfect the mouth with olive oil, or with spirit in oil. . . . Take care that the sucking person has no wound in his mouth or rotten teeth. . . . should there be no man available to do the sucking, apply cupping-glasses, with or without fire; the heated ones have a much better effect because they combine the advantages of sucking and cauterizing at the same time. . . . Then apply the great theriac. . . . Apply some medicine to the wound that will draw the poison out of the body.

In his book on poisons, Maimonides also describes the long incubation period for rabies (up to forty days). Numerous Arabic, Hebrew, and Latin manuscripts are extant.[38] A German translation was published in 1873 by Steinschneider.[39] A French translation appeared in 1865 by Rabbinowicz and was reprinted in 1935.[40] An English translation of Steinschneider's German version is that of Bragman in 1926.[41] The definitive Hebrew edition of Muntner appeared in 1942,[42] and Muntner's English version was published in 1966.[43] I commented on this work[44] and subsequently published a

38. F. Rosner, "Moses Maimonides' Treatise on Poisons."
39. M. Steinschneider, "Gifte und ihre Heilung."
40. I. M. Rabbinowicz, *Traité des poisons.*
41. L. J. Bragman, "Maimonides' Treatise on Poisons."
42. S. Muntner, *Moshe ben Maimon: Samei ha-Mavet ve-ha-Refuot ke-Negdam.*
43. S. Muntner, *Treatise on Poisons and Their Antidotes.*
44. F. Rosner, "Moses Maimonides' Treatise on Poisons," reprinted as chap. 3 of this book.

fully annotated new English translation with commentary and bibliography.[45]

The eighth book is the *Regimen of Health* (*Regimen Sanitatis*), which Maimonides wrote in 1198 during the first year of the reign of Sultan al-Malik al-Afdal, eldest son of Saladin the Great. The sultan was a frivolous and pleasure-seeking man of thirty, subject to fits of melancholy or depression due to his excessive indulgence in wine and women and his warlike adventures against his own relatives and in the Crusades. He complained to his physician of constipation, dejection, bad thoughts, and indigestion. Maimonides answered his royal patient in four chapters. The first chapter is a brief abstract on diet taken mostly from Hippocrates and Galen. The second chapter deals with advice on hygiene, diet, and drugs in the absence of a physician. The extremely important third chapter contains Maimonides' concept of "a healthy mind in a healthy body," one of the earliest descriptions of psychosomatic medicine. He indicates that the physical well-being of a person is dependent on his mental well-being, and vice versa. The final chapter summarizes his prescriptions relating to climate, domicile, occupation, bathing, sex, wine drinking, diet, and respiratory infections.

The whole treatise on the *Regimen of Health* is short and concise but to the point. This is the reason for its great success and popularity throughout the years. It is extant in numerous manuscripts. A Hebrew translation from the original Arabic was made by Moses ben Samuel ibn Tibbon in 1244, and this version was reprinted several times in the nineteenth century (Prague, 1838; Jerusalem, 1885; Warsaw, 1886). Two Latin translations were made in the thirteenth century. Several fifteenth-century incunabula and sixteenth-century editions of these Latin versions exist. One of the first Hebrew editions was that of Bloch in 1838.[46] An annotated German translation by Winternitz was published in 1843;[47] and Rus-

---

45. Rosner, *Moses Maimonides' Treatises on Poisons, Hemorrhoids, and Cohabitation.*
46. S. Bloch, "Mikhtav ha-Rav Rabbenu Moshe ben Maimon be'ad ha-Sultan."
47. D. Winternitz, *Das Diatetische Sendschreiben des Maimonides an den Sultan Saladin.*

sian and Spanish translations in 1930 and 1961, respectively.[48] The Arabic text with German and Hebrew translations was published by Kroner in 1925,[49] although he had already published the all-important chapter 3 dealing with psychosomatic medicine eleven years earlier in 1914.[50]

English translations of chapter 3 have been published by Bragman, Savitz, and Butterworth, and of the first two chapters by Skoss.[51] The definitive Hebrew edition is that of Muntner, dated 1957,[52] although the Maimonidean bibliographer Dienstag cites several additional Hebrew editions.[53] Two English translations of the entire work have been published: in 1958 by Gordon and in 1964 by Bar Sela, Hoff, and Faris.[54] Another German translation by Muntner appeared in 1966.[55] These numerous editions in many languages attest to the importance and popularity of Maimonides' *Regimen of Health.*

The ninth medical writing of Maimonides is the *Discourse on the Explanation of Fits.* This work has been called Maimonides' swan song, as it was thought to be the last of his medical works, having been written in the year 1200, four years before his death. It was also written for the Sultan al-Malik al-Afdal and is sometimes considered to represent chapter 5 of the *Regimen of Health.* The sultan persisted in his overindulgences and wrote to Maimonides, who was himself ill, asking advice about his health. Maimonides con-

---

48. I. K. Shmukler, *Pismo Moishe Maimonida k Egipetskomu Sultanu*; E. Chelminsky, "La Preservación de la Juventud de Maimonides, Version Castellana."

49. H. Kroner, *"Fi tadbir as sihhat,* Gesundheitsanleitung des Maimonides für den Sultan al-Malik al-Afdhal."

50. H. Kroner, *Die Seelenhygiene des Maimonides.*

51. L. J. Bragman, "Maimonides on Physical Hygiene"; H. Savitz, "Maimonides' Hygiene of the Soul"; C. E. Butterworth, "On the Management of Health": S. L. Skoss, "The Treatises of Maimonides on Health Care."

52. S. Muntner, *Moshe ben Maimon: Hanhagat ha-Beriyut.*

53. J. I. Dienstag, "Translators and Editors of Maimonides' Medical Works."

54. H. L. Gordon, *Moses ben Maimon, The Preservation of Youth: Essays on Health* (*Fi Tadbir as-Sihha*); A. Bar Sela, H. E. Hoff, and E. Faris, *Moses Maimonides' Two Treatises on the Regimen of Health.*

55. S. Muntner, *Regimen Sanitatis oder Dietetik für die Seele und den Korper mit Anhang der Medizinischen Responsen und Ethik des Maimonides.*

firms most of the prescriptions of the sultan's other physicians regarding wine, laxatives, bathing, exercise, and the like, and, near the end, gives a very detailed hour-by-hour regimen for the daily life of the sultan. The original Arabic was edited and published with Hebrew and German translations by Kroner in 1928.[56] Also available are English editions by Bar Sela, Hoff, and Faris in 1964 and myself and Muntner in 1969,[57] another German version by Muntner in 1966,[58] and another Hebrew edition by Muntner in 1966.[59] The most recent and best edition is that by Leibowitz and Marcus, entitled *On the Causes of Symptoms*, in which the text is presented in four languages (Arabic, Hebrew, Latin, and English) and is accompanied by a running commentary, explanatory essays, and a comprehensive catalogue of drugs.[60]

The final authentic medical book of Maimonides is the *Glossary of Drug Names*. This work was discovered by Max Meyerhof, an ophthalmologist in Egypt, in the Aya Sofia library in Istanbul, Turkey, as Arabic manuscript no. 3711.[61] Dr. Meyerhof edited the original Arabic and provided a French translation with a detailed commentary, which he published in 1940 in Cairo.[62] A Hebrew edition by Muntner appeared in 1969,[63] and my English translation was published in 1979.[64] The work is essentially a pharmacopoeia and consists of 405 short paragraphs containing names of drugs in Arabic, Greek, Syrian, Persian, Berber, and Spanish.

In summary, Maimonides' medical writings are varied, comprising extracts from Greek medicine, a series of monographs on health in general and several diseases in particular, and a more

---

56. H. Kroner, "Der Medizinische Schwanengesang des Maimonides."
57. Bar Sela, Hoff, and Faris, *Moses Maimonides' Two Treatises on the Regimen of Health*; Rosner and Muntner, *Treatise on Hemorrhoids and Maimonides' Answers to Queries.*
58. Muntner, *Regimen Sanitatis.*
59. S. Muntner, *Moshe ben Maimon: Hanhagat ha-Beriyut.*
60. J. O. Leibowitz and S. Marcus, *Moses Maimonides On the Causes of Symptoms.*
61. M. Meyerhof, "Sur un glossaire de matière arabe composé par Maïmonide" and "Sur un ouvrage médical inconnu de Maïmonide."
62. J. Meyerhof, *Un glossaire de matière médicale, composé par Maïmonide (Sarh Asma al'Uqqar).*
63. Muntner, *Moshe ben Maimon: Biyur Sheimot ha-Refuot.*
64. F. Rosner, *Moses Maimonides' Glossary of Drug Names.*

recently discovered pharmacopoeia demonstrating Maimonides' extensive knowledge of Arabic medical literature and his familiarity with several languages. Some people feel that Maimonides' medical writings are not as original as his theological and philosophical writings. However, his medical works demonstrate the same lucidity, conciseness, and formidable powers of systematization and organization so characteristic of all his writings. The *Book on Poisons*, the *Regimen of Health*, and the *Medical Aphorisms* of Maimonides became classics in their fields in medieval times.

I would like to conclude by citing a paragraph from my first paper on Maimonides:

> Maimonides died on December 13, 1204 [Tebet 20, 4965 in the Hebrew calendar] and was buried in Tiberias, Palestine. The Christian, Moslem and Jewish worlds mourned him. His literary ability was incredible and his knowledge encyclopedic. He mastered nearly everything known in the fields of theology, mathematics, law, philosophy, astronomy, ethics, and, of course, medicine. As a physician, he treated disease by the scientific [as opposed to the empiric and/or popular] method, not by guesswork, superstition, or rule of thumb. His attitude towards the practice of medicine came from his deep religious background, which made the preservation of health and life a divine commandment. His inspiration lives on through the years and his position as one of the medical giants of history is indelibly recorded. He was physician to Sultans and Princes, and as Sir William Osler said, "He was Prince of Physicians." The heritage of his great medical writings is being more and more appreciated. To the Jewish people he symbolized the highest spiritual and intellectual achievement of man on this earth; as so aptly stated, "From Moses to Moses there never arose a man like Moses," and none has since.[65]

---

65. F. Rosner, "Moses Maimonides (1135–1204)."

# ❧ 2 ❧

# The Treatise on Asthma

Moses Maimonides' *Treatise on Asthma*, like all his medical works, was originally written in Arabic, under the title *Maqalah Fi al-Rabo*. An original Arabic version with Arabic lettering is manuscript No. 601[9] in the Madrid library (formerly Escorial No. 888). Additional Arabic manuscripts but in Hebrew letters are manuscript No. 1211 of the National Library in Paris and Bodleian (Neubauer) manuscript No. 1202 in Oxford.[1] The Parisian catalogue lists this work with the notation "a few pages are not in proper order," but in reality Paris manuscript No. 1211 also contains three other Maimonidean medical treatises: the *Treatise on Poisons*, the *Regimen of Health*, and *Medical Responsa*.

Maimonides' *Treatise on Asthma* was twice translated into Hebrew and once into Latin. However, the extant manuscripts in the various libraries throughout the world have not all been adequately studied.

The first Hebrew translation, in 1320, apparently prepared from the Latin version (see below), was that of Samuel Benveniste, a Spanish physician from Saragossa. He was physician in the house of Don Manuel, brother of King Diego IV of Aragon. Benveniste's

---

1. M. Steinschneider, *Die Arabische Literatur der Juden*, p. 215; idem, *Die Hebraeischen Uebersetzungen des Mittelalters und die Juden als Dolmetscher*, pp. 767–68; S. Muntner, *Rabbenu Moshe ben Maimon: Sefer Ha-Katzeret o Sefer ha-Misadim.*

translation is extant in the following manuscripts: Parma–Rossi No. 1208, Bologna No. $20^5$, Paris No. 1173, Paris No. 1175, Paris No 1176, Vienna No. 151 (fol. 163, Gold fol. 86). There are differences among these manuscripts. In only one of the six manuscripts is the name of the translator (Benveniste) mentioned in chapter 12.[2] The Vienna manuscript is briefer than the others, and the Paris manuscripts are incomplete. The Bologna manuscript has the additional title *Sefer ha-Misadim* (lit., Book of Nourishments), probably because the unknown patient for whom the book was written asked for and was given nutritional advice in regard to which foods he should select and which he should avoid, and which regimen he should follow to be cured of his asthma. Steinschneider points out that the *Treatise on Asthma* contains parallel phrases and verbatim wording of various sections of Maimonides' *Regimen of Health*.[3] Steinschneider also points out that a fragment of Benveniste's translation was extant in the private library of Joshua H. Schorr.

The second Hebrew translation of Maimonides' *Treatise on Asthma* was that of Joshua Shatibi from Xativa (Játiva), Spain, about the end of the fourteenth century. He translated directly from the original Arabic into Hebrew. Shatibi was called "the scholar in every field of knowledge, especially medicine." A copyist's note in Munich manuscript No. 280 states that Shatibi translated this treatise for an unknown Jewish apostate of high standing at the court of King Juan I of Castile, who reigned from 1379 to 1390. The translator did not translate the title nor much of the Arabic text except for the names of therapies. Only two manuscripts of Shatibi's Hebrew version of Maimonides' *Treatise on Asthma* are extant today: Munich manuscript No. 280, fol. 35 (copy also in Munich manuscript No. 43 from the middle of the sixteenth century) and Steinschneider manuscript No. 30, fols. 66–92b. The latter is now in the National Library in Berlin as manuscript No. 232 and also contains several other Maimonidean medical treatises, including *Commentary on the Aphorisms of Hippocrates, Regimen of Health, Treatise on Sexual*

---

2. Steinschneider, *Die Hebraeischen Uebersetzungen des Mittelalters.*
3. Ibid.

*Intercourse, Treatise on Hemorrhoids, Medical Responsa,* and *Medical Aphorisms of Moses.*

Maimonides' *Treatise on Asthma* was translated into Latin by Armengaud de Blaise, a French scholar, in May 1302. The Latin version exists in Cambridge (Smith Catalogue, p. 92) as manuscript St. Peters, Cambridge 209[8] under the title *Tractatus Contra Passionem Asthmatis* or *De Regimine Egrorum et Sanorum et Specialiter de Asinate* (should be *asthmate*). An additional Latin manuscript is described by Friedenwald, who states that this work is "not found elsewhere in Latin translation. . . . This anonymous translation differs from that of Armengaud and is otherwise unknown."[4] It would thus appear that this manuscript, which is now part of the Friedenwald Collection of the Hebrew University in Jerusalem, differs from the Cambridge Latin manuscript described above.

Muntner writes that Dr. L. Bertolot in the Vatican discovered a fifteenth-century Latin manuscript containing translations of six of Maimonides' medical writings, including his *Treatise on Asthma.*[5] The others are his *Regimen of Health, Medical Responsa, Poisons and Their Antidotes, Treatise on Hemorrhoids,* and *Treatise on Sexual Intercourse.* This Latin manuscript is probably identical to the Friedenwald manuscript, which also contains the other five Maimonidean medical works in the same sequence. The Vatican and Friedenwald manuscripts begin and end with the same phrase: *Inquit Moyses filius Maymonis filii Abdelle cordubensis yspanus—Narravit nobis dominus rex . . . Finis. Explicit Tractatus Alrabo idest asmatis.*

Maimonides' *Treatise on Asthma* remained dormant for several hundred years until the early part of the twentieth century, when Dr. Herman Kroner, rabbi in a small town in Germany, began editing this work and translating it into German. Unfortunately, he died in 1930 before the task was completed.[6] Ten years later, Suessman Muntner published the first critical Hebrew edition of the *Treatise on Asthma,* based mainly on Paris Hebrew manuscript No.

---

4. H. Friedenwald, *Jewish Luminaries in Medical History*, pp. 99–100.
5. Muntner, *Rabbenu Moshe ben Maimon: Sefer Hakatzereth o Sefer Hamisadim*, p. 10.
6. F. Rosner, "Moses Maimonides' *Treatise on Asthma*," pp. 1227–30.

1173, which represents Benveniste's Hebrew translation.[7] Muntner's edition is complete with introduction, bibliography, remarks, commentary, and Hebrew, Arabic, Greek, and Latin indices. Also included are an analysis of Maimonides' *Treatise on Asthma*, a lengthy discussion on Maimonides the physician, an essay on "Asthma in Ancient Hebrew Literature," and a brief chapter devoted to "Modern Views on the Pathology and Treatment of Asthma." For the non–Hebrew reader, there is also an English summary of this Maimonidean book. Muntner's Hebrew edition was commented upon by Levy and reviewed by Nemoy.[8]

During the preparation of an English edition of Maimonides' *Treatise on Asthma* (see below), Muntner discovered numerous typographical and textual errors in his Hebrew edition. He, therefore, published a revised and corrected Hebrew edition in 1963. This second Hebrew edition is limited solely to the Hebrew text, and the reader is referred to the first edition for the profuse commentaries mentioned above. Since only three hundred copies of the second edition were published, Muntner published a third edition of only the Hebrew text but containing additional corrections. This edition is bound together with critical editions of two other Maimonidean medical works, the *Treatise on Hemorrhoids* and the *Treatise on Cohabitation*.

Muntner's English translation of the *Treatise on Asthma* was published in 1963[9] and contains a preface by the famed pediatrician Bela Schick, who says: "I was impressed by the depth of Maimonides' knowledge of the disease [i.e., asthma], by the clarity of the discussion of its cause and of the influence of the environment, as well as of the general health of the individual, upon the disease." In an introduction to the English version, the noted allergist M. Murray Peshkin points out that "in spite of spectacular modern advances made in the theoretical and practical aspects of the allergies, the studies of the asthmatic state, written in the 12th century by Maimonides, still merit our attention."

---

7. Muntner, *Rabbenu Moshe ben Maimon: Sefer ha-Katzeret o Sefer ha-Misadim.*
8. A. J. Levy, *He'arot le-Sefer ha-Katzeret le-ha-Rambam,* pp. 129–32; L. Nemoy, "Rabbenu Moshe ben Maimon: *Sefer ha-Katzeret.*"
9. S. Muntner, *The Medical Writings of Moses Maimonides: Treatise on Asthma.*

Shortly after the appearance of the English edition of Maimonides' *Treatise on Asthma*, Muntner, in collaboration with Isidore Simon, founder and editor of the Paris-based *Revue d'histoire de la médicine hébraïque*, published a French version but without notes, commentary, or index.[10]

From the time of the Greeks to the era of Maimonides to the present time, the significance of the name asthma has changed several times. The disease itself has changed even more, as physicians looked for different sets of symptoms that changed with their theoretical concepts of causality. It is, therefore, possible that Maimonides' *Treatise on Asthma* may not refer to what is today known as asthma. All one can say is that asthma was a difficulty of breathing or a pain in the chest.

In the introduction to this work, Maimonides praises his benefactor for having asked him to write the book. Maimonides points out that asthma should be treated according to the various causes that bring it about. He further states that one can only manage the disease properly if one has thorough knowledge of the patient's constitution and individual organs, the age and habits of the patient, the season and the climate. Maimonides asserts that in this book he intends to include general principles which might be useful to all people to preserve their health and to prevent disease. He then lists the thirteen chapters and their headings:

Chapter 1 advises on the best course of personal conduct in general.

Chapter 2 deals with dietary measures that should be adopted or avoided when one is afflicted with the disease under consideration.

Chapter 3 deals with foods to be taken or eschewed, with special emphasis on foods of familiar origin.

Chapter 4 deals with the preparation of the dishes commendable in this disease.

Chapter 5 deals with the quantity of food the patient may safely consume.

Chapter 6 deals with the number of meals to be taken in a given period of time.

Chapter 7 deals with beverages.

Chapter 8 deals with respiration and emotional processes.

Chapter 9 deals with bowel movement, eventually of holding back of evacuation.

---

10. S. Muntner and I. Simon, "Le traité de l'asthme de Maïmonide (1135–1204)."

Chapter 10 deals with habits of sleep and waking up, of bathing, massages, and coitus.

Chapter 11 deals with simple remedies and their use in this disease.

Chapter 12 deals with the composition of drugs which might be called for in treating this disease in line with the present treatise.

Chapter 13 includes short summaries which might be useful to any man desirous of preserving his health and administering to the sick, in the form of concise admonitions.

At the beginning of each chapter I also give a preview of its contents. May God assist me in this labor.

In the first chapter, Maimonides gives general advice regarding illnesses which are characterized by acute attacks, such as arthritis, migraine, asthma, kidney stones, and the like. He cites Galen, who recommends dietary means to treat and even to prevent these maladies. Maimonides states that hygienic principles can be grouped into seven categories, of which the first six are obligatory and the seventh is commendable: clean air, correct eating and drinking, regulation of one's emotions, exercise and rest, sleep and wakefulness, excretion or retention of wastes, and bathing and massaging. To these he adds the regulation of coitus as an important factor in a general health regimen. These are discussed in detail in the subsequent chapters.

Chapter 2 deals with nutritional and dietary measures to be adhered to or avoided by the patient suffering from asthma. Maimonides recommends that food be consumed in moderate amounts and be easily digestible. He states that a fattening diet is objectionable and may endanger life, especially in an asthmatic patient. Gas-generating foods and scalding-hot food should also be avoided.

In chapter 3, Maimonides lists a variety of poorly digestible foods, such as grossly sifted wheat flour, flour pudding, macaroni, and spaghetti, especially when these are fried in oil or treated with cane sugar or dipped in honey and fried, since all flour dishes which fatten the body are detrimental because they generate thick juices which block the body's vessels and passageways. Rather, flour should be finely ground and unadulterated. One should avoid gas-producing foods, such as black beans, peas, rice, lentils, nuts, onion, and garlic. Maimonides also describes the virtues and detriments of a variety of other foods, such as different types of meat and fowl, cheese, eggs, fish, vegetables, and fruits. Chicken soup is recommended for patients suffering from asthma, as is freshwater fish. Also efficacious for asthmatics are fennel, parsley, mint, penny royal, origanum, watercress, and radish, whereas lettuce, pumpkin, cauliflower, and turnip are harmful. Figs, quinces, and raisins in moderate amounts are beneficial, whereas watermelon, peaches, apricots, cucumbers, and fresh dates should be avoided.

Chapter 4 presents numerous recipes for the preparation of dishes helpful to the asthmatic patient. One example is a soup made from rue, beets, and chicken, cooked with or without beans.

Chapter 5 deals with the quantity of food one should consume. This quantity varies from person to person and from season to season. A person should cease eating before experiencing a sense of repletion or fullness. Overeating is one of the prime causes of many diseases and maladies, such as heartburn, diarrhea, and fainting. One should also not consume a large variety of foods during a single meal. Not only are the quality and quantity of food consumed important but also the sequence of consumption. Galen is cited as recommending that light dishes be consumed before heavy ones. Other authors are of the opposite view. Maimonides suggests that a single uniform dish, not too light or heavy, is preferred. He then points out the virtues of moderate exercise prior to eating and advises against such exercise immediately following a meal. He regards sexual intercourse, bloodletting, and the taking of hot baths immediately after eating as offenses against one's health because they involve strenuous physical and emotional exercise. Finally, Maimonides enumerates a variety of ailments which occur in people who insufficiently or inadequately digest their food: heartburn, loose stools, impotence, insomnia, lethargy, depression, urinary retention, fever, inflammation of the kidneys, spleen, liver, or joints.

Chapter 6 deals with the timing and number of meals one should eat. Maimonides suggests that healthy people should eat a single meal daily, and that the elderly and debilitated and those convalescing from illness should consume small quantities at frequent intervals. One should only eat when the stomach is empty. The time to eat again is when the food has left the stomach, when there is no aftertaste from eructation, and when one feels real appetite and salivates in the mouth—even then one should wait another half-hour. Maimonides then recounts his personal eating habits. He customarily ate only once in twenty-four hours, except on the Sabbath. In the winter he drank a little wine, depending on the degree of cold, before going to bed. For Moslems, to whom wine is prohibited, Maimonides suggests a fine honey drink.

Chapter 7 deals with beverages. Excessive imbibition of wine is said to be injurious in that it makes the drinker feel heavy, affects his brain and hearing, gives rise to severe diseases, and aggravates others, such as asthma. However, a small quantity of wine during or after meals is useful in the diet of the healthy and an excellent cure for many disorders in that it aids digestion, increases natural body warmth, and removes superfluities in the form of sweat and urine. Maimonides again offers a substitute for wine for Moslems, to whom wine is forbidden: honeyed drink (i.e., mead) seasoned with spices. He also lists spices which stimulate urination: lentils, borax, mint, anise, ginger, mastic, muscat nuts, and nard. Recommendations regarding the drinking of water include the following: it should be sweet, clear, and pure, boiled a little, and drunk from a clean vessel after it cools down. The best time to drink water is about two hours after eating.

Chapter 8 is concerned with rules of conduct regarding fresh air and psychic or emotional moods. Not only should air be fresh and clean but its temperature is important. On hot days, the air should be conditioned by spraying and sprinkling the floor with aromatic water, by flowers, heat-abating leaves, and draft. Conversely, on cold, rainy days, the air should be fumigated with perfumes which warm the body. Maimonides asserts that if a person is emotionally upset or mentally agitated, his physical well-being suffers and eventually he becomes physically ill. This statement is perhaps an early description of psychosomatic medicine, indicating that a deranged psyche can profoundly affect the somatic or physical well-being of an individual. Conversely, continues Maimonides, gaiety and joy gladden the heart, and stimulate the blood and mental activity. Excessive indulgence in the pursuit of pleasure, however, is injurious to one's health. The avoidance of illness induced by such excesses is by conducting oneself according to ethical and moral principles.

In chapter 9, Maimonides discusses constipation, urinary retention, and other forms of retention of body superfluities. A variety of oral cathartic preparations and antidiarrheal concoctions are described. One should try to regulate one's bowels by maintaining a regular and normal diet. Very potent cathartics should be avoided. Numerous types of enemas to cleanse the bowels are cited, and various emetics to cleanse the stomach are listed. The conditions under which all these remedies are to be used are clearly enunciated. For example, vomiting is best effected when the patient is in a raised position, so that nothing remains in the stomach. Maimonides then describes a series of experiments that he conducted on himself to regulate his bowels. Finally, he posits that urine stimulation, bloodletting, and purgation do not preserve health and should not be done on healthy people but reserved for cases of illness.

Chapter 10 deals with the effects of sleeping, waking, bathing, massage, and coitus on asthma. Sleeping immediately after meals is said to be harmful, as is washing with cold water. Sleeping after bathing is efficacious. The bath water should be warm and contain some salt. Massaging the body upon awakening in the morning and before going to bed at night is highly recommended. Several types of massaging are described, as are certain forms of exercise for the young and the elderly. The final portion of this chapter is devoted to a discussion of coitus, an excess of which is injurious even to healthy people. A man who indulges excessively in coitus suffers from memory lapses and decline in mental capacity, faulty digestion, and defective vision. Coitus should be avoided soon after a bath, soon after physical exercise or bloodletting, at daybreak, and when a person is hungry or fully satiated, or seriously ill.

In chapter 11, Maimonides discusses simple medicinal therapy for asthma. He advises the patient to use an experienced and expert physician who develops a rational treatment plan and implements it. He counsels against the use of "empiricists who do not think scientifically" but who succeed or fail purely by chance in treating patients. He cites the following parable: A patient who puts his life in the hands of a physician who has practical experience but lacks scientific training is like a mariner who places his trust in good luck, relying on the sea winds, which sometimes blow in the direction he desires but sometimes spell his doom. Maimonides is obviously cautioning against consultation with and treatment by medical quacks. In support of his position, he cites Galen and Hippocrates, who assert that medicines should be compounded scientifically and logically, according to the individual qualities of the patient. Specifically for asthma, Maimonides recommends enemas to drain the thick juices, and aromatic herbs "to fortify the brain and dry out any humidity therein." These should be employed once or twice a year. During an acute attack, chicken soup is advised if the patient is afebrile, and sweetened barley porridge if the patient has fever. Should these be insufficient to allay the attack, an enema should be used. For the most severe cases, an emetic may be necessary. The patient should sleep as little as possible and in a sitting position. Excessive bathing and strenuous physical exercise should be avoided, but light exercise may be beneficial.

Chapter 12 describes compound remedies for asthma in ascending order of potency. The mildest remedy is made from liquiritia, althaea, fleabane, and fennel boiled and strained into freshly made rose-water syrup. Maimonides endorses a remedy of Rhazes' to clear the lungs of moisture, ease respiration, and eliminate the cough: soak wheat bran overnight in hot water, filter, and add sugar and almond oil; place on the fire until it resembles a julep and drink when lukewarm. A mild remedy of Galen's for asthma consists of equal parts of seeded raisins and fenugreek cooked in clear water, sifted, strained, and left standing for a prolonged period. More potent remedies of Galen's are also described.

Maimonides cautions against the use of opiates except for severe cases of asthma. He details at some length the case of one of his patients who suffered from asthma, a young, thin, unmarried woman with a moderately warm constitution, for whom he prepared a remedy containing numerous ingredients. His purpose was "to cleanse her lungs, fortify her brain, and stop her catarrh." He states that no mention of this remedy is found in any of the medical texts written by ancient or modern physicians but that he had great success therewith. Maimonides again asserts that chicken soup assists in the expectoration and expulsion of pulmonary phlegm.[11] He points out that Ibn Zuhr preferred powders to oily pastes for "fortifying the brain" in asthmatic patients. Various formulas for ointments, fumigations, enemas, and purgatives are then described, and their varying degrees of potency are cited. Most of these formulae were taught to Maimonides by "Western [i.e., Moroccan] Masters," and only a few are recorded in medical books. He concludes this chapter by stating that he has only listed those remedies for asthma whose ingredients are easily available and whose preparation is simple.

The last and most important chapter of Maimonides' *Treatise on Asthma* is concerned with concise admonitions and aphorisms which he considered "useful to any man desirous of preserving his health [i.e., the patient] and ministering to the sick [i.e., the physician]." The chapter begins as follows: "The first thing to consider . . . . is the provision of fresh air, clean water, and a healthy diet." Fresh air is then described in some detail:

> . . . city air is stagnant, turbid, and thick, the natural result of its big buildings, narrow streets, the refuse of its inhabitants . . . one should at least choose for a residence a wide-open site. . . . living quarters are best located on an upper floor . . . and ample sunshine . . . toilets should be located as far as possible from living areas. The air should be kept dry at all times by sweet scents, fumigation and drying agents. Concern for clean air is the foremost rule in preserving the health of body and soul . . .

These air-pollution control measures, advocated by Maimonides about eight hundred years ago, seem appropriate indeed to the twentieth-century reader of this essay.

Maimonides maintains in this treatise that the healing of illness is dependent not only upon the therapeutic measures prescribed by

---

11. For further details, see below, chap. 19.

the physician but also the nature and constitution of the patient. In mild cases of illness, the physician should not interfere but allow nature to heal. If the physician errs and prescribes a therapy which is contrary to the course of nature, he may impede the cure or even aggravate the illness. Even if the physician prescribes correctly, and even if the patient follows the prescription precisely, it is possible that cure will not be effected because nature may not cooperate. The same may happen to the farmer; he does everything that is expected of him yet the seed brings forth no fruit if nature does not cooperate. Maimonides then quotes the famous aphorism of Rhazes, who said:

> When the disease is stronger than the natural resistance of the patient, medicine is of no use. When the patient's resistance is stronger than the disease, the physician is of no use. When the disease and the patient's resistance are equally balanced, the physician is needed to help tilt the balance in the patient's favor.

This rule of *primum non nocere* was already enunciated centuries earlier by Hippocrates, who said that the physician should help the patient and not harm him; if one cannot help, at least do no harm. Maimonides then criticizes "famous physicians who commit grave errors on patients who later succumb." Maimonides says that he has often observed physicians prescribe the use of strong purgatives for patients who did not even need a mild one. Some physicians commit gross blunders, according to Maimonides, yet the patient survives; others commit seemingly small errors and the patient dies. Anyone with common sense should keep this in mind. The genuine physician is always beset with doubts, whereas the charlatan thinks that everything is clear.

Maimonides cites Rhazes' aphorism which considers medicine to be an art, and Galen's assertion that "The medical art seems easy and simple to men of limited vision, but how profound and far-reaching was this art in the eyes of a man like Hippocrates." Maimonides makes reference to his *Commentary on the Aphorisms of Hippocrates*.[12] He also quotes Aristotle, who said that most people

---

12. See below, chap. 5.

die of the remedies given them, a clear reference to iatrogenic disease. Maimonides warns, however, that this observation should not lead to the abandonment of appropriate remedies. Medicine is an essential science at all times and in all places, not only for the ill but also for the healthy. However, one should seek out and consult with expert physicians who have complete mastery of theoretical and practical knowledge. Unlearned physicians should be avoided; if an expert physician is not available, one should rely only on nature, confirming Hippocrates' assertion that "nature cures disease . . . she takes no orders from man . . . nature does all that is necessary." Where a diagnosis is in doubt, it is best to rely on nature to cure the illness.

Maimonides then addresses himself humbly to the sultan for whom he wrote his *Treatise on Asthma*, saying:

> Do not assume that I am the right person in whose hands you might place your body and soul for treatment. Heaven be my witness that I myself know well that I am one of those who are not perfect in this art [of medicine] and who shrink from it because it is enormously difficult to attain its vastness.

The chapter continues with the observation that therapeutic measures developed by practical experience are more frequently employed than those arrived at by theoretical reasoning. Maimonides again warns against the use of "experienced" quacks. The genuine physician has at his disposal not only his own experience but that of all physicians over many generations up to the time of Galen and Hippocrates, as recorded in medical books. Another cardinal rule is that the physician should not treat the disease but the patient who is suffering from it.

The case of a young Moroccan patient who was wrongly treated and whose care was then taken over by one of Maimonides' teachers is cited in detail. Other cases of erroneous treatment with fatal outcome are also mentioned. Another case described in detail is the illness of Sultan Amrael Muselmin in Marrakesh, Morocco, treated by four of the greatest professors of medicine: Abu Ali ibn Zuhr, Serapion, Abu Alchassan ibn Kamniel of Saragossa, and Abu Ayub ibn al-Muallim of Seville. The strong young sultan recovered from his illness but later died, probably of an incorrect dosage of medicine. Maimonides investigated the circumstances surrounding the sultan's death and comments thereon at some length. He expresses admiration for the fundamental rules of medical practice in Egypt and enumerates several reasons for his admiration. Finally, he lists the circumstances where multiphysician consultations should be avoided.

Chapter 13, and thus the entire treatise, ends with the following prayer: "May God the Gracious and Truthful guide us on the right path to our salvation in eternity. Praise be to God forever and ever."

Maimonides' logical and systematic approach to the prevention, diagnosis, and treatment of illness in this treatise is typical of all his medical and other writings. His allusions to psychosomatic medicine and his discussion of iatrogenic disease, seemingly modern concepts, are especially noteworthy. His teachings that a bad physician is worse than none, that it is necessary to treat patients, not diseases, and that *primum non nocere,* should be taken to heart by all present-day students of medicine and medical practitioners.

# ⸨ 3 ⸩

# The Treatise on Poisons

The original Arabic version of Maimonides' *Treatise on Poisons and Their Antidotes* is available in Arabic script in the following manuscripts: Bodleian Uri No. 578, beginning missing, and No. 608, Escorial No. 884, written in 1312; Florence Medicea No. 253; Gotha No. 1986; Paris No. 2962, possibly lost; and Paris No. 1094.[1] The Arabic text with Hebrew lettering is extant in Manuscripts Bodleian Neubauer No. 1270-5; Bodleian Uri No. 78, middle part missing; Paris No. 1211, missing in the catalogue and perhaps should be No. 411; and Sassoon No. 573-10.

Maimonides' *Treatise on Poisons* was translated into Hebrew in the thirteenth century by Moses ibn Tibbon under the titles *Ma'amar ha-Nikhbad*, the literal meaning of which is "The Important Treatise" or "Treatise to the Honored One," and *Ha-Ma'amar be-Theriac*, the literal meaning being "Treatise on the Theriac," and is extant in more than a dozen manuscripts.[2] These include Bologna No. 20-2; Florence Medicea Plut No. 88, Codex No. 29; Munich No. 111-2, fol. 936; Paris No. 1124-7, incomplete; Paris No. 1173-4; Parma de Rossi No. 1280; Vienna No. 152, Gunzburg Number 165-b54; Steinschneider No. 30, fol. 104–Berlin No. 8:36; and Bodleian Neubauer No. 2585, fol. 16.

---

1. M. Steinschneider, *Die Arabische Literatur der Juden*, p. 213.
2. S. Muntner, *Samei ha-Mavet ve-ha-Refuot ke-negdam*, pp. xx, 236; M. Steinschneider, *Die Hebraeischen Uebersetzungen des Mittelalters und die Juden als Dolmetscher*, p. 764.

A second Hebrew translation of only the foreword of this work, probably by Zeraḥiah ben Yitzḥak ben Shealtiel Ḥen, is extant in Munich manuscript No. 280-2, fol. 37b, and copied in Munich manuscript No. 43-5, fol. 86.

The *Treatise on Poisons* was translated from the original Arabic into Latin by Armengaud de Blasius of Montpellier. Five Latin manuscripts are extant: Oxford Corpus Christi No. 125; Cambridge College St. Petrie No. 209; Vienna Tabula IV, 95 No. 5306-1; Parma de Rossi Latin No. 59, incomplete; and Bibliot. Medicini Practic I, No. 399.[3]

Friedenwald describes an additional Latin manuscript which Muntner states is the translation of John de Capua.[4] This manuscript is probably identical to the one that Muntner states was discovered by L. Bertalot in the Vatican.[5] Friedenwald mentions that Maimonides' *Treatise on Poisons* is also found in Latin in Manuscript Palat No. 1298, fols. 189–205 in the Vatican Library, and in Codex No. 2280, fols. 89–99 of the National Library in Vienna.[6]

A German translation of this work, based on the unedited Bodleian Hebrew manuscript, was published by Steinschneider in 1873.[7] Steinschneider's translation is annotated and is followed by a brief essay on the family of Ibn Zuhr. The latter essay has no relationship to the Maimonidean treatise.

A French translation of Maimonides' work on poisons, based on the Hebrew version but in consultation with the Arabic text, was published by Rabbinowicz in 1865 and reprinted in 1935.[8] Rabbinowicz had access to the three manuscripts in the National Library in Paris: one Hebrew, one Arabic in Arabic letters (now lost), and one Arabic in Hebrew letters. Although Rabbinowicz's

---

3. M. Steinschneider, "Gifte und ihre Heilung," p. 62; S. Muntner, *The Medical Writings of Moses Maimonides. Treaise on Poisons and Their Antidotes*, vol. 2, pp. xxxviii, 77.

4. H. Friedenwald, *Jewish Luminaries in Medical History*, p. 99; Muntner, *Medical Writings of Moses Maimonides*, vol. 2, p. 10.

5. S. Muntner, *Sefer ha-Katzeret*, p. 10.

6. Friedenwald, *Jewish Luminaries in Medical History*, p. 99.

7. Steinschneider, "Gifte und ihre Heilung."

8. I. M. Rabbinowicz, *Maïmonide (Abou-Amram Moussa Ibn-Maimon, 1135–1204): traité des poisons*.

version is not annotated, it is preceded by a brief historical essay on poisoning and is followed by an alphabetic table of Arabic and Hebrew pharmaceutical names mentioned in Maimonides' *Treatise on Poisons* interpreted according to the *Traité des synonymes* of M. Clement-Mullet. Rabbinowicz's French edition stimulated the writing of two articles which outline and briefly comment on this medieval work on poisons.[9] Other articles deal in general with the natural sciences, particularly zoology, in the writings of Maimonides and specifically in his *Treatise on Poisons*.[10]

In 1926, Steinschneider's German translation was translated into English by Bragman.[11] No commentary was provided, and the translation is quite poor. There are numerous errors in translation, the translation is quite loose, and phrases or words which Bragman could not understand in the German are totally omitted.

A definitive Hebrew edition, based on Paris manuscript No. 1173, complete with introduction, bibliography, extensive commentary, numerous illustrations, appendices, and indices was published by Muntner in 1942.[12] Muntner also cites the books on poisons and their antidotes which preceded Maimonides' treatise; discusses the history of knowledge of poisons; describes the snake and its venom in the religion, poetry, and art of various peoples and snakes in the Bible and Talmud; and discusses poisonings in general and the poisons transmitted by snakes and mushrooms in particular. Shortly thereafter, Muntner wrote a brief article describing this work.[13]

In 1966, an English translation, said to be based on the Arabic original from Paris manuscript No. 1211, was published by Muntner, together with a photostatic reproduction of the entire Paris manuscript.[14] Muntner's English edition, which was reviewed by

---

9. L. Perel,"Sur quelques idées modernes dans le *Traité des poisons* de Maïmonide"; H. Herscovici, "Le traitement des morsures venimeuses d'après Maïmonide."

10. J. Aharoni, "Maimonides the Zoologist"; J. Theodorides, "Les sciences naturelles et particulièrement la zoologie dans le *Traité des Poisons* de Maïmonide."

11. L. J. Bragman, "Maimonides' *Treatise on Poisons.*"

12. See above, n. 2.

13. S. Muntner, "Maimonides' Book for Al-Fadil."

14. See above, n. 3.

DiCyan,[15] contains a preface, bibliography, illustrations, appendix, and index. The text itself is not annotated, and the translation is very loose, with errors of omission and commission, The translation often follows Rabbinowicz's French version, which was based on a Hebrew manuscript. In 1968 I wrote an article describing Maimonides' *Treatise on Poisons*, with emphasis on Muntner's English version.[16]

The *Treatise on Poisons and Their Antidotes* was written by Moses Maimonides, at the request of his lord protector, the Vizier Qadi al-Fadil, also known as Abu-Raḥim ibn 'Ali al-Baisani, in the Moslem month of Ramadan in the year 595, corresponding approximately to July, 1198. Maimonides himself states this in the introduction to his work, where he also mentions that he entitled his discourse *Treatise to the Honored One* or *Treatise of Fadil*.

> It was thus in the month of Ramadan in the year 595 that our Master addressed his humble servant as follows: "It occurred to me yesterday that someone could be bitten by a poisonous animal and die before he was able to reach us and take the theriac because the poison would already have disseminated throughout his body. . . . therefore, I command you too prepare a treatise, short in length and concise in style, indicating what the bitten person should begin to do." . . . I began to comply with your command and your request, and composed this treatise. I called it *The Treatise to the Honored One.*

The text is divided into an introduction and two main parts or sections, In the introduction, Maimonides praises Vizier al-Fadil for his modesty, his deeds of charity, his preserving of holy places from destruction, his diplomacy in peace and heroism in war, his redemption of prisoners and education of children, and his distribution among his people of all the blessings of wealth and riches which God had bestowed on him.

Maimonides then describes al-Fadil's orders to him to import from distant lands drugs which were lacking in Egypt for the preparation of the great theriac and the electuary of Mithridates. These costly remedies were to be distributed to any person suffering from

---

15. E. DiCyan, *"Treatise on Poisons and Their Antidotes* by Moses Maimonides."
16. F. Rosner, "Moses Maimonides' *Treatise on Poisons.*"

a poisonous bite or sting. Following this, al-Fadil asked Maimonides to compose a short treatise on the treatment of cases of poisoning by venomous animals prior to the arrival of a physician or until the patient could be brought to the dispensary to receive the theriac antidote.

## First Section

The first section of Maimonides' *Treatise on Poisons*, in six chapters, deals with the bites of snakes and mad dogs and the stings of scorpions, bees, wasps, and spiders. Chapter 1 concerns the conduct of the victim in general. Maimonides states as follows:

> When someone is bitten, strive to immediately tie and bind a ligature above the site of the bite as tightly as possible so that the poison does not disseminate throughout the body. . . . another person should make incisions with a knife at the site of the bite and suck with his mouth as strongly as he is able. He should spit out all that he sucks. He should first rinse his mouth with olive oil or wine and oil . . . and if there is no one available to do the sucking, strive to apply cupping glasses, either without fire or with fire; the latter are stronger. . . . empty the victim's stomach with a mild emetic . . . then take the great theriac . . . then, on the site of the bite, apply a medication which draws out the poison, either a simple or a compounded medication.

The Maimonidean description of emergency care for a victim of snakebite is as up to date as any twentieth-century textbook on toxicology or poisoning. We still apply ligatures proximal to the wound, incise the bite, and suck out the poison. Maimonides also recognized the need for the person sucking the wound to avoid absorbing any of the poison by first coating his mouth and palate with oil. Furthermore, Maimonides appreciated the value of cautery when he stated that cupping glasses with fire are more efficacious than those without fire.

Chapter 2 of section 1 deals with simple and compounded remedies which draw out the poison when applied to the bite or sting. Maimonides describes various efficacious preparations and names the easily procured, well-tolerated ingredients.

In Chapter 3, Maimonides provides information on the efficacy of simple remedies to be taken internally that are helpful to the snakebite victim. An apparent distinction is made between hematotoxic or hot and neurotoxic or cold effects of the particular poison when Maimonides states:

> I have not found any cooling remedy which is beneficial against a bite except for the mandrake root. It is not improbable that the hot or the cold remedy is beneficial for every poisoning. . . . if the patient is very hot, as occurs in someone who is bitten by a viper, it is best for him to choose from those remedies which are taken in milk or in vinegar. If the patient is very cold, as occurs in someone bitten by a scorpion, he should choose from those remedies which are taken in wine.

Aware that wine is prohibited to Moslems, Maimonides offers an alternative when he states: "If wine is forbidden to a person, these remedies should be taken in a decoction of anise." The preparation of the various simple remedies as well as the dosages for adults and children are then detailed,

Chapter 4 consists of descriptions of the various theriacs and electuaries, including the great theriacs, the asafoetida theriac of Rhazes, the nut theriac, the onion theriac of Ibn Zuhr, the electuary of Avicenna, and the antidote of Galen.

Chapter 5, still in the first section of the book, deals with specific remedies against the bites of certain animals. It first describes the treatment for a scorpion sting:

> Begin with the general therapeutic measures, as mentioned above, of incisions, sucking, and bandaging, followed by the application of a plaster to the site of the bite. Then take those non-compounded remedies specific for scorpion bites . . .

These specific remedies are detailed as follows:

> Drink three drachmas of the leaves of *bandranguya*, which is *herba citrina*, and rub the site of the bite therewith. Ethrog [citron] seeds and colocynth root constitute an exceptionally good remedy for a scorpion bite The maximum amount to take is two drachmas, and make a plaster thereof to place on the site of the bite. If it is fresh, pulverize it and rub the site [of the bite]. If it is dry, knead it in vinegar and apply a plaster thereof on the wound. Boil an ounce of *nanachah* seed in two liters of water until its strength has been extracted and wash therewith the site of the bite. So too, one part each of sulfur and fennel and two parts of garlic, all kneaded together and a plaster made thereof [and applied] on the site of the bite. Similarly, one part each of salt and flax seed and two parts of garlic all kneaded and a plaster made thereof [and applied] on the site [of the bite]. Similarly, the theriac of the

four [ingredients] is more efficacious than anything else for scorpion bites; take one to four drachmas thereof.

Chapter 5 continues with descriptions of the stings of various spiders, bees, and wasps and specific remedies for them. For snakebite, the best remedy is the great theriac. If not available, substitute the electuary of Mithridates.

Amazing in this chapter is Maimonides' recognition of the long incubation period for human rabies incurred from the bite of a mad dog.

> An old man who was a famous physician related to me that he once saw the son of a weaver in the weavery bitten by a dog. There was no sign to indicate that the dog was mad. As a result, the physicians said that it was a domesticated dog and they closed the wound after a month or a little more. The child recovered, much time elapsed, and he performed activities like a healthy person. Later, symptoms became apparent, he developed fear of water and died. Beware of this [type of situation] because there is no analogy to the virulence of poisons.

The final chapter of the first section deals with diet in general, and in particular for the bitten person, together with a few appropriate specifics. Dishes rich in salt, honey, and butter, and strong wine are recommended. The popular belief that unleavened bread is efficacious for someone bitten by a poisonous animal or for someone who has swallowed some poison is rejected by Maimonides as being without rational, scientific, or traditional basis.

## Second Section

The four chapters of the second section of Maimonides' *Treatise on Poisons* describe vegetable and mineral poisons and their antidotes. In the first chapter, dealing with precautionary measures against poisons, Maimonides seems too allude to the fact that since poison is a common means used to eliminate undesirable enemies or competitors, rulers and prominent people should beware of colored foods, thick broths, and astringent aliments with strong odors. He calls for exacting examination of all sharp and bitter foods before their ingestion. He also cautions against the ingestion or imbibition of foods or beverages with altered taste, odor, or color. He also discusses premeditated poisoning.

Be careful about [foods with] altered tastes and about various types of bad odors and about everything whose nature is not known. Also be careful about colored foods which we commonly use, such as thick soups like the Egyptian ones, and foods to which lemons have been added or whose appearance is altered, such as foods containing sumac or pomegranate juice or foods cooked in fishbrine or foods in which an apparently sour or styptic or extremely sweet taste predominates or which have a bad odor, such as those prepared with vinegar or those containing onions or those cooked with garlic. Only eat these [types of] foods if they were prepared by a reliable person about whom you have not the slightest doubt, because the cunning of those who wish to do harm by poisoning is only accomplished through foods in which the taste or the odor or the appearance of the poison is assimilated. On the other hand, such cunning is impossible with any foods cooked in water alone, whether meat or fowl, or roasted, because the slightest tampering therewith changes its taste or its appearance or its consistency or its odor. Similarly, such cunning cannot succeed in the case of pure water.

The second chapter deals with general rules for those who have either taken or believe they have taken poison. Emesis should be induced by means of hot water with *Anethum* and much oil, followed by fresh milk, butter, and honey, all of which should be vomited. Then the specific antidote should be administered.

Chapter 3 of the second section deals with simple and compounded remedies effective for the person who has swallowed one of the general varieties of poisons. Universal antidotes consist of the great theriac, the electuary of Mithridates, and the small theriac, composed of only four ingredients.

Ibn Zuhr is described as one of the greatest toxicologists, possessed of "vast experience, for he was the greatest tester of these remedies and occupied himself with them more than all other [physicians]. He was able to do so because of his great wealth and his expertise in the practice of medicine."

The final chapter of Maimonides' *Treatise on Poisons* details the treatment for one who knows what kind of poison he took. Here is described the wicked habit of women who strew poison, i.e., menstrual blood, into their husband's food and the difficulty with which the physician is faced in arriving at the correct diagnosis. Maimonides gives an excellent description of the symptoms of belladonna poisoning: "redness and a sort of excitation..."

Equally vividly described are the symptoms following ingestion of cantharides, or Spanish fly: "wounds in the bladder, hematuria, severe colic, and inflammation. Death intervenes after a few days."

## Comment

The *Treatise on Poisons* shows Maimonides to be a scientist who did not abide by medical dogma but experimented for himself or accepted the valid investigations of others. His originality, conciseness, and lucidity are reflected in every chapter. His recommendations in the twelfth century concerning first aid for poisoning still have much validity. For this reason, Maimonides' *Tractatus de Venemis* was one of the foremost textbooks of toxicology and therapeutics throughout Europe and the Near East in the Middle Ages. The age-old adage that an ounce of prevention is worth a pound of cure is evident from Maimonides' emphasis on preventive or prophylactic measures. Perhaps most interesting of all in this work is the distinction he makes between "hot" and "cold" poisons, which, according to Muntner, are equivalent to the modern hemolysins and neurotoxins. The latter are exemplified by the scorpion's poison, which "cools" and paralyzes the victim's respiratory center, with fatal outcome. Hemolysins, or "hot" poisons, are found in adder's poison, as from certain vipers, and produce hemorrhage, intravascular hemolysis, hypertension, fever, and death.

It is hoped that this brief exploration into the *Treatise on Poisons* will stimulate the reader to examine the entire work and evaluate for himself the genius of Moses Maimonides.

# ⁎ 4 ⁂

# Maimonides' Medical Aphorisms

The *Aphorisms of Moses* (*Fusul Musa fial tibb* or *Fusul el Qortobi* in Arabic; *Pirkei Moshe* in Hebrew; *Aphorismi Rabi Moysi* in Latin) was written by Moses Maimonides between 1187 and 1190. It is the most voluminous of all his medical writings and comprises twenty-five chapters, each dealing with a subspecialty in medicine. Each chapter or treatise is subdivided into aphorisms which follow a logical sequence. Most of the approximately fifteen hundred aphorisms in this work are based on the writings of Galen, including the latter's commentaries on the works of Hippocrates. Some years ago, Muntner commented upon the ninety works of Galen quoted by Maimonides in the *Aphorisms of Moses*, some of which are no longer available in the original.[1] However, Maimonides also refers to such famous Arabic physicians as al-Tamimi, Ibn Wafid, Ibn Zuhr, Ḥunain ibn Isḥaq, Rhazes, Avicenna (Ibn Sina), and many others. At the end of each aphorism, Maimonides cites his source. This he did not do in his earlier theological and philosophical writings, an omission for which he was severely criticized both during his lifetime and for many years thereafter. Most of the aphorisms

---

1. S. Muntner, "Reexamination of Galen's Books Listed by Maimonides in *Pirkei Moshe*."

are annotated and commented upon by Maimonides, and not an insignificant number are original with him. Maimonides' own statements always begin with "Moses says."

The *Aphorisms of Moses* was originally written in Arabic, as were all of Maimonides' medical works. A complete Arabic manuscript exists in the Gotha library in Germany. Maimonides' *Aphorisms* were translated into Latin in the thirteenth century, and there are at least two different versions extant in many editions.[2] One of the Latin translations was by John de Capua. It appeared as an incunabulum in Bologna in 1489 and Venice in 1497, and was rapidly followed by numerous Latin editions.[3]

Two Hebrew translations appeared almost simultaneously around 1277, one by Rabbi Nathan ha-Me'ati, the other by Rabbi Zerahiah ben Yitzhak ben Shealtiel Hen, both in Rome. The Hebrew translation of Rabbi Nathan ha-Me'ati was first published in Lemberg, Poland, in 1834, incomplete and with many errors. A second printing of this same poor edition appeared in Vilna in 1888.[4] A totally new Hebrew edition, with commentary, preface, English and Hebrew indices, bibliography, and appendix, was published by Muntner in 1959.[5]

Until fairly recently, Maimonides' medical aphorisms were not available in any vernacular other than the original Arabic and the Hebrew and Latin translations. In 1934 the foreword to the book was translated into German,[6] nine aphorisms from the twenty-fifth chapter were translated into English in 1939,[7] and the fifth and sixteenth chapters and other brief excerpts were published in American medical journals.[8] A complete English translation by Rosner

---

2. J. Leibowitz, "Maimonides' Aphorisms."
3. J. O. Leibowitz, "The Latin Translations of Maimonides' Aphorisms."
4. Z. Magid, *Pirkei Moshe.*
5. S. Muntner, *Moshe ben Maimon: Pirkei Moshe bi-Refuah.*
6. P. Kahle, "Maimonides Aphorismorum Praefatio et Excerpta."
7. J. Schacht and M. Meyerhof, "Maimonides Against Galen on Philosophy and Cosmology."
8. F. Rosner and S. Muntner, "Moses Maimonides' Aphorisms Regarding the Analysis of Urine"; W. Steinberg and S. Muntner, "Maimonides' Views on Gynecology and Obstetrics"; F. Rosner and S. Muntner, "The Surgical Aphorisms of Moses Maimonides"; F. Rosner, "Maimonides and Diseases of the Chest"; idem, "Geriatrics in the Medical Aphorisms of Moses Maimonides"; idem, "Ophthalmology in the Medical Aphorisms of Moses Maimonides."

and Muntner was published in two volumes in 1970 and subsequently reprinted.[9]

The *Aphorisms of Moses* are a rich collection of medical rules and regulations, selected mainly from the abundant works of Galen and the latter's commentaries on Hippocrates. Later works of Arabic physicians and others are also frequently quoted. Maimonides displays an exemplary knowledge and erudition of contemporary and less recent medical literature. What others could not express in lengthy treatises, he clarifies in concise and lucid phrases. With the systematic exactitude and meticulous methodology characteristic of all his writings, medical and otherwise, Maimonides presents in twenty-five chapters or treatises some aspects of various subspecialties in medicine, such as anatomy, physiology, surgery, balneology, gynecology, pharmacology, hygiene, and many others. He attempts to eradicate preformed opinions and dictated dogmas from the minds of students and physicians alike. He encourages them to experiment and observe for themselves, and to develop an attitude of keen criticism and skepticism toward accepted traditions and teachings even if these originate from so renowned a medical scholar or authority as Galen. Maimonides himself takes issue with many of Galen's views in the most important twenty-fifth treatise. The book is based almost entirely on rational medicine, independent observation, and the scientific method. Rule of thumb, guesswork, and superstition have no place in this work or in Maimonides' thinking, although an occasional "specific therapy" which he advocates may have no rational basis. A brief description of each chapter with some direct quotations and excerpts translated into English are the subject of this chapter.

Maimonides' reason for writing the *Pirkei Moshe*, the format used, the source material available at the time, and a general outline of the contents of the book are given in the foreword to the work, which follows in English translation. Words in brackets are additions to clarify the meaning but are not part of the original text.

---

9. F. Rosner and S. Muntner, *The Medical Aphorisms of Moses Maimonides.*

Thus speaks the author, Moses, the son of God's servant, the Israelite, from Cordova:

Many authors have written works in the form of aphorisms in various fields of knowledge. The science most in need of this [approach] is medicine, and this is because medicine contains precepts which, because of their multitudinous learning facets, are difficult to comprehend. It is further composed of tenets which contain basic knowledge, the latter already being difficult to understand, such as logic and grammar. Verily, medical knowledge does not delve into its contents with as much thoroughness as other subjects of learning, and, indeed, perseverance in this field is most difficult in many ways because of the necessity for learning and remembering innumerable facts; not only remembering the general principles but also paying heed to the details. Another reason [for the need for aphorisms in medicine] is to alleviate studying for the less knowledgeable individuals in this field of learning, as has already in actuality been demonstrated.

These works, written in the form of aphorisms, are undoubtedly easy [to grasp] and help the reader thoroughly understand their contents and remember them by heart. For this reason did Hippocrates, the greatest of physicians, write his famous work entitled *Aphorisms* in this fashion. Similarly, many physicians followed in his footsteps and composed aphorisms, such as the *Aphorisms of Razi*, the *Aphorisms El Susi* [probably referring to Ibn Sina, author of *Aphorismi de Anima*], and the *Aphorisms Ibn Messue*.

It becomes clear at first glance to the observant reader that anyone who writes aphorisms in any field of knowledge encompasses its fundamental principles. A further reason for authors to compose their works in the form of aphorisms is to commit the facts to memory so as not to forget them, either because they are easily forgotten or because they have practical application. In general, the intent of a writer of aphorisms is not to impart all the facts in his field of knowledge. Nor was this the intent of Hippocrates in his *Aphorisms* nor of Abu Nasser al-Farabi in all the works that he composed in the form of aphorisms, and certainly not other famous authors.

I have purposefully commenced with these preliminary remarks in order to state that the aphorisms collected in this book are to be understood in this light. Of this collection of aphorisms I shall not say that I have compiled [lit. authored]; rather, I have selected and collected from the words of Galen, out of all his works, meaning from his original works as well as from his commentaries on the works of Hippocrates.

I was not as zealous in the reproduction of these aphorisms as I was in the reproduction of the *Compendium Mukhtazareth* [another of Maimonides' medical writings]. In the latter I reproduced Galen's text word by word, whether it represented his own words or the original words of Hippocrates, both being inseparably interspersed in the commentaries of Galen on the works of Hippocrates. Some of the aphorisms contain partly the original words of Galen and partly my own words. Other aphorisms are completely my own as a result of independent research whenever I took issue with a statement of Galen's. What prompted me to this is the lack of clarity in certain propositions requiring elucidation from many scattered sources among the works of Galen. In such a case, I collected the intent of the aphorism in question and subjected it to critical analysis to determine its correctness. It is known to me that many people who cite previous authors' statements do so after thorough research. However, incorrect quotations are more numerous than correct ones. Therefore, at the end of each aphorism I have seen fit to cite the source chapter and book of Galen to which the particular aphorism in question has reference. Then, should anyone question the language or the intent of Galen, he can refer to the aphorism in question and find the original contents without deletion or addition. As soon as he becomes convinced, all doubts will disappear. No one in the world can criticize me for not mentioning that a given precept is mentioned in another article or that it is repeated in several places for didactic purposes, because, had I supported my contention with references to these places, I would still have been criticized and censured. To mention all source references would be superfluous, with no advantage, and would only have been an amassing of words. I explored the subject matter in question, mention of which is made in many places, and remained with my initial reference citation. I should also not be censured and criticized by people who say: "Why did you select an aphorism on this topic and not on another topic?" because our intent is as that of any writer of aphorisms; not to include everything. In examining any of these aphorisms, someone may object and say: "What was the intent of mentioning this aphorism to the exclusion of another, mention of which would have shown reliability and trustworthiness, since it is so famous?" It is precisely its widespread renown to practitioners of the art of medicine which obviates the necessity for repeating or even mentioning it.

In regard to another aphorism which I mention, one might say: "What you consider important is to me unimportant." To yet another, he might say: "What is incomprehensible to you is quite clear to all other physicians." The answer to these objections, then, is that a person does not select to the satisfaction of his neighbor but according to his own taste and inclination.

Therefore, I have selected the following aphorisms for myself to facilitate remembering them. Similarly, anyone who is at my level of learning, or who is less knowledgeable than I, can benefit from them. I have not selected and explained them for the use of someone at the level of Galen or close to it. I am, without a doubt, convinced that many of these aphorisms are already well known and do not need to be mentioned or learned by heart. Further, I do not think that what appears unfamiliar to me should be not at all strange to another. Similarly, I do not think that something which required much contemplation on my part should not require the same from another. Where I believed that I removed doubts, be it in substantiating the correctness of a subject or in clarifying a concept, I found some people who had no doubts initially. This is due to their complete knowledge of medicine.

In these aphorisms, I include some personal opinions, only the essences of which are stated. These are mentioned as my own, in the first person. In these aphorisms, I also bring the opinions of some modern scholars. These are mentioned according to their names.

I have subdivided these aphorisms into a number of treatises in order to facilitate remembering them or to use them to greatest advantage in what I have tried to disclose. The number of treatises is twenty-five.

The first treatise contains aphorisms pertaining to medical themes; specifically, morphological features of the organs of the human body, their activities and energies.

The second treatise contains aphorisms pertaining to bodily humors.

The third treatise contains aphorisms pertaining to basic methods, principles, and foundations of medicine.

The fourth treatise contains aphorisms pertaining to the pulse and its signs [i.e., its interpretation].

The fifth treatise contains aphorisms pertaining to urine and its signs.

The sixth treatise contains aphorisms pertaining to other symptomatology.

The seventh treatise contains aphorisms pertaining to some known and unknown etiological factors which are in dispute.

The eighth treatise contains aphorisms pertaining to general methods of treatment of disease.

The ninth treatise contains aphorisms pertaining to the treatment of special diseases.

The tenth treatise contains aphorisms pertaining to fevers.

The eleventh treatise contains aphorisms pertaining to the periods and stages of diseases and their crises.

The twelfth treatise contains aphorisms pertaining to purgation with laxatives and enemas.

The thirteenth treatise contains aphorisms pertaining to emptying [of the body] by means of laxative medications and enemas.

The fourteenth treatise contains aphorisms pertaining to emetics.

The fifteenth treatise contains aphorisms pertaining to general surgery.

The sixteenth treatise contains aphorisms pertaining to gynecology.

The seventeenth treatise contains aphorisms pertaining to general rules of health.

The eighteenth treatise contains aphorisms pertaining to physical exercise.

The nineteenth treatise contains aphorisms pertaining to bathing.

The twentieth treatise contains aphorisms pertaining to food and drink.

The twenty-first treatise contains aphorisms pertaining to general pharmacology.

The twenty-second treatise contains aphorisms pertaining to special remedies.

The twenty-third treatise contains aphorisms pertaining to definitions of diseases and of technical medical terms perhaps familiar to the physician but unfamiliar to the general public. Our intent is to do this reliably.

The twenty-fourth treatise contains aphorisms pertaining to medical curiosities which occasionally occur and are noted in medical books. These are only rarely found.

The twenty-fifth treatise concerns problematical statements in many places in the books of Galen which attracted my attention.

Chapter 1 of Maimonides' aphorisms is devoted exclusively to anatomy and physiology. First is a description of nerves, tendons, ligaments, and blood vessels. Maimonides distinguishes sensory and motor nerves and subdivides blood vessels into arteries, veins, and capillaries: ". . . arteries in the entire body communicate with veins and interchange some blood and air through these anastamoses which are so narrow as to be invisible to the eye." Arteries and veins are called pulsating and non-pulsating vessels respectively. The circle of Willis is described, as is the lamina cribrosa; "the bone, which protects the brain from the inside and the palate, is hollow. Anatomists call it the sieve." Maimonides recognizes that "the spinal cord . . . is surrounded by the same two membranes that surround the brain." The morphological and physiological descriptions of many body structures and organs, such as the eyeball, the larynx, the spleen, the kidneys, and the gallbladder, are provided. Muscle action is described in its various phases, including voluntary contraction and passive relaxation. The physiology of respiration and the relationship of the diaphragm and accessory muscles of respiration are vividly and accurately described: "The diaphragm alone is responsible for the ease of inhalation and exhalation. However, when exhalation becomes difficult, then intercostal muscles, pectoral muscles, shoulder and neck muscles participate as well." The physiology of sleep is compared to one's state of mentation during intoxication.

Maimonides hints at the lesser (pulmonary) circulation by emphasizing the connection between the right ventricle and the lung when he states: "The right chamber of the two chambers of the heart was created for the benefit of the lung. . . . Should the lung die, the right chamber of the two chambers of the heart also dies." He also subscribes to the three Galenical phases of digestion to explain the physiology of nutrition and adds a fourth of his own.

"The first stage is digestion in the stomach. . . . The second stage is the transition to the intestines, where it adds to . . . the liver substance. The third stage . . . the metabolism that occurs in every one of the organs. There is an additional metabolic phase, a fourth, which is called assimilation." The development of individual organs as well as the human organism as a whole is dependent upon several forces, the procreating force (*vis generationis*), the developmental force (*vis alterationis*), the structure-forming force (*virtus auctrix*) and the nutritive force (*virtus nutrex*). The latter is composed of four powers: attraction, retention, expulsion, and alteration (digestion or assimilation or metabolism). The first chapter ends with an aphorism describing the two types of stomach muscles, longitudinal and transverse: "The stomach has some threads which are stretched lengthwise with the function of attraction [of food] and some that are stretched widthwise with the function of squashing [food]."

Chapter 2 is devoted to the ancient concept of physiology dealing with the four humors: blood, white bile or phlegm, red (or yellow) bile, and black (melancholy) bile. The sites of production of these various substances are described and their various characteristics are outlined. Blood is considered the best, and black bile the worst. Disease consists of derangements in the normal qualities, quantities, or interrelationships of the bodily humors. Maimonides, quoting Galen, states: "The illnesses which occur as a result of black bile are cancer, elephant skin, psoriasis, quartan fever, confusion [depression], and thickness of the spleen." The etiology of peptic ulceration seems to be alluded to in two aphorisms: "The stinging liquid which is in the stomach . . . will sink into the folds of the stomach. . . . A sharp liquid which descends on one side and is retained [in the stomach] causes nausea and cannot be expelled. This liquid then returns and reascends, causing a burning in the stomach."

Chapter 3 is a lengthy treatise dealing with various basic ideas and teachings of ancient and medieval medicine. Heart disease is described as being compatible with long life but sometimes fatal: "Should the heart muscle dry out even a trifle, then the strength will rapidly wane. However, one can live many years in such a state.

He whose heart muscle completely dries out, however, is in a condition which leads to rapid wasting and weakness, and he will shortly expire." The relationship of the vascular arterial system to the heart under pathological conditions is portrayed as follows: "It is indeed impossible for the arteries to undergo a complete change without the heart being involved and suffering concomitantly."

Seasonal and climatic influences on disease are repetitively discussed throughout Maimonides' medical writings. Excerpts from this chapter include: "Bodily secretions are less in the winter because the cold makes them rigid, whereas in the summer they are plentiful because the heat dissolves them. . . . Semen and blood are of one constitution in the summer and a different constitution in the winter. . . . The worst [climate] in any country is that which is closed to easterly winds and where raw and cold winds prevail." Maimonides observed and describes cerebrospinal fluid and synovial fluid but considers them to be one and the same: "Between the vertebrae, should they separate somewhat, is a white sticky fluid similar to that which effluxes in other joints. Around the spinal cord, too, flows a sticky liquid similar to the fluid which flows around the ligaments which unite the vertebrae."

Further observations regarding the normal and pathological physiology of nutrition, digestion, and assimilation are recorded. A direct quotation from Galen is cited here without comment, whereas elsewhere Maimonides expresses amazement at such statements: "You should not be astonished that the right testicle in males has more warmth [than the left] and the right womb [in females] more than the left, and thus it is not strange why male fetuses develop on the right side and females on the left side."[10] Urinary sediments and their significance are mentioned briefly and are discussed in greater detail in chapter 5.

Amazing in aphorism 52 is the recognition by Maimonides that the cornea and chambers of the eye are completely avascular and nourished from retinal and other vessels: "There are no vessels

---

10. S. Muntner, *Moshe ben Maimon: Commentary on the Aphorisms of Hippocrates*, p. 109 (chap. 5, aphorism 48).

whatever in the crystalline, albugineous, and vitreous humors as well as in the corneal tunica. Even so, the crystalline humor is nourished from the vitreous humor through osmosis, and the vitreous [receives its nourishment] from the retinal tunica, which has abundant arteries and veins. The cornea, too, is nourished by osmosis from the uveal covering because the uvea also contains an abundant vasculature."

Of further interest is the description of the terminal branches of the nerves in the skin and the fact that loss of sensation in the skin overlying a muscle does not affect the movement of that muscle: "It should not be astonishing that if skin overlying a muscle loses its sensation, the movement of that muscle will not be abolished, because the nerve that grows and divides within that muscle has not been damaged, whereas that part [of the nerve] which sprouts and spreads into the skin was damaged." The following quotation from one of Maimonides' aphorisms is self-explanatory: "The most important [thing] in treating most illnesses is [the reestablishment of] homeostasis." The response of an individual to a noxious stimulus depends on his age and body condition or state of health, as is illustrated in the following aphorism: "A person who is constantly and regularly in good health can tolerate great stresses without causing a change in his body. However, the elderly, or those convalescing from illness or those actually ill, are subject to great changes in their bodies from even the weakest stimuli. Similarly, if an elderly person or one convalescing from an illness should veer even slightly from his [prescribed] diet, either in amount or type, great harm may ensue as a result. However, young people react only slightly even to very strong stimuli."

The theory of otitis media is outlined as follows: "Discharges originating from the roots of the ears which begin to dissolve spontaneously should not be squeezed, nor drawing salve applied. The fundamental principle under these conditions is that everything should be left to nature. If a pus blister forms, then it should be pierced, the fluid extruded or pressed out, and medication applied for resolution."

The following two aphorisms are as true today as they were in the twelfth century when Maimonides wrote them: "The following lesson is of great and important significance, worthy of committing to memory, namely, in arranging the composition of medications one should pay careful attention and direct one's willpower, because many times antagonistic medicines become mixed in which are useless and inappropriate for their intended use"; and "It is impossible to put together a single prescription that will cure all ailing bodies."

The fourth chapter deals with the pulse in health and disease. Thus, Maimonides states: "The sign which points to strong, unfailing health is a uniform pulse which is also totally regular." He further says: "The pulse of a newborn during the neonatal period is very rapid . . . the pulse of old people is rather slow . . . the pulse is fullest and strongest in the prime years of youth." Maimonides goes on to describe the different types of pulses, strong and feeble, slow and rapid, regular and irregular, and so on, with the causes leading thereto and the effects resulting therefrom. He also points out, however, that "regularity of the pulse cannot be used as a reliable prognostic sign." He recognizes the fact that the pulse accelerates secondary to fever, heartburn, nausea, eructation, hiccups, or aggravation of illness. Toward the end of chapter 4, in aphorism 44, is an unbelievable description of blood circulation refuting the to-and-fro theory several centuries before Harvey. Maimonides claims to have found this information in the seventh treatise of Galen's *Megapulse*. The translation is purposefully word for word: "Do not consider arterial movements in three dimensions as movement of a cubic form or a pointed shape called a cone and the like, but consider it as a movement in one direction as the movement of a ball so that the movement of the artery which produces sensation makes a complete revolution."

The fifth chapter contains aphorisms with lessons pertaining to the urine and its examination. Hints are provided regarding the possible relationship of disease states to the color, odor, and particulate matter or sediment of urine. Diabetes as an illness is mentioned by name in this chapter: "When urine resembling water is micturated repeatedly, as occurs in people with the illness diabetes."

Diabetes is described in greater detail in later chapters, including the symptoms of acidosis, which are enumerated in chapter 6. Hemoglobinuria is alluded to when Maimonides states that "black urinary sediments signify either fiery heat or extreme cold. Every urine which turns black is extremely malignant. I have never seen anyone who urinated black urine who survived." The fifth chapter ends with an aphorism in which Maimonides summarizes all of Galen's statements on urine signs and concisely outlines the four basic types of urine in his own characteristically clear and lucid manner.

The sixth chapter is concerned with various prognostic signs. At the outset Maimonides speaks of cerebrovascular disease: "One can prognosticate regarding a stroke, called apoplexy. If the attack is severe, then he will certainly die, but if it is minor, then cure is possible, though difficult. . . . the worst situation that can occur following a stroke is the completely irreversible suppression of respiration."

Undoubtedly, Maimonides is describing diabetes when he states: "Individuals in whom sweet white [humor] occurs are very somnolent [ketoacidosis or hyperglycemia?]. To those who have an excess of sour white [humor], hunger occurs [hypoglycemia?]. If an excess of salty white [humor] occurs, they become extremely thirsty. When this white liquid is neutralized, the thirst will disappear." Later, in chapter 8, we are told that Galen mentioned that he only saw two cases of diabetes. However, Maimonides explains that diabetes mellitus was seldom seen in "cold" Europe, whereas it was frequently encountered in "warm" Africa. He also reports this disease to be associated with the imbibition of sweet water of the Nile. (Maimonides lived in Fostat, or Old Cairo.) Below is the English translation of this most important aphorism, no. 69, from the eighth treatise: "Moses says: I, too, did not see it in the West [Spain and/or Morocco], nor did any of the teachers under whom I studied mention that they had seen it [diabetes]. However, here in Egypt, in the course of approximately ten years, I have seen more than twenty people who suffered from this illness. This leads to the conclusion that this illness occurs mostly in warm countries. Perhaps the waters of the Nile, because of their sweetness, may play a role in this."

Continuing in chapter 6, we find a description of the signs of inflammation and pus formation. Psychiatric illnesses, including manias, phobias, and depression (melancholia), are also precisely depicted. Polycythemic bleeding was already recognized by Maimonides, as he states: "Sometimes epistaxis can occur during [apparent] health secondary to an excess of blood." Prognostication from the appearance of the tongue is related in aphorism 19. Further prognostication is delineated in aphorism 27: "If the illness is stronger than the resistance [of the patient], then the patient will certainly die. . . . The longer the disease persists, the more certainly do the signs indicate a fatal outcome." An excellent description of unilateral headaches or migraine headaches follows. An erroneous statement of Galen's is perpetuated by Maimonides: "Movement of the tongue is mediated through the seventh pair of the cranial nerve pairs" (should be the twelfth or hypoglossal). A very accurate description of obstructive emphysema is provided during a lengthy discussion of respiratory disease: "the reason [for respiratory embarrassment] is narrowing of the organs of respiration, then the breast will be seen to greatly expand. This expansion will produce rapid and cut-off [respirations]."

Clubbing of the fingers associated with bronchiectasis is beautifully depicted in aphorism 51: "With the illness affecting the lungs called *hasal*, namely phthisis, there develops rounding of the nail as a rainbow. If the tongue becomes cyanotic . . ." The signs and symptoms of pneumonia are remarkably accurately depicted in aphorism 54: "The basic symptoms which occur in pneumonia and which are never lacking are as follows: acute fever, sticking [pleuritic] pain in the side, short rapid breaths, serrated pulse and cough mostly [associated] with sputum." Hepatitis is just as beautifully described: "The signs of liver inflammation are eight in number, as follows: high fever, thirst, complete anorexia, a tongue which is initially red and then turns black, biliary vomitus initially yellow egg yolk in color, which later turns dark green, pain on the right side which ascends up to the clavicle. . . . Occasionally a mild cough may occur and a sensation of heaviness which is first felt on the right side and then spreads widely." The value of palpation as part of the physical examination is stressed as being vital in making a correct diagnosis of intraabdominal pathology: "Arriving at a diagnosis of a process which is below the hypochondrium and is causing spasm is by palpation and light massage. Thus, one will know whether a hot [acute] inflammation or a hard inflammation [abscess or tumor] or flatulence or pus or fecal impaction lies therein. When one knows what illness [is causing the abdominal signs], one can plan ways to eradicate it."

A pearl of wisdom comes near the end of this chapter, where we find the following quotation: "From the medical theoretical standpoint, it suffices to deliberate and speculate regarding most illnesses. However, therapeutically, speculation is not adequate, and true and correct knowledge is imperative." The next-to-last aphorism is a lengthy dissertation by Maimonides on the pathogenesis of disease. Body homeostasis or health is that situation in which "there is complete harmony between the various activities of the body." This is all dependent upon the body's spiritual, physical, and natural powers (*virtus spiritualis, animalis,* and *naturalis,* respectively).

The seventh treatise (chapter) deals with etiologies of disease. Moderation in eating, drinking, exercise, and emotional extremes is among "the things which cause an increase and invigoration of bodily strength. . . . The things which weaken bodily strength and diminish it are of eight etiologies: fasting, insomnia, anxiety . . ." Next follows a description of the effect of emotions on health. The causes which may lead to shock, or "collapse," are related by Maimonides after he strongly criticizes Galen for disorganization and lack of completeness in discussing this topic. Maimonides enumerates and explains twenty-one types of collapse falling into six major categories. A clear and concise statement regarding psychosomatic medicine is expressed in this chapter: "Just as bodily humors influence man's moods [or temperaments], so, too, do moods influence humors."

The causes of pruritis, tremors, skin sores, osteoporosis [lit. wasting of bones], mental confusion, headache, and many other maladies are related. Even arteriosclerosis was already recognized, as evidenced by this statement: "The causes leading to hardening of arteries are one of the following three: either they become dry or congealed from the cold or stretched." Parasitic disease was also well known to Maimonides: "Worms called gourd-grains or cucumbers [ascaris or tenia] consume all that an individual has eaten, and thus the body will become slender." Later, in chapter 23, filariasis and dracunculus medinensis worm infestation are described. Sneezing is considered a good prognostic sign. Chills, fever, shivering, "goose pimples," trembling, tachypnea, hoarseness, and similar physical phenomena are explained and their causes depicted.

The etiology of duodenal ulcer is strongly alluded to in aphorism 53: ". . . food remains undigested in the stomach. Proof that heat prevails in that location is that some relief is obtained from cold things and also from the pyrosis which occurs." The cause of "pain in the right shoulder blade" in hepatitis and cirrhosis is elucidated. A description suggestive of Addison's disease erroneously places the cause in the spleen rather than the adrenal, as follows: "If his spleen is weak, then his appearance will be dark brown, the reason being dissolution and combination with black biled blood." Visual disturbances are depicted, including the visual *mouches volantes*, or "mosquitoes," one sees flying about secondary to vitreous opacities or following intoxication. The following aphorism speaks for itself: "Laughter that occurs during tickling of the axillary region and the soles of the feet, as well as the laughter that occurs when seeing comical things or when hearing comical things, has no practical diagnostic significance." The final aphorism in this chapter differentiates living creatures from plants "on five levels," in that the former are endowed with the senses of touch, taste, smell, hearing, and vision.

Chapter 8 contains aphorisms "pertaining to general therapeutic methods for [various] diseases". Here, three general stages of illness are described, including aggravation, crisis, and defervescence. "All illnesses are weaker during the initial and final stages, and are strongest during the acme." Death occurs during the crisis of an illness

and not at the outset or defervescence of the malady. The importance of physical examination, including observation and palpation,
is stressed: "One should note all findings as they are." The rule *primum non nocere* ("first do no harm") is strongly advocated. Maimonides states that therapy for a chronic illness may be prolonged
and require several changes in medication depending upon the
patient's response to the treatment employed. Purgation and bloodletting are part of the physician's armamentarium. Medications
should not be used when diet alone suffices: "[Patients with]
chronic illnesses need bland diets. Indeed, in many instances, this
therapy alone is sufficient for healing. . . . Measuring food in regard
to time, quality, and quantity is [often] sufficient to [aid] nature to
heal illnesses." Maimonides quotes Galen regarding the efficacy of
certain foods, such as barley gruel, *sela* fish in water, porret, anise
salt, and oil, in certain maladies. A most interesting aphorism
expresses the following: "Anxieties represent pain of the soul
[psyche]. Thoughts and meditations are the physical exercise of the
soul. All emotions [lit. movements of the soul] give rise to biliary
liquids." Thus, as in the previous chapter, Maimonides recognizes
the fact that "mental exercise," or emotions, can have a profound
effect on bodily organs and their functions. This certainly represents the modern concept of psychosomatic medicine.

Next follow rules regarding drug therapy. Firstly, the importance
of individualization for each patient is stressed. Secondly, the
strengths of medications should be commensurate with the severity
of the problem, as he states: "Medications which alleviate pain,
namely those which contain sedative [analgesic] and somniferant
drugs, should only be taken in cases where pain is unusually strong
and severe, causing the patient to cry out [in agony], such as severe
colic or [kidney] stones or unbearable insomnia. . . . For any [ill-
ness] that is less serious than those we have just enumerated, it suffices to use non-sedative medications." The aims of such therapy are
threefold: ". . . sensation should be numbed; secondly, no residual
damage should remain in the affected limb after therapy, and
thirdly, the afflicted limb should receive great benefit therefrom."
Maimonides cautions against prescribing strong laxatives or purga-

tives for patients with intraabdominal pathology. Compound drugs are sometimes worse than individual ones: "Composite medications made up from many individual drugs will not always be beneficial in an illness where a single drug would be effective: rather, the individual drug will work better for that particular illness."

Quotidian and quartan fevers are mentioned for the first time here, but numerous additional references to these and other types of fever occur in later chapters. "Fever which has its time daily is thought to occur only with stomach illnesses, just as four-day fevers are thought only to occur with splenic illnesses."

The two important aphorisms in this chapter dealing with diabetes mellitus have already been described above. A careful search for the causative agent of disease is the primary aim in attempts at its ultimate elimination, as is related: "The first rule that one must follow when beginning therapy, and that one must pay heed to [as long] as one is engaged in treatment [of an illness] is the elimination of the agent which is dissolving body strength and weakening it." Maimonides, quoting Galen, teaches us that when one is in doubt regarding the therapy of a particular illness, leave the healing to nature, since "nature knows the constitution of organs and sends to each organ the best nutrition which it needs from that which maintains the health of all living beings and thus heals it from its illness [*vis medicatrix natural*]."

The ninth treatise or chapter contains aphorisms pertaining to specific disease entities. Thus epilepsy, epistaxis, migraine headaches, respiratory infections, depression (black confusion or melancholia), meningitis, and many other problems are discussed. An allusion to what today is tube feeding for a comatose patient is found in aphorism 11: "In people who are found to be in a stupor, we grasp the tip of the tongue and depress it downward as far as possible. Then we insert an instrument at the side of the mouth into which we place some free-flowing liquid food. Then we push it [backward] to the base of the tongue and its contents will pour into the esophagus."

An eye disease, possibly trachoma, is said to be more common in warmer climates than in colder ones. "People who live in cold lands seldom suffer from ophthalmia, but when it does occur, it is strong and hard and produces ulcers in the eye." An incredibly accurate description of tuberculosis seems to be the gist of aphorism 39 in this chapter: "He who is afflicted with sores of the lung cannot be healed save after a long time, [that is,] until the liquids have become localized and the ulcers and boils have dried up and become hard or putrefied. The surrounding areas will decay until the entire lung caseates [and the patient dies]."

Lengthy accounts of gastrointestinal disturbances follow, including eructation, flatulence, diarrhea, abdominal pain, nausea, indigestion, anorexia, and the like. Dietary and medicinal remedies of various sorts are prescribed. Hepatic and splenic illnesses are considered next. Intestinal worms are considered to be of three types. "One resembles an arrowhead and resides in the perianal region [oxyuris?], another resembles gourd seeds and is found in the large intestine [taenia?], and the one resembling snakes is in the small intestine [ascaris?]. They produce pain in the stomach [abdomen] when they ascend in an upward direction. Worms develop in the abdomen from a bad, irritating liquid." The last phrase is consistent with medieval medical thinking.

Several aphorisms are devoted to renal disease, one of which precisely describes acute renal shutdown: "Sometimes, no urine at all comes to the bladder because the function of the kidney has ceased and becomes suspended. The urinary bladder is empty in this case; nothing at all is retained in it." Skin disorders such as eczema and psoriasis are mentioned next, followed by a description of joint inflammation, possibly rheumatoid arthritis: "Liquids within joints have the appearance of mucin [lit. paste or jelly]. If these increase ... then a moist inflammation will develop. ... many physicians consider that there is pus therein to the point that they cut into them and nothing is expelled ... the joint ... full of mucin."

An excellent regimen for weight reduction is prescribed in aphorism 101, including "much walking in the sun . . . bathing in the sea . . . foods which are not very nourishing, such as vegetables . . . and onions and garlic and sea fish . . . drink little." Concerning surgery, Maimonides states that "a hernia in which the membrane which covers the intestine [peritoneum], the stomach, and the omentum is caught, is a serious and severe illness even though its size may not be large. The hernia which encloses water [hydrocele] is a [relatively] mild illness, although it may reach a large size."

Interesting in aphorism 107 is the quotation from Galen in which he states that leprosy and cancer are curable if diagnosed and treated early in the course of the disease. However, no one has survived following the appearance of the full-blown disease. These illnesses, he further states, were quite common in Alexandria (Egypt), rare in the land of Germania, and never observed in the land of Scythia, "where the nutrition is [mainly] milk [and milk products]." Paroxysmal palpitations of the heart do not necessarily indicate heart disease, as is noted in aphorism 113. "We have seen many healthy people suffer from sudden heart palpitations. This is in people whose health lacked nothing, young boys as well as the elderly."

The tenth chapter is devoted entirely to aphorisms pertaining to fevers. Maimonides recognizes that fever is only a symptom and not a disease, and that both symptom and underlying cause should be treated after careful search for the latter. "It is important to know the precise differentiation between the fever of a septic process and the cause for that septic process. It is important to know which remedy to use to treat a fever, which therapy to employ to treat a septic process, and which medicine to use to treat the cause for the septic process." There is clear separation of fevers into tertian, quotidian, and quartan varieties, although the causes given for these are not correct according to modern medical thought. Thus, Maimonides quotes Galen as follows: "Intermittent fevers which cease during specific intervals are of three types, and these are: tertian fever; that which comes daily, called permanent or quotidian; and quartan fever. Tertian fever occurs from red bile which putrefies. Quotidian fever is produced from biles which begin to decay and are of the white type. Quartan fever develops as a result of the deterioration of black bile." Various features of the three types of fever are then described. Much faith is placed in theriac as a therapeutic drink for quartan fevers preceded by imbibition of absinthium juice. Phlebotomy is advocated for chronic fevers.

Chapter 11 is a brief treatise dealing with the stages of illness. These are four in number, as related in the first aphorism: "The periods of an illness in general consist of four stages: the onset [beginning], the crescendo [lit. increase], the acme [maximum or status], which is called the end stage, and the decline [descendo]. It is only with great difficulty that one can precisely know at any given moment in what stage [of illness] the patient finds himself." In some cases, the stages may overlap: "Thus, it becomes clear that there are many illnesses in which neither time of onset nor crescendo is noticeable." Several types of crises during an illness are described and their characteristics delineated. Acute illnesses are distinguished from chronic ones.

Chapter 12 treats the subject of bloodletting, or venesection. Specific indications and contraindications are spelled out. Maimonides states that "One should not phlebotomize a youth below age fourteen nor anyone over the age of seventy. One should not only be guided by the number of years [of age of any particular patient] but should examine his facial appearance. This is because many people who are only sixty years old cannot tolerate phlebotomy at all, whereas others who are seventy years old can tolerate it well because their blood is plentiful and their strength is great." He further states: "The conditions and complications that mitigate against bloodletting . . . are as follows: convulsive disorders, severe insomnia, anginal-type pain . . . someone who is extremely obese, or someone who is inordinately anxious, or a youngster or an elderly person or someone who is very fearful and cowardly, or someone who is not accustomed to giving blood . . . or someone plagued by diarrhea and colitis." The frequency, timing, and site of venesection, the quantity to be removed, and other facets of bloodletting are discussed. "During [the procedure] . . . most important of all is to examine the status of the pulse. If the pulse changes either in largeness [fullness] or evenness [rhythm], [immediately] terminate the phlebotomy. It is obviously unnecessary for me to mention [that venesection should cease immediately] if a patient becomes faint."

The thirteenth chapter deals with laxative purgatives and enemas.

Avoidance of their use, wherever possible, is recommended: "In most instances, purgation by means of cathartics or emetics is not appropriate. This type of emptying should be reserved only for him who needs a drastic type of emptying." Maimonides states that Hippocrates and Galen instructed their patients to consume barley soup to rinse the alimentary tract in order to wash down residue of a laxative medication that might adhere to the stomach wall. Maimonides' own observation was that only the Greeks could tolerate this, and that the peoples of Egypt and other countries in which he had traveled would regurgitate the aforementioned medication. He, therefore, recommends julep or althea. Later in the chapter, Maimonides relates his experiences with the larch fungus [or agaricon] in wine as a body-cleansing or depoisoning agent.

In aphorism 10 of this chapter, Maimonides speaks of "unripe liquids" which, "due to their thickness and viscosity," occlude coronary arteries. This seems to be a clear description of coronary thrombosis and myocardial infarction. A good laxative pill is obtained by compounding aloe, colocynth, larch fungus, blue bdellium, and gum arabic. Differences in individual patients' reactions to laxatives are recognized: "There are some people in whom cathartic action is difficult to effect, and there are others in whom a small quantity of laxative will produce a marked purgative action." Most interesting is the diagnosis that poisoning due to quail eating is due to the fact that quail feed on the poisonous hellebore with impunity. This fact was already recorded in the Old Testament (Exod. 16:13, Num. 11:31, Ps. 105:40). A long discussion of enemas and clysters follows. The chapter ends with quotations from Abu Ali ibn Zuhr and Al-Tamimi describing some of the purgatives they recommended.

The fourteenth chapter is extremely brief, comprising only thirteen aphorisms pertaining to emesis. The onion of the narcissum (a member of the daffodil family) is characterized as a good emetic. Also of aid to induce vomiting is bodily movement, and this is analogized to seasickness, where movement induces or contributes to emesis: "Bodily activity in the form of physical exercise after the imbibition of the emetic [medication] is helpful to the vomiting process because movement stimulates the liquids upwards, as occurs to sea voyagers on ships in the ocean."

The fifteenth treatise is the chapter devoted to surgery (lit. handcraft). Principles of sterility and cauterization are laid down, and the danger of infecting open wounds is indicated, as depicted in aphorism 8: "If one expels pus from a site [of infection] by cauterization, one should be most careful at that time and for some period thereafter not to utilize oil or water [to wash the wound]. If the wound needs lavation, then it is proper to wash it with honey water or diluted vinegar or wine mixed with honey." The recognition of gangrene and the necessity for surgical intervention are described two aphorisms later: "A limb which dies to the point of not sensing when it is pricked or cut or burned with fire will undoubtedly become black. In such a case one should hasten to amputate it next to the demarcation site where healthy tissue is connected. . . . Having amputated the limb, one should cauterize the stump, as I have often done for wounds."

Surgical cure of cancer in its early stages by wide excision is advocated: "[Concerning] cancer, this is an illness I have treated many times at its inception and [the patients] were cured . . . through surgical methods in which one excises the tumor and uproots the entire tumor and its surroundings up to the point of healthy tissue. . . . If the tumor also happens to be situated in close proximity to any major organ, then excision is dangerous because one will not be able to cauterize the root of the wound because of its proximity to the major organ." Surgical principles pertaining to a variety of disorders, including varicose veins, nasal polyps, peritonsillar abscesses, tumors of various sorts, colitis, and many others, are outlined. Ligatures to effect hemostasis are recommended for bleeding vessels: "If a severed vessel from which blood flows is a pulsating vessel [i.e., artery], then the blood can be stopped. . . . it can be fastened by tying." External compression to effect hemostasis as well as hemostatic drug preparations are also depicted. Incision and draining of abscesses is pictured in aphorism 48: ". . . to incise it . . . one lets the pus flow out, and then one applies a drying [agent]."

The last few aphorisms in this chapter are devoted to orthopedics. The time for various fractures to heal is related: "If the nasal bone is broken . . . it will heal and unite in ten days. However, the maxillary bone and the clavicle reunite in twenty days, the arm in thirty days, and the thigh bone [femur] and calf bone [tibia] in forty days. Bones of young people unite earlier than those of children." The splinting of fractures, application of casts, and positioning of broken limbs during and after reduction are all described.

Chapter 16 is devoted to obstetrics and gynecology, or, to use Maimonides' own language, to "women." Menstruation, pregnancy, amenorrhea, dysmenorrhea, anatomical features of the genitalia, and related subjects are discussed. The increased blood volume during pregnancy is recognized: "During pregnancy, the pulse is greater, the beat is stronger and also more rapid. However, other [bodily] functions remain in their same condition." Maimonides, quoting Galen, states that "A woman may abort because of [exertional] activity or because of steambathing." The stages of fetal growth are outlined as follows: "The time for complete formation of the fetus is thirty-five or forty-five days, and in twice that many days movement is created. In three times the [amount of] time from the onset of quickening, birth will occur."

Chapter 17 is devoted to general principles of hygiene. It consists entirely of quotations from Galen and Hippocrates and conforms nearly exactly to the hygienic principles enumerated by Maimonides in his rabbinic works[11] and the two treatises on hygiene which he wrote for Sultan al-Malik al-Afdal, eldest son of Saladin the Great of Egypt.[12] The reader is referred to the English, Hebrew, and German translations of Maimonides' hygienic principles.

Chapter 18 is a brief treatise on physical exercise and, together with chapters 19 and 20, which deal with bathing and nutrition, is probably a continuation of the general principles outlined in chapter 17. Maimonides here states that exercise before meals is beneficial for bodily health, and that exercise of the "soul" is salutary for

---

11. F. Rosner, "The Hygienic Principles of Moses Maimonides."
12. A. Bar Sela, H. E. Hoff, and E. Faris, *Moses Maimonides' Two Treatises on the Regimen of Health*; S. Muntner, *Hanhogat ha-Beriyut*; idem, *Maimonides: Regimen Sanitatis oder Diätetik für die Seele.*

emotional health. Ball playing and hunting are examples cited of gymnastic enterprises. Complete and constant immobility predisposes to illness. A shower following physical exercise should precede meals.

The nineteenth treatise, as already mentioned, deals with bathing. Indications, contraindications, and timing of bathing are discussed. The contents of the bath, the temperature of the water, the duration of the bath, and things to do before and after the bath are described.

The twentieth chapter contains aphorisms dealing with foods and beverages and their usages. The second aphorism in this treatise summarizes the importance of nutrition in both health and disease: "A knowledge of dietetics [lit. strengths of foods] is practically one of the most helpful things in the field of medicine because of the constant, never-ending need for food during health as well as during illness." The remainder of the chapter elaborates at length on this principle. A few excerpts from the various citations in this chapter will suffice to impart the general flavor of the treatise: "Soft food is more easily and rapidly digested. . . . It is not proper for us to gorge ourselves full of food . . . the quantity consumed should not overburden [the patient]. Putrefied foods and beverages produce decay [i.e., toxins] similar to that produced by deadly poisons. Some foods soften the stool. . . . The most valuable and most appropriate bread for someone who does not perform any physical exercise or for the elderly is bread which has been well baked in the oven and which contains a large quantity of sourdough. Wine to which an equal quantity of water has been added warms the entire body and stimulates all limbs. . . . Drinking cold water before meals damages the food and the liver. Milk nourishes a defective body. . . . Cheese . . . harms patients with hydrops. Cow's milk is the thickest of all milks and the fattest of all." A host of foods, including fruits, grains, and meats, their properties and characteristics are then enumerated. A lengthy quotation on dietetics from Abu Marwan ibn Zuhr (one of Maimonides' teachers) follows. The chapter ends with several citations on nutrition and foods from Al-Tamimi, author of the book *Al-Murshid*.

Chapter 21 is devoted to aphorisms pertaining to medications. It is a veritable pharmacopoeia of materia medica. Several hundred drugs, simple and compounded, are described, and it is beyond the scope of this chapter to do more than review some of them very briefly. The value of alcohol in the form of wine as a diuretic and soporific is mentioned at the outset. Milk mixed with honey is said to be "valuable against pains in the chest and lung. However, it is ... harmful ... for the spleen and liver." The benefits and contraindications of oxymel (a mixture of honey and vinegar) are outlined. Astringents, such as extracts of blackberry bushes or wine bushes, are recommended for stomach ailments. Regarding exogenous poisons and endogenous toxins, Maimonides states: "Milk, garlic, boiled [distilled] wine, vinegar, and salt are of value against [animal] poisons or against substances that develop [in the body] which are similar to poisons." Caper is reported to be an appetite stimulant and purgative. The actions and indications for a variety of medications, such as saffron, Ceylon cinnamon, spikenard, andropogon, aromatic calamus, spicknel, aloe, wormwood, and bdellium, are stated.

Immunization against disease is strongly suggested by the following citation: "Someone who is about to undertake a long journey should drink an amount of theriac [almonds pulverized in diluted wine] equal to a large bean in six ounces of warm water prior to eating, in order to immunize against [lit. to repulse or expel] the damage of [toxic] waters [that he might drink on the road]." Furthermore, "A knowledgeable physician related to me that once a devastating pestilence occurred ... and he recommended to people to take this theriac because no medicine was effective against the aforementioned illness. . . . He who drank it [prophylactically] prior to the onset of the illness was saved from developing it. This is not surprising, because this medication is an antidote against all [types of] poison."

Next follows a classification and categorization of drugs according to various parameters. Sweetness, saltiness, bitterness, and sharpness are indicators of different drug effects. The properties of drugs which are astringent or sour or sharp or bitter or tasteless or sweet or oily are described. The remainder of this chapter enumerates hundreds of drugs which fit into these various categories. This list is by no means exhaustive, as Maimonides himself states: "I therefore [only] intend to describe the properties of drugs that are universally commonly used, whose names are well known and which are employed internally." A sample excerpt from one of these aphorisms depicting one group of medicaments follows: "Cooling drugs which moisten to the first degree are ten [in number]. These are pears, spinach, violets, chicory, lotus, fenugreek, wormwood, mangold, mallow, and liquiricia."

Chapter 22 contains aphorisms pertaining to specific remedies. The first half of the chapter consists of quotations from Galen, the latter half, citations from Ibn Zuhr and al-Tamimi. They are mostly of historical interest only, although occasionally a modern therapeutic regime is described, such as the treatment of gout with colchicine. The following are a few excerpts for the reader's interest: "Mouse excrement, if pulverized in vinegar, is beneficial for alopecia. The brain of a camel, if dried, prepared in vinegar and imbibed, is of value against epilepsy. If one rubs the gums of children with brains of an ewe lamb, it will facilitate growth of the teeth without pain. Earthworms, if pulverized, [dissolved,] and imbibed by a patient with icterus will immediately cleanse his body. Cattle's milk is of aid against intestinal ulcers. . . . The spleen of a wild donkey or the spleen of a wild horse should be dried and pulverized and given to drink to a patient with illness of the spleen. . . . The consumption of rabbit heads, as much as one is able to eat, helps against tremors. A lotion made of the liquid of roses and sugar strengthens vision. . . . the gillyflower [*Eugenia caryophyllata carnefolium*], pulverized and filtered [and placed] on the forehead during the winter is a reliable remedy for preventing catarrhal colds. The ingestion of radish or cabbage eliminates hoarseness. Hedgehog meat, if dried and some of it imbibed in oxymel, is beneficial for pain in the kidneys. . . . if one takes pulverized, dried snakeroot and three parts of wheat flour and places all this in sesame oil and kneads it with leavening and salt and bakes it and dries this bread and pulverizes it and snuffs about ten drachmas of its dust every morning in a spiced honey drink, then hemorrhoids will be obliterated in three days."

The twenty-third chapter attempts to elucidate some of the mechanisms or pathophysiology of well-known illnesses and also to define and explain various technical terms used in medicine. Maimonides first speaks of plethora or hypertonia as representing an excess of blood. Rusty (hyperbilirubinemic) blood is distinguished from watery (anemic) blood. The differences between chyle and chyme, epidemic and pandemic, shaking and trembling, paralysis and paresis, continuous fever and intermittent fever, inflammation and abscess, carbuncle and furuncle, and many others are described. He recognizes that pitting and non-pitting edema represent different signs of illness. Thus he states: "The difference between a swelling [edema] and a soft inflammation is that if one presses on a swelling with one's hand, it will not remain depressed. . . . If one presses on the loin of a patient with soft inflammation, it remains depressed and sunken." Further terms, such as varicocele and hydrocele, intestinal hernia and omental hernia, stupor and lethargy, benign ulcer and malignant ulcer, amnesia melancholia, and amentia, are all discussed. An astonishingly accurate description of conjunctivitis, trachoma, and other ophthalmological diseases is found in aphorisms 69–72 in this chapter: "The waters which accumulate in the eye [produce] what physicians call [ocular] tension. These accumulate between the crystalline lens and the corneal membrane. If a hemorrhagic inflammation occurs to the membrane known as sclera–conjunctiva, which is the white of the eye, this is called ophthalmia. This damages one's visual ability and hinders its normal use. . . . If a site on the cornea becomes corroded and part of the uveal tunic protrudes, this is called a staphyloma. The pus that develops beneath the corneal membrane is called hypopyon. If the eyelids become thickened and hardened on their inner sides, this is the illness called trachoma [lit. grape scab]. Eyelids whose appearance is red and whose celia are lacking [occur in] the illness called blepharitis [Arabic *sulak*], meaning swelling of the lids. A lack of flesh on the large cornea of the eye, which is also called the large [inner] canthus, is an illness spoken of as epiphora [dacryocystitis]."

Asthma, a disease concerning which Maimonides wrote a separate essay,[13] is concisely and precisely described: "If someone has rapid breathing . . . without being febrile, then physicians have long been accustomed to call this occurrence asthma. They have also named it upright breathing because the patient with this ailment has an erect chest during respiration. This illness arises because of constriction that occurs in the chest and abdomen." Various gastrointestinal and genitourinary illnesses and technical terms are then delineated. The chapter ends with a consideration of certain nutriments and drugs and their effects on the human body.

Chapter 24 comprises aphorisms on medical curiosities, strange occurrences, and unusual and rare happenings. One example is the statement that in Sicily, following a total solar eclipse, women gave birth to bicephalic monsters. Another is the remarkable description of teratomas: "Inflammations that are called tumors are found to be of varying types when cut open. Sometimes, objects resembling mud, urine, feces, honey, excrement, stone, teeth, and flesh are found therein. Sometimes one even finds living creatures therein that arise from putrefaction." The last sentence seems to indicate a belief in spontaneous generation, an accepted fact in the Middle Ages until Spallanzani disproved it in the eighteenth century.

Maimonides also cites the eggplant (*Solanum melongena*; Arabic *bading'an*) from one of Galen's works even though Galen did not mention it by name. He adds that this word crept into Galen's book only as a conjecture on the part of the translator or copyist, who thought that a black-and-reddish fruit could be nothing but eggplant. Many interesting customs and qualities of various peoples are described in this chapter, where we hear of Greeks, Romans, Scythians, Germans (Slavs), and Berbers. We also hear of diseases in Rome, Athens, Ethiopia, Alexandria (Egypt), and Maimonides' own Spanish homeland when he states: "In our land . . .". Famous physicians encountered in this chapter include Galen, Hunain ibn

---

13. See above, chap. 2.

Isḥak, Ali ibn Rodwan, Hippocrates, Batrik, Aristedes of Mysia, and Plato.

The twenty-fifth chapter is known as the "Sacred War for Independent Investigation in Science Against Galen," and, unlike the other chapters, does not deal with practical medicine but contains a sharp attack on Galen, whose views were accepted as dogma throughout the Middle Ages. It shows Maimonides' ability and courage as a profound critic, and demonstrates his astounding knowledge of the spiritual world of the ancient Greeks. Aphorism 59 in this chapter is outstanding in this respect, for it presents Maimonides as an exponent of Aristotelian philosophy in its Arabic-Jewish garb conforming with the principles of Judaism. The peak of his greatness is revealed in aphorism 69, where he challenges conventional views in general, and exposes Galen's falsifications and errors in particular. Maimonides demands research through experimentation and recognizes the influence of ecology on the human organism. He disputes Galen's views on life. He cannot comprehend how a man like Galen could pay attention only to "material" things to the exclusion of the spirit. Whereas to Galen, knowledge without experience sufficed, to Maimonides, both are necessary to make a good physician. This final chapter of Maimonides' medical aphorisms is of such importance that the reader is referred to the full report describing his scholarly attack against dogmatism.[14] A sample excerpt therefrom is as follows: "If any man declares to you [that he has found] facts that he has observed and confirmed with his own experience, even if you consider this man to be most trustworthy and highly authoritative, be cautious in accepting what he says to you. If he attempts to persuade you to accept this opinion which is his viewpoint or any doctrine that he believes in, then you should think [critically] and understand [what he means] when he declares that he has observed it, and your thoughts should not become confused. . . . Rather, investigate and weigh this opinion or that hypothesis according to the requirements of pure logic . . . [critically appraise] even a statement of the great sage Galen."

---

14. See Rosner and Muntner, *Medical Aphorisms of Moses Maimonides.*

Sir William Osler aptly stated that Moses Maimonides was not only physician to princes, but also "Prince of Physicians." There is little question, from his aphorisms as from his other works, but that Maimonides takes a place as one of the all-time giants of medicine.

I readily admit that I have on occasion read modern ideas into Maimonides' aphorisms and have sometimes extrapolated from some of the remarkable things he said, thus somewhat "modernizing" this great medieval author. I hope that critical historians will not consider this approach to be too ahistorical. The English-reading medical bibliophile and reader now has available to him this classic work rendered into his own language.[15]

---

15. M. Etziony, "Apropros of Maimonides' Aphorisms."

# ❧ 5 ❧

# The Introduction to the Commentary on the Aphorisms of Hippocrates

Maimonides' *Commentary on the Aphorisms of Hippocrates* should not be confused with the *Medical Aphorisms of Moses*, discussed in the preceding chapter. The famous *Aphorisms of Hippocrates* were translated from the Greek into Arabic by Ḥunain ibn Isḥaq in the ninth century, and Maimonides wrote his commentary on this translation. An excellent medieval translation into Hebrew was made by Moses ben Samuel ibn Tibbon, and was soon followed by renderings into Latin and numerous other languages

A brief description of Maimonides' *Commentary on the Aphorisms of Hippocrates* with sample aphorisms appeared in 1935.[1] The entire work was published in Hebrew by Hasida in 1935 and again in a definitive edition by Muntner in 1961.[2] The various Arabic and Hebrew manuscripts of this work are listed by Steinschneider, Brockelmann, and Muntner.[3]

---

1. L. Heilperin, "Perush Pirkei Abukrat le-Rabbi Moshe ben Maimon."
2. M. Z. Hasida, "Perush le-Pirkei Abukrat shel ha-Rambam"; S. Muntner, *Moshe ben Maimon: Commentary on the Aphorisms of Hippocrates.*
3. M. Steinschneider, *Die Hebraeischen Uebersetzungen des Mittelaelters und die Juden als Dolmetscher,* C. Brockelmann, *Geschichte der Arabischen Literatur,* Muntner, op. cit.

The introduction to this work was edited in the original Arabic with two Hebrew translations and one in German by Stein-schneider in 1894.[4] Bar Sela and Hoff published Maimonides' interpretation of the first aphorism of Hippocrates.[5] This is the famous aphorism which has been called the motto or credo of the art of medicine: "Life is short, and the art long, the occasion fleet-ing, experience fallacious and judgment difficult. The physician must not only be prepared to do what is right himself, but must also make the patient, the attendant, and the externals cooperate."

This first aphorism of Hippocrates has been commented upon by many writers in several languages.[6] This is not surprising in view of the enduring value of the precepts therein, which set forth, as a background for the teaching of the practice of medicine, the diffi-culties and hazards which the physician faces.

Maimonides describes his comments on the first aphorism as being more detailed than those on the rest of Hippocrates' work. As pointed out by Rosenthal in his discussion of the first aphorism of Hippocrates, Maimonides also disregards his own conception of what he considers the task of a commentator, since he says that he is not concerned with elucidating Hippocrates' intentions, and merely wishes to give some worthwhile additional information. Indeed, Maimonides does not reproduce any of Galen's comments on the first aphorism, although elsewhere, throughout his com-mentary, he relies upon Galen's commentary for the general drift of his remarks. As a result, according to Rosenthal, Maimonides' lengthy comments on the first aphorism of Hippocrates are most remarkable for their lack of dependence on Galen, which distin-guishes them favorably from the remainder of Maimonides' com-mentary, and further indicate his rare independence of mind and breadth of knowledge.

---

4. M. Steinschneider, "Die Vorrede des Maimonides zu Seinem Commentar. . . ."

5. A. Bar Sela and H. E. Hoff, "Maimonides' Interpretation of the First Aphorism of Hippocrates."

6. R. E. Schlueter, "The First Aphorism of Hippocrates as Explained by Paracelsus"; D. W. Richards, "The First Aphorism of Hippocrates"; F. Rosenthal, "'Life Is Short, the Art Is Long': Arabic Commentaries on the First Hippocratic Aphorism."

Maimonides' introduction to the *Commentary on the Aphorisms of Hippocrates* provides interesting historico-literary remarks which prompted Steinschneider to translate and publish it separately. In his introduction, Maimonides discusses the virtues and shortcomings of commentaries in general. He challenges Galen's commentary in a tone that Ibn Zuhr and Averroes before him had not dared to adopt. However, Maimonides never indulges in the aggressive type of criticism found in the twenty-fifth chapter of his own medical aphorisms.[7] He states that Galen could not, or would not, admit that Hippocrates was guilty of making an erroneous statement. Thus, Galen would attribute misstatements of fact to "another Hippocrates, not the famous Hippocrates." Alternatively, Galen would attempt to justify Hippocratic assertions by interpreting them in a manner exactly opposite to what was stated. For example, Hippocrates clearly says that "the earth surrounds the water," to which Galen comments: "Perhaps Hippocrates meant to say that the water surrounds the earth." Maimonides claims that Galen did this to save the honor of Hippocrates.

There follows my English translation of Maimonides' *Introduction to the Commentary of Hippocrates*, based on the German and Hebrew versions of Steinschneider and Muntner, respectively. Words in brackets are my own additions to help clarify the meaning of the text.

ও ও ও

Thus speaks the great Rabbi, our Master and Teacher, Moses, son of the servant of the Lord, the Israelite, from Cordova:[8] I do not believe that any scholar who composes books would write a book in any field of learning with the intent that the words in his work not be understood unless a commentary were provided. If any did so intend, then the purpose of his composition would be thwarted, because a writer does not compose a book in such a manner that he alone understands the contents. Rather, he composes his book

---

7. See above, chap. 4.
8. This entire phrase was added by the copyist.

so that others also comprehend it. If, however, his book is incomprehensible without another book [to explain it], then his book will be neglected.

In my view, the reasons that later generations found it necessary to explain and to comment upon the works of earlier generations are four [in number]:

The first reason concerns the perfection of the level [of knowledge] of the author, who, because of his excellent understanding, speaks a few words of deep and hidden matters, difficult to grasp, but which are clear to him and require no elaboration. When someone in a later generation tries to understand these matters [written] in abbreviated form, he finds it extremely difficult. Then the commentator must add words to the treatise so that the thoughts which the original author intended to impart can be clearly understood.

The second reason concerns the omission in a book of certain premises which the author takes for granted. For an author sometimes composes an incomprehensible book, because he thinks that the reader is already familiar with certain assumptions without which the book cannot be understood. It then becomes necessary for the commentator to briefly mention these assumptions to compensate for their lack. For the same reason, the commentator must also explain certain ideas totally omitted by the author.

The third reason concerns the [proper interpretation of the] various expressions in the treatise. For most treatises in any language are subject to varying interpretations, and it is possible that certain statements in that treatise are understood in different ways, some opposite and some contradictory. The result is that confusion and controversy arise among those who delve into the treatise. One person extracts one meaning [from the text] and states that the author only intended that one, whereas another person extracts a different meaning. The commentator on the treatise must then make the decision as to which of the interpretations is the correct one, and must cite evidence for its correctness and therewith annul the other interpretation.

The fourth reason concerns ideas [or uncertainties] which occur to the author but which have not been carefully thought out, or the repetition of a thought, or that which has no utility at all. The commentator must then allude to such a statement and must cite evidence for its invalidity, or its lack of utility, or its repetition. In reality, this should not be called a commentary but a refutation and annotation. It is, however, common practice for people to examine a book [in the following manner]. If most of the contents of the text are correct, then the annotations to the few [erroneous] statements therein are considered as part of the commentary, and the latter states that "the author made a pronouncement without giving it any thought, but the truth is such and such," or "this needs no mention," or "this statement is repetitious," and thus all is explained [in the commentary]. However, if most of what is said in the book is erroneous, then the later work, which exposes the errors, is called a refutation, not a commentary. When the work of refutation cites a correct expression from the original book, it will state: "That which he says such and such is in fact correct".

It seems to me that all the commentaries written on the books of Aristotle were composed because of the first and third reasons. All the commentaries on mathematical books were composed for the second reason, although some mathematical works also had commentaries written for the fourth reason. For the book *Al-Majesti* [written by Ptolemy], in spite of the extreme authority of its author, contains certain ideas [or uncertainties] not well thought through and concerning which many of the Andalusians[9] made annotations and composed books.

On the other hand, all the commentaries written on the books of Hippocrates were mostly composed for the first, third, and fourth reasons. However, a few were composed for the second reason. Galen does not admit this, however, and under no circumstances does he consider any statement of Hippocrates to be erroneous; he [Galen] offers explanations which cannot be sup-

9. Although Maimonides wrote this work while living in Egypt, he still considered himself a Spaniard or Andalusian, after his birthplace. Spanish Arabists were strong critics of the Ptolemaic system.

ported by the text and gives interpretations which are not at all alluded to in the [Hippocratic] statement. This he did, for example, in his commentary on *The Book of Humors*, although he was even in doubt whether this book was written by Hippocrates or by someone else. He was induced to do this by the confusion which he found in this book, and the fact that it resembles the writings of the alchemists or even worse. In my opinion, it would have been much more appropriate to call this work "The Book of Confusion." Since the book is generally attributed to Hippocrates, Galen composed this odd commentary thereon. That which Galen advances in this commentary is medically correct; however, the explanation has no relationship to the statement being explained. Thus, [Galen's] commentary should in reality not be called a commentary, because a commentary brings out *in actu* that which is potentially interpretable from the statement [to be explained]; so that if one rereads the [explained] passage after one understands the interpretation, one sees hints in the text to support that interpretation. The latter is what I would call a true commentary. A commentary does not consist of someone enunciating true statements, asserting that they are the explanation of what someone else had said, as Galen did for some of the treatises of Hippocrates.

The same applies to those who draw conclusions from the statements of an individual and call [their conclusions] a commentary. In my opinion, such is not a commentary but another type of work, like the major portion of the commentary of al-Nairizi on Euclid. I do not call the latter a commentary.

Similarly, we find that Galen, in his commentaries on the writings of Hippocrates, explains certain statements in the exact opposite of their intended meaning in order to justify the correctness of the statements. He did this in the *Book of Heptaden*, where Hippocrates states that the earth surrounds the water. Galen explains this assertion by saying that it is possible that Hippocrates meant to say that the water surrounds the earth! He [Galen] does all this in order not to have to say that Hippocrates erred in his statement or espoused an erroneous viewpoint. If the matter became too difficult for him, however, in that the error was very obvious, leaving him no outlet, he [Galen] would assert that the [error] had been interpolated into the statement of Hippocrates and thus was attributed to him; or Galen would say that the [erroneous] statement had been made by another Hippocrates but not the famous Hippocrates. This is what he [Galen] did, for example, in his commentary on the book *The Nature of Man*. All this was done to justify Hippocrates; although he is without doubt one of the greatest of physicians, the justification of misstatements, even of a great man, is not admirable.

It is known that not everything in a book which has already been explained or which is still to be explained requires explanation. There are undoubtedly [certain] very clear assertions therein which need no explanation. However, the intent of the commentators in their commentaries varies, as do the methods of authors in their compositions. Some authors strive for brevity and maintain this approach, so that if, for example, it is possible to fulfill the purpose of the composition in 100 words, they would not use 101 words. Other authors prefer length and verbosity, and prepare a book of voluminous size and a great number of subdivisions even if the total content is quite meager.

The same applies to commentators: some explain the matter to be elucidated in the briefest possible manner and avoid the other [lengthy] approach; others expand [their commentary] and explain that which requires no explanation or explain that which does, but unnecessarily verbosely.

I thought that Galen was one of those who stretched out his commentaries in most of his works until I saw the following remark by Galen at the beginning of his commentary on Plato's *Laws*, where he [Galen] states: "I have observed that a commentator explained the following statement of Hippocrates in more than 100 skins [pages] without cause and without substance: 'When the illness reaches its climax, then the [therapeutic] regimen must be maximally minimized.'"

Moses [Maimonides] says: when I saw this statement of Galen's, I began to defend his works and his commentaries, and recognized that he wrote very briefly indeed in comparison to his contemporaries. One finds considerable verbosity in the latter, which can only be denied by a distorter [of the truth]. I am only speaking, however, to one who is free of passion [or bias], and who only seeks the truth in every matter. In the sixth tractate of *Therapeutics*, Galen [also] mentions that contemporaries expanded greatly in their commentaries thereon.

It is because I saw that the book of aphorisms of Hippocrates is of greater value than all his other books that I decided to explain them. These are aphorisms which every physician, and even non-physician, should know by heart. I also saw that children memorize them in school, so that non-physicians also know many of them by heart, like schoolchildren who learn from their teacher.

Among the aphorisms of Hippocrates are some which are doubtful and require explanation, some which are self-evident, some which are repeated, some which are not useful for medical therapeutics, and some which are absolutely erroneous viewpoints. Galen, however, denies such statements and explains them as he wishes. But I will explain them in the manner of brevity; namely, I will only explain those [aphorisms] which require explanation. I will follow the opinions of Galen, with the exception of a few aphorisms where I will state my own opinion in my own name. That which I mention anonymously is a statement of Galen's with which I agree. For my intent is not an explanation according to his wording, as I did in the *Compendium*.[10]

In this commentary, my sole intent is brevity, so that the meaning of those aphorisms which require explanation is easily remem-

---

10. Maimonides wrote another medical book entitled *Extracts from Galen* or *Compendium Galeni*. Galen's medical writings consist of over 100 books, and two volumes were required just to catalogue and index them all. Maimonides extracted what he considered the most important of Galen's pronouncements and compiled them verbatim in a small work which was intended primarily for the use of students of Greek medicine. This work, like all of Maimonides' medical books, was originally written in Arabic. No complete Arabic manuscript exists today, but several Hebrew manuscript translations are available. Until recently, only extracts therefrom, in both English and Hebrew, appeared in a Hebrew periodical in 1955; see U. S. Barzel, "The Art of Cure." Eventually, the entire text was published in English by Barzel (Maimonides Research Institute, Haifa, 1992).

bered. I thus strived for brevity of words as much as I could, with the exception of the first aphorism, where I dwell a little longer. To be sure, the latter is not in the manner of a true commentator, but I did so to describe something useful, whether Hippocrates so intended it or not.

And now I will begin the commentary.

# Medical Topics

# ❧ 6 ❧

# Ophthalmological Aphorisms

The most voluminous and famous of Maimonides' medical writings is *Pirkei Moshe bi-Refuah*, known in English as the *Medical Aphorisms of Moses*.[1] Most of the aphorisms that Maimonides cites in this work are culled from the writings of Galen, Aristotle, Hippocrates, Rhazes, al-Farabi, and Avenzoar. Some are original with him, and these he always prefaces with the phrase "Moses says . . ." In this chapter I present the aphorisms dealing specifically with ophthalmology. The source on which each aphorism is based is given at its conclusion.

The reader is asked to take into consideration that the English translation of this twelfth-century work was performed by a twentieth-century physician. Hence, due to the modern medical outlook of the translator, certain interpretations may not necessarily coincide with Maimonides' understanding and knowledge of ophthalmology. Words in brackets are additions by the translator meant to help clarify the meaning of particular phrases or aphorisms.

## Aphorisms

Chap. 1:48. The inner part of the covering of the eyeball [choroid] has soft and moist hairs [cilia] to gather the fine liquid [aqueous], similar to the soaking of a sponge. It is covered by a moist

---

1. See above, chap. 4.

thin [membrane], the albuginea, which lies flat on the fine liquid. The covering of the eyeball [cornea] is shiny and transparent as a mirror as it covers the fine liquid on the outside, originating from the fluid of the glass [vitreous]. *De Usa Partium X*

Chap. 3:52. There are no vessels whatever in the crystalline, albugineous, and vitreous humors [of the eye], as well as in the corneal tunica. Even so, the crystalline humor is nourished from the vitreous humor through osmosis, and the vitreous [receives its nourishment] from the retinal tunica, which has abundant arteries and veins. The cornea, too, is nourished by osmosis from the uveal covering because the uvea also contains an abundant vasculature. *De Usa Partium X*

Chap. 3:78. If the covering of the uvea [of the eye] is severely torn, the albugineous humor will escape and egress outside the uveal tunica and meet the corneal tunica. Through this, afflictions will occur; one of these is that the uveal tunica will fall on the crystalline humor, and another is that air will penetrate and escape through this wound. *De Morbis et Symptomis IV*

Chap. 6:13. If a scale forms on the face from conjunctival secretions or sweat which has evaporated and become like dust, this is a bad sign. Similarly, darkening of vision in acute illnesses signifies the death of the power of vision. *Comment. Epidemiarum III*

Chap. 6:18. The eyes reflect a true picture of the measure of bodily strength, providing that vision and lid opening are normal. *Comment. Epidemiarum VI, 4*

Chap. 6:34. The vision of someone who suffers from vertigo and confusion in the head will become darkened [scotomata] and lost, and he will vomit from the slightest stimuli. He who suffers from vertigo and confusion in the head secondary to a stomach ailment will primarily have palpitations and nausea. *De Locis Affectis III*

Chap. 7:69. If the albugineous humor of the eye is present in greater or lesser than normal amounts, vision becomes damaged. If it becomes thick, then outgoing vision is diminished [vision was thought to "go out" from the eye rather than light rays "coming into" it], so that objects at a distance can no longer be seen, and even close objects cannot be clearly differentiated. If this humor becomes extremely thick, as occurs in the loss of the liquid which gives rise to vision [aqueous humor opacifies to form a cataract], and if because of this thickness a part of the eye near the pupil becomes covered and only a small opening remains, then one only sees every item through that opening, but cannot see many objects simultaneously [tubular vision?]. If only a small amount of thick liquid accumulates in the center of the pupil and everything surrounding it remains clear, then one sees everything [opaque] as if one were looking through a focusing screen. If the substances are massive, spread out, and separated in that place [pupil], then the affected individual seems to imagine that he sees a mosquito flying about [*mouches volantes* secondary to vitreous opacity]. This occurs to many people upon awakening from sleep and appears as [dancing] figures. This often occurs to young people [deliriums] and in those whose heads are filled with wine or some other, similar type of [intoxicating] beverage. *De Morbis et Symptomis IV*

Chap. 9:8. Sparks and lightning which a man sees before his eyes are due to liquids whose substance and appearance are transformed into albugineous liquids which gather between the crystalline and vitreous humors of the cornea. *Comment. Peri Chymon I*

Chap. 9:22. For eye pain, it is appropriate to apply to the eye a sponge soaked in water in which melilot and buckshorn clover have already been cooked. If the pain is mild, this should be applied only once or twice a day, whereas if the pain is severe, it should be applied many times, especially in the long [summer] days. *Miamir IV*

Chap. 9:26. It is important that all ocular medications should be of an even luke-warmness; for this we use breast milk and separate egg whites. Regarding medications to tranquilize earache produced by irritating liquids, we customarily use the same as for eye pain. *Miamir III*

Chap. 9:30. al-Tamini [an eleventh-century Arab physician] says: *Elbalach elsini*, a white, round, glittering stone, zinc oxide [cadmium], gold and silver [cadmium], [the dried milk substance of] *convulvulus scammonia*, types of vitriol of cyper, tortoise excrement, shells of turtle dove eggs, and *terra rubra* [silicates and iron oxides]—

all these ingredients should be in specific doses [finely pulverized]. One takes [and uses] this as [eye] powder because it purifies the white of the eye [conjunctiva] extremely well, and when dissolved in liquid, it cleanses [the eye] without irritation and without damage. *Comment. de Vintis I*

Chap. 9:31. People who live in warm countries often suffer from ophthalmia which is rapidly cured. People who live in cold lands seldom suffer from ophthalmia, but when it does occur, it is strong and hard and produces ulcers in the eye. So, too, is the analogy regarding the ophthalmia which occurs in the summer versus that which occurs in the winter. *Comment. de Vintis I*

Chap. 12:38. For illnesses of the head or chronic ailments of the eyes, one sometimes bleeds the pulsating vessels of the temples and those behind the ears [temporal or occipital arteries]. This is done if the cause of the illness is a warm, soft material, especially if it originates in the membranes [meninges]. The patient feels as if he was stabbed, after which the pain spreads out, but the stabbing [sensation] remains in the center of that site. However, bloodletting from pulsating vessels [i.e., arteries] entails great danger because sometimes one cannot stop the [flow of] blood, or heat might occur with the blood. For this reason, physicians are very reluctant to phlebotomize a large or even small [artery]. A small incision into them is of little benefit. If a vein is severed in its width into two halves, there is no danger, since each end will constrict to the side it is in. *De Phlebotomia [VI]*

Chap. 15:24. Cornification of the eye [lids], as long as it is small, [can be treated] with warming medications that liquefy, just as the remedies for *al garab* of the eye. If this [cornification] increases and hardens, then it should be treated with the scalpel [by excision]. *Finis Megatechne*

Chap. 15:25. Hail in the eye [chalazion] requires excision. The same applies to pus collected in the [anterior chamber of the] eye in the illness *hypopion*. Most of this should be treated with dissolving medications, not with something that will effect a strong drying action. When the major portion [of the pus] will have been expelled, the remainder will congeal. It will also be eliminated [eventually] by [outward] movement [out of the eye], just as occurs in head illnesses, until the entire pus will have descended downward [out of the eye]. *Finis Megatechne*

Chap. 15:28. The eye is the most sensitive of organs. Therefore, it is proper that one drip medications into it extremely gently, after having slightly raised the upper eyelid. One should dissolve these medications in liquids that are usually non-irritating. Ancient physicians found egg albumen to be of great benefit [as a base for eyedrops]. *Megatechne XIII*

Chap. 15:29. A moistening medication that flows [drops] has no effect [on the eye] unless a bandage is applied. Therefore, for eye diseases, one should use medications as dry pastes, because a bandage has to cover the entire eye [preventing vision]. The eye cannot tolerate being bound with a bandage that is not removed for many days, because a fistula will develop. *Miamir V*

Chap. 15:30. If the liquid [eye medicine] trickles down the face of the patient, then one should hold a vessel [eye cup] for a long time over the place where one wants the washing, so that [the liquid] can be reasborbed into the eye. *Katagenes I*

Chap. 15:31. If the horny tunic [cornea] bursts, then a thin, clear liquid will pour and flow out, and will first cause softening [of the eye]. This is the liquid that one sees in many people, flowing out from a hole where one punctured the eye [ocular paracentesis] in order to remove the [excess] water therefrom [early therapy of glaucoma?]. Following this, a generalized contraction of the eye occurs, and it becomes constricted and sunken. *De Usu Partium X*

Chap. 19:16. When ophthalmia of the eye begins to ripen, and when its ripening terminates, if the body is pure, then bathing is one of the best remedies for these [patients]. That is, the pain will subside immediately, the deposition of [bad] liquids that heretofore flowed to the eye will cease, and the liquids will distribute themselves and mix equally [throughout the body]. *Megatechne XIII*

Chap. 21:9. In barley we find a cooling force for an [inflamed] eye, if it [the barley] is consumed in the form of bread or gruel or roasted kernels. Even if one does not remove the outer shell, the gruel made therefrom is still useful for its cleansing effect, which cannot be attained in any other manner. Indeed, it is because the power of barley gruel counteracts the strength of lentils, so that if one mixes equal quantities [of these] together, then between them a food is produced which is among the most nutritious of all foods. *De Alimentorum Virtutibus III*

Chap. 22:4. The brain of a bat, prepared with honey, is valuable against ophthalmia. The same is accomplished with the brain of *etaia* [lamb or sheep]. *De Theriako ad Pisonem*

Chap. 22:5. Bile of the ostrich, the *al adaga*, mixed with honey and applied to the eye, is of value for ophthalmia. If it is cooked in oil of lilies, however, it is beneficial for weakness of vision. *De Theriako ad Pisonem*

Chap. 22:37. Staring at the eyes of a wild donkey permanently [guarantees] healthy vision, and helps against tearing of the eyes. He [Ibn Zuhr] further states that this is absolutely true, and without doubt. *De Usu Partium X*

Chap. 22:39. If one paints [the eyes] with a gold lotion, one's vision is strengthened. *De Usu Partium X*

Chap. 22:69. Kidney and bladder stones should be burned [and pulverized], and if [they are then prepared as a liquid] and painted [on the eye], they liquefy a cataract [lit. white in the eye], whether the latter is old or recent. Similarly, shiny-white porcelain, burned and pulverized and dried [i.e., used as a powder] and mixed with some dissolving drugs [liquefies a cataract]. *De Usu Partium X*

Chap. 23:69. The waters which accumulate in the eye [aqueous humor] [produce] what physicians call [ocular] tension. These accumulate between the crystalline lens and the corneal membrane. *De Usu Partium X*

Chap. 23:70. If a hemorrhagic inflammation occurs to the membrane known as scleraconjunctiva, which is the white of the eye, this is called conjunctivitis. This inflammation damages one's visual ability and hinders its normal use. However, if [ophthalmia] due to red bile develops therein, then, because of its burning, it leads to "darkening of the vision" [blindness]. This is not just possible, [but is the general rule]. *De Morbis et Symptomis IV*

Chap. 23:71. If a site on the cornea becomes corroded, and part of the uveal tunic protrudes, then this is called a staphyloma. The pus that develops beneath the corneal membrane is called *hypopion*. If the eyelids become thickened and hardened on their inner sides, then this is the illness called grape scab [trachoma?]. Eyelids whose appearance is red, and whose cilia are lacking, [occur in] the illness called blepharitis [Arab. *sulak*], meaning "swelling of the lids." A lack of flesh on the large corner of the eye [medial canthus], which is also called the large canthus, is an illness spoken of as *epiphora* [dacryocystitis?]. *Miamir IV*

Chap. 23:72. A fistula in the canthus of the eye is called a lacrimal fistula [Arab. *gharab*]. The hard membrane which is on the inner aspect is called *nabilath*. *Miamir V*

Chap. 24:35. I have already observed an exceptional situation, which is not usual, and which is as follows: A young boy received a blow with the end of a knife, near the pupil. Liquids and fluids flowed out from the opening, and the pupil of his eye became smaller, and the corneal membrane contracted completely. After one had engaged in his therapy, he saw well again, because the liquids which had suddenly flowed out all at once, reaccumulated slowly. Such a situation occurs only rarely. *De Morbis et Symptomis IV*

Chap. 24:20. If one observes a man who has conjunctivitis, and if one is not accustomed to seeing this, then one's eyes will at first begin to fill with liquid [tears]. If one continues to stare, then conjunctivitis will also occur in oneself. Similarly, sometimes a man sees his friend urinating or defecating or yawning or eructating, and this seems to force him to perform the same activity. *De Motu Liquidis*

# ❧ 7 ❧

# Surgical Aphorisms

The fifteenth chapter of the *Medical Aphorisms of Moses*, dealing with the principles of surgery, is presented here, translated from Hebrew Manuscript No. 1173, a copy of which was obtained from the Bibliothèque Nationale in Paris. Words in brackets are my own additions to aid the clarity of the translation. As in the preceding chapter, the source of each aphorism is given at its conclusion.

The reader is particularly directed to the modernity of the concepts advanced by Maimonides. The principles of sterility and cauterization are outlined in aphorism 8, in which Maimonides cautions against infecting open wounds. In aphorism 10, the recognition of gangrene and the necessity for surgical intervention are pointed out. Early cure of "cancer" by wide excision is advocated in aphorism 13. The surgical approach to varicose veins, nasal polyps, peritonsillar abscesses, various tumors, and many other conditions is described. That effective hemostasis requires the application of ligatures to bleeding vessels was recognized and advocated by Maimonides in aphorism 40. Incision and drainage of abscesses is depicted in aphorism 48. The final several aphorisms in this chapter are devoted exclusively to orthopedics. Splinting of fractures, cast application, positioning of limbs, and healing time are all described. Many other interesting insights into medieval medicine can be found by the perceptive reader.

The Fifteenth Treatise contains aphorisms pertaining to surgery [lit. handcraft].

1. Putrefied boils [skin ulcers] which spread and expand into the surrounding tissues require very strong remedies. Quite often [lit. many times] cauterization with fire is necessary as part of the treatment. *Katagenes V*

2. There is a boil called carbuncle [anthrax?] which arises at a site that appears as though branded with fire. The inflammation [lit. abscess] seems to involve the surrounding area and leads to fever and great danger. One should apply a very strong remedy from the available medications upon the site of the burn and [also] apply a plaster bandage on the surrounding inflammation. Into this [plaster bandage] compound [drugs] that will arrest and prevent further spread and extinguish and dissolve that which is in the inflammation. *Katagenes V*

3. Do not use a corrosive agent [lit. cauterization] on an organ which has depth or hollowness, and there is no organ in the body that does not have depth or hollowness except the hands, legs, and soles of the feet. *Comment. Aeres II*

4. If the accumulated humor resides between the chest and the lung, making it impossible for it to be eliminated through expectoration, apply a caustic agent to the chest. *Comment. Aphorismorum VI*

5. Moses says: Consider the [warning] not to apply [caustic to the chest] unless no other means is available [lit. after despondency]. Therefore it does not contradict the aforementioned [in aphorism 3].

6. Cauterization with a red–hot iron or with corrosive medications should be employed at sites where a great deal of bad humors exude from the patient, as occurs in virulent boils. *Comment. Epidemiarum V, 6*

7. Do not hasten to puncture the abdomen of a patient with ascites. However, this is unavoidable if the humors increase until they weigh heavily on the patient and weaken him. But one should hasten to cauterize the chest in patients with virulent boils before such a boil becomes metabolized [i.e., decayed]. *Comment. Epidemiarium VII, 7*

8. If you expel pus from a site [of infection] by cauterization, be most careful at that time and for some period thereafter not to utilize oil or water [to wash the wound]. If the wound needs lavation, wash it with honey water [alcohol?] or diluted vinegar or wine mixed with honey.[1] *Ad Glauconem II*

9. Malignant ulcers which become infected [lit. bad boils which have putrefaction in them] require medications which have maximum sharpness so that their power is nearly as strong as the power of fire, such as vitriol and *galaktar* and the two types of arsenic [white and brown][2] and chalk [calcium]. The burning of these medications is like the burning of fire. Quite often we use fire itself for the aforementioned boils if these medications fail and their action is unsuccessful. These medications are also of benefit if applied to the "fireplace," meaning the central crater of the illness that resembles a carbuncle, because this is the site where putrefaction is stimulated. They should not be applied to the surrounding area [of the carbuncle]. *Ad Glauconem II*

10. A limb which dies to the point of one's not sensing when it is pricked or cut or burned with fire [anesthesia of a limb] will undoubtedly become black [necrotic or gangrenous]. In such a case, hasten to amputate it next to the demarcation site where healthy tissue is connected. *Ad Glauconem II*

11. The medications which are salutary [when applied] to the sites of putrefaction are vetch flour [*Vicia ervilia*, a herbaceous twining plant] in vinegar, darnel flour [*Lolium tumulentum*, a genus of grasses characterized by many two-ranked flowered spikelets] in honey, and bean flour [*Vicia faba*] in vinegar and honey. Add salt to these and similar preparations according to the constitution of the patient. *Ad Glauconem II*

12. If you amputate a limb which has already putrefied or which is already necrotic [lit. dead], be most careful and cautious, and employ the medications that I have mentioned after first examining the constitution of the patient to be healed and the nature of the

---

1. Excellent concept of asepsis and sterility long before Paré and Lister.
2. See also chap. 23, aphorism 101.

limb [in question]. Having amputated the limb, cauterize the stump [lit. root] as I have done for wounds. *Ad Glauconem II*

13. Cancer [Heb. *sartan*] is an illness I have treated many times at its inception and [the patients] were cured. However, if the situation becomes prolonged [lit. established] and the tumor [lit. abscess] greatly enlarged, then I have not observed even one such patient who was cured except through surgical methods [lit. therapies of iron, i.e., therapy with the scalpel] in which one excises the tumor and uproots the entire tumor [mass] and its surroundings up to the point of healthy tissue, except if the tumor contains large vessels, especially if these are pulsating [i.e., arteries], because then one cannot with assurance immediately stop the flow of blood. If the tumor also happens to be situated in close proximity to any major organ, excision is dangerous, because you will not be able to cauterize the root of the wound because of its proximity to the major organ. *Ad Glauconem II*

14. Patients with dizziness and spells of giddiness, which is called scotoma, or [patients with] vertigo or various types of severe headaches, such as migraine [lit. split head] and cephalalgia, sometimes derive benefit from bloodletting from the pulsating arteries behind the ears [branches of the external carotid artery]. Sometimes they are not benefited by this [procedure] because the vapors which produce the illness rise to the brain through other pulsating arteries [branches of the internal carotid artery or vertebral artery] which are not visible on the surface substance and which rise to the base of the brain [to the circle of Willis or cerebral plexus]. *De Locis Affectis III*

15. Any wound at any site of the body, if that site happens to be a tendon or nerve or vessel not covered with much flesh or where bone [protrudes], the patient is in danger, and insomnia, pain, cramps meaning spasms, and mental confusion can easily occur. *Megatechne IV*

16. If you are dealing with a sensitive organ, treat it with a medication that is completely painless. Organs which are less sensitive can be treated with medications which have greater potency, if the patient is in need of such a strong medication. *Megatechne IV*

17. If someone suffers from a sting or stab directly into any nerve, then absolutely, without doubt, alleviate the pain and hinder the formation of an inflammation, because the nerve is the most pain-sensitive [organ of all]. This is effected by leaving the wound open so that it does not stick together. And pour an appropriate oil thereon or enlarge [the wound] by cutting [lit. tearing] the skin, and phlebotomize if the [patient's] strength is adequate and he can tolerate this. However, if the pain is caused by bad humors, eliminate the detrimental humors through purgative medications. You should [also] pour extremely thin oil on the site of the sting, meaning heated oil. Be extremely cautious that no warm water come in contact [with the wound] because it will putrefy the nerves and the patient will die. *Megatechne VI*

18. If you wish to treat a cancer through surgery, commence [lit. commence your beginnings] by eliminating the black biles through purgation. Then excise the entire site of the illness until no residue thereof remains. Let the blood flow [from the operative site] and do not hasten to stop it. Then compress the surrounding vessels and press the thick blood out therefrom [local phlebotomy, or possibly the expression of residual clots of blood]. Then treat the wound. *Finis Megatechne*

19. Scrofula [Heb. ḥarizim] is a hard inflammation [tumor] that arises in soft flesh [lymph glands]. If it develops in weak flesh [secretory glands] which was created for an important function, such as that which was created to produce sputum [salivary glands] and the like, and if these [tumors] compress pulsating arteries, then their therapy should be similar to the treatment of other tumors [lit. hard abscesses]. However, if such [a swelling] develops in soft flesh which was created to fill empty space, and if it presses on arteries, it is healed by complete excision of the diseased organ. This can be done either by surgery [lit. cutting with a knife], as is done for cancer, or by letting it putrefy [and the pus drains out spontaneously]. *Finis Megatechne*

20. Skin tumors most commonly arise on the surface of the body. The three general goals to strive for in their therapy are: dissolution [by systemic therapy], or putrefaction [with expulsion of

pus],[3] or excision with a knife. For exostoses, only one of these [forms of therapy] [i.e., surgical excision] can be utilized. Those [swellings] that contain material that resembles groats [lit. flour] cooked in water can either be excised or allowed to putrefy. On the other hand, fatty tumors [lipomas] can only be treated by surgery; they cannot be putrefied or dissolved. *Finis Megatechne*

21. The excess flesh on the edges of the eyes called *mak*[4] and the excesses around the anus which are hemorrhoids require surgical excision. *Finis Megatechne*

22. If you consider excising something from the body, devote your attention to three things. The first [lit. one of these] is to complete one's work in the shortest possible time; the second is that no pain should be felt at all during the surgery; and the third is that you are convinced of the outcome [i.e., that the patient will survive and/or be cured]. The latter, however, has three prerequisites. The first is that it should be clear that your intent can be absolutely completed [i.e., that you are capable of doing the surgery in question and that the patient will benefit therefrom]; secondly, if your intent is not fulfilled, the patient should not suffer any damage from other causes; and thirdly, you should be convinced that the illness will not return. If you pay heed to these conditions, you will clearly see that sometimes surgical intervention is more salutary, whereas other times the use of medications is preferable. *Finis Megatechne*

23. If the vessels of the thigh or testicles become broadened [varicose veins, and varicele of the pampiniform plexus, respectively], they should be excised and uprooted. Similarly, excessive flesh in the nose [nasal polyps] should be excised, with the covering internal membrane [nasal mucosa]. Also completely excise the nasal conchi. *Finis Megatechne*

24. As long as cornification of the eye [lit. nail in the eye] [lids] is minor, [it can be treated] with warming medications that liquefy, as do the remedies for *al garab* [Arabic: eczema? or other illness of the

---

3. This mode of therapy is only applicable to inflammatory tumors. Neoplastic tumors require one or both of the other two modalities.

4. Arabic word; probably refers to verrucae or xanthalasma or milia (retention cysts of sebaceous glands or hair follicles) or mollusca (cutaneous tumors of various types).

eye] of the eye. If it [cornification] increases and hardens, it should be treated with the scalpel [i.e., surgical excicision]. *Finis Megatechne*

25. Hail in the eye [chalazion] requires excision. The same applies to pus collected in the [anterior chamber of the] eye in the illness *hypopion*. Mostly use dissolving medications, but not those that strongly dry, because when the major portion [of the pus] is expelled, the remainder will congeal. It is also eliminated by [outward] movement, as occurs in head illnesses, until the entire pus descends downward [out of the eye]. *Finis Megatechne*

26. At the beginning of the treatment of an illness associated with pain, it is proper to employ remedies that moisten and also exert a slight warming effect. Then use [pain-]alleviating [lit. softening] medications, and these are those that loosen the stretching of organs. *Katagenes* IV

27. If an illness develops around the uvula [peritonsillar abscess] and markedly weakens [the patient], but without an abscess [i.e., without pus formation], medications that warm and cleanse white [bile] [i.e., pus] are of benefit. However, if in that case [lit. at that time], as in most instances, there is a tendency to whiteness as if lacking in blood [pale or anemic, i.e., yellow-white due to pus], we would usually excise it. *Miamir VI*

28. The eye is the most sensitive of organs [lit. has the most sensation]. Therefore, drip medications into it extremely gently after slightly raising the upper eyelid. Dissolve the medications in liquids whose nature is non-irritating [lit. far from biting]. Ancient physicians found egg albumen to be of great benefit [as a base for eyedrops]. *Megatechne XIII*

29. A moistening medication that flows [i.e., liquid drops] has no effect [on the eye] unless a bandage is applied [lit. only if tied]. Therefore, for eye diseases use medications as dry pastes, because a bandage has to cover the entire eye [preventing vision]. The eye cannot tolerate being bound with a bandage that is not removed for many days, because a fistula might develop. *Miamir V*

30. If the liquid [eye medicine] trickles down the face of the

patient [lit. the one who sees], hold a vessel [eye cup] for a long time over the place where you want to wash, so that [the liquid] remains in the eye. *Katagenes I*

31. If the horny tunic [cornea] bursts, a thin, clear liquid will pour and flow out and will cause softening [of the eye]. This is the liquid that one sees in many people, flowing out from a hole where one punctured the eye [ocular paracentesis] in order to remove the [excess] water therefrom [possibly early therapy of glaucoma]. Following this, a generalized contraction of the eye occurs, and it becomes constricted and sunken. *De Usu Partium X*

32. The most salutary and appropriate medication for nerve injuries is one which dries while exerting a slight warming effect or one in which the warming effect is not noticeable but which dries just the same. Further, everything that draws liquids from the depths of the body to the outside is of benefit for nerve injuries [such as lukewarm compresses in vinegar]. *Katagenes III*

33. For nerve injuries, I [Galen] used medications in which I put crude sulfur [lit. sulfur that fire has not found] with oil until it looked like thick bathhouse mud [used for mudpacks]. Sometimes, for young persons and those of similar constitution, use either turpentine resin [*Pistacia terebinthus*] alone or with spurge [euphorbion] for dry body constitutions. Similarly, use honeycomb dung [beeswax] alone or with spurge kneaded in old oil. For people with strong bodies, use sagapenum [*Ferula persica*, a bitter oleo gum resin] mixed either with oil or with turpentine resin. So too opopanax. Also mix oil and washed lime [chalk, calcium] therein. *Megatechne VI*

34. If a nerve lies exposed from trauma, do not treat it [lit. do not approach it] with any medication, but apply lime mixed in dilute oil thereon. *Megatechne VI*

35. If a large abscess develops in any organ, it is dangerous to empty the pus therefrom all at once, since the patient may immediately develop syncope and loss of strength. This is because the pus acts as if it obstructs the openings of pulsating vessels, and if the entire pus is expelled [at once], much air is suddenly released all at

once [either respiration is interrupted or shock ensues due to loss of volume in the peripheral circulation]. *Comment. Aphorismorum VI*

36. The elimination of water accumulated in the abdomen of a patient with ascites is effected either through diuretics [lit. dissolving drugs] or by puncturing with a knife the membrane that covers [the intestines] called peritoneum. On the other hand, liquids accumulated in the water-flowing [system], called hydrocele [lit. hernia in the hanging organ, i.e., scrotum], should be emptied by a catheter [drainage pipe] inserted therein. Sometimes, a part of the membrane must be excised in [treating] illness of the water-flowing [apparatus] which is called hydrocele. And excise the mesentery. But do not hasten to excise them [i.e., perform surgery for hydrocele] until they have existed for some time. Then astringe [the area] with lime water and operate. *Finis Megatechne*

37. In abdominal injuries, pay careful attention to suture [lit. unite] the side of the injury somewhat higher than the opposite side. If the injury is on the right side, place the patient on the left side; if on the left, place him [lit. lean toward] on the right. After suturing the wound, apply bandages as appropriate. *Megatechne VI*

38. For any ulceration of any type in the abdomen [ulcerative bowel disease?], it is appropriate that blood exude from the wound itself, whether little or much, because if blood flows therefrom, the abscess develops there, but less so in the surrounding [tissues] [i.e., the infection remains localized]. *Megatechne IV*

39. In a wound from which blood is gushing [lit. the exit of blood is maximal] because of compression [lit. strangulation] on the [blood] vessels, the blood can be stopped by cauterization or by drugs whose strength is equal to cautery or by something that closes and coagulates or by its [the blood's] transfer to the closest neighboring site or by its attraction to the opposite side [i.e., phlebotomy] or by cooling the entire body, and in particular by cooling the organ in which the wound is situated. Many times, the drinking of cold water mixed with vinegar or an astringent, acidic wine, or other substances that cool and constrict, if poured on externally, stops the bleeding. *Megatechne V*

40. If [during surgery] a severed vessel from which blood egresses

is a pulsating vessel [artery], then the blood can be stopped by one of two methods; either it [the artery] can be fastened by tying or it can be [completely] severed and separated into two halves so that each part constricts and contracts back to its side and becomes covered with flesh [hemostasis is effected by tying off the vessel or by external compression]. Sometimes, it is necessary to do the same for a nonpulsating vessel [vein] if the vessel is large or the organ is a major one where there is great danger. It is most correct to use both methods simultaneously; namely, tie the root of the vessel proximal to the heart or liver and sever it into two halves [distally]. *Megatechne V*

41. Cauterization becomes necessary in a situation where blood is flowing because of corrosion [lit. digestion] in an organ or because of a putrefactive [septic?] process that has developed in the organ. We [Galen] would cauterize the proximal root [of the vessel] with fire or would sear it with cauterizing, constricting resins, such as vitriol and its various types. *Megatechne V*

42. It is appropriate that either little or much blood flow from ulcers [or boils or wounds]. If the diseased organ turns green or black or red [necrosis or resolving hematoma], we would scarify it to expel its blood, and place a dry sponge thereon. Then we would treat it with drying medications. If it became necessary to expel blood therefrom a second time, we would empty it again. *Megatechne IV*

43. If you see that only the border of an ulcer changes its appearance or becomes indurated, it is proper to operate and "uproot" it until you reach healthy flesh. If this change has already spread over a large area, it should be extirpated or treated with medications for a prolonged period. *Megatechne IV*

44. If a fistula from which nothing has flowed for quite some time develops material which is withheld, it is proper to incise it [lit. open it]. *Comment. Epidemiarum VI, 2*

45. For the inflammation [lit. abscess] called *machabo* [either colitis or dysentery] in which [the stool] is very watery [alternative trans. unclear or dirty], one should give an enema of dust water which is called *el quatir* [pulverized resin of *Dracaena draco l.*] or [an

enema] of water and honey. If it becomes less watery and the urge
to defecate [lit. need] diminishes, then later also clysterize with
wine mixed in honey and honey water. For stronger cleansing [of
the bowels], wine is more beneficial to solidify [the stool] after the
cleansing. And apply a plaster [*bolus alba*, a type of white clay] that
customarily adheres from above, and put a new sponge dipped in
wine thereon and bind it thereon from above. Begin tying it from
the bottom of the abscess and complete it at its opening so that it
[the knot or tying] presses on the abscess. Within three days change
the bandage once daily and place a small cloth with a plaster on the
opening [of the abscess]. If the bottom of the abscess and its opening are both above and you cannot change it, leave it alone. In such
a case, split it from below so that its contents may flow out.[5] *Ad
Glauconem II*

46. If much blood gushes forth, we concern ourselves with the
artery and sever it in its width, and although this [arterial stump]
will never completely seal off, at least the patient will survive this
dangerous [hemorrhage]. Similarly, if a nerve is afflicted with a bite,
then not infrequently we would be forced to cut it breadthwise.
This abolishes the movement [of the affected organ or limb but is
necessary] to save the patient from convulsions [lit. spasm] or mental confusion or both. In this manner [lit. according to this exam-
ple] we treat inflammation [lit. boil] of a large joint which is also
associated with a luxation; namely, we treat the inflammation
which in most instances produces a contracture [lit. spasm]. Thus,
we treat the more dangerous condition [first]. *Megatechne III*

47. The following medication will arrest blood flow that gushes
out from arteries, even large arteries. Take frankincense [olibanum
from *Boswellia carterri birdu*, a tree of Northern Africa and India having triangular, three-celled fruit with winged seeds] or pulverized
frankincense and aloe, and mix these in egg white until the entire
[mixture] develops the consistency of honey. Roll rabbit hairs

---

5. This aphorism is unintelligible. The first half seems to be dealing with a gastrointestinal
problem, whereas the latter half seems to be dealing with an external abscess, carbuncle, or
tumor.

therein and place this [remedy] on the torn artery and on the entire wound. Then bind a tight bandage over it. Beware of pain, because there is nothing in the world that is more irritating in provoking hemorrhaging of blood than pain. After three days remove the bandage. If the medication is firmly adherent to the wound, do not remove it but rather apply more of the same medication thereon. If the rabbit hairs which you mixed in fell out, replace them and apply the bandage again. Do not cease repeating this until the wound heals [lit. until the flesh sprouts]. *Megatechne V*

48. If you see that the medications are unable to completely dissolve the abscess, and pus develops and prevails, cover the abscess called an "expulsion," and incise it at its highest and thinnest point [i.e., incise the head of the abscess]. Let the pus flow out and apply a drying [agent] that will not irritate. If part of the organ has already putrefied, the putrefaction will have to be excised. Sometimes it is necessary to excise from the skin of the extremities [elbows], an amount equivalent [in size] to a myrtle leaf because of the slackness of the skin in these places. Be careful that the direction of the incision be in the width of the vessels and not in their length [i.e., transverse or perpendicular to the vessel and not parallel to it]. After the incision, fill the site with pulverized olibanum [see aphorism 47 above]. *Megatechne XIII*

49. If humors become entangled in any of the nonessential parts of an organ [e.g., muscle, skin, bone], and no way exists to expel them from that organ, apply medications on that organ to displace that which flows to it. The emptying is effected by an incision and by dissolving medications, especially if you think that an exudate [lit. something held back] exists in those sites that are near the nonessential parts. *Mikrotechne I*

50. Phlegmatic abscesses that develop without an external cause lead to great affliction in those affected, in particular if you perform scarification at the outset. However, if the illness is prolonged, then there is no danger in scarification. The same applies to the abscess called *chomra* [erysipelas?]; that is, if its condition is one of lividness or greenness or blackness, scarification should be done. *Ad Glauconem II*

51. The abscess known as a carbuncle should be punctured at the outset when the fever subsides and its boiling ceases, because then scarification is beneficial. And apply a compress thereon made from watery barley flour. *Ad Glauconem II*

52. If an abscess is difficult to convert into pus, meaning it is hard to dissolve, the liquids which are adherent in the organ are of a thick, viscous consistency. Therefore it is appropriate to do a deep [lit. sinking] scarification. Also beneficial for these abscesses are compresses made of figs. These should be such that the figs are cooked until the water develops the consistency of honey. Mix this once with barley flour and another time with wholemeal flour. *Ad Glauconem II*

53. You will note [lit. find] that a superficial [lit. non-sinking] scarification has no great value and has only moderate efficacy for inflammations. But a deep incision which extends lengthwise produces marked emptying [of pus] to the point that the patient feels faint. This type of scarification itself needs specialized medications. An intermediate incision which is in between the two aforementioned ones is the safest and [least likely to produce] afflictions. Therefore, I [Galen] myself have seen fit to always employ this [intermediate type of incision] except in a case where it is difficult to ripen and dissolve the abscesses. Then I made the deep incision. *Ad Glauconem II*

54. Two obligatory superfluities are secreted in the body. One [probably sweat] is of thin consistency and becomes dissolved in an imperceptible [lit. hidden] manner. The second [probably the secretions of the sebaceous glands] is thick, and this is the filth that accumulates on the [surface of the] body. The thin [secretion] in a boil [alternative trans. ulcer or wound] is called "rust" [seborrhea], and the thick [secretion] develops into a rash, it is called "filth" [exanthem?]. The boils might become moist [e.g., herpes, miliaria, sudamina, or pemphigus] or dirty [e.g., impetigo] because of an excess of one of these two secretions. Therefore, because of its moistness, the rash requires something that dries without burning, and because of its dirtiness it needs something that cleanses. In deep

boils the production of these two secretions does not cease even for a minute.[6] *Megatechne III*

55. A deep wound always needs a drying and cleansing medication. A medication that induces granulation tissue formation [lit. sprouts] should be on the first order of dryness [should have very potent drying powers], equal in its cleansing and drying actions. For example, a mixture of olibanum and pulverized beans [*Vicia faba*, lit. bean flour], and pulverized bitter vetches [*Vicia ervilia*], and pulverized white lilies [*Lilium candidum*], and blossoms of opopanax and zinc-oxide [cadmium, Heb. *tutiya*], and wine, constitutes an excellent remedy for all wounds. *Megatechne III*

56. A binding medication [dessicant] should have a more powerful drying action than one which induces granulation of flesh. The former should not have any softening or cleansing [disinfectant] action, as is necessary for the one which induces granulation tissue growth, but should bind and constrict. The medication which seals and cures [the wound] should have a much more potent drying action than the one which binds and constricts, because the former must dry the surface of the flesh [skin] until it becomes viscous and hard [a crust forms] and dry, and this [crust] replaces [the normal] skin. Examples of this [type of medication] are moist [fresh] gall-nuts, skins of pomegranates, aloe, licorice [*Liquiritia*, *Glycyrrhiza glabra*], pomegranate blossoms [*Punica granatum* or *Mesua ferrea*], and the like. *Megatechne III*

57. Wild flesh [*caro luxurians*. lit. extra flesh] that grows around a boil needs a very strong drying medication that also softens and digests, such as verdigris. *Megatechne III*

58. For many people in whom one wishes to induce sneezing, act according to the following example: Take black caraway [*Nigella sativa*] and finely pulverize it, mix it in old oil, and atomize it well. Have the patient fill his mouth with water and then tilt his head back as far as he can. Instill the oil into the nostrils and the patient will sneeze from the medication. Instruct the patient to take deep

---

6. The nature of the rashes described in this aphorism is not clear.

breaths so that the medication will penetrate more strongly. *De Olfactorio VI*

59. A man once related to me that he had a chronic boil [or ulcer or wound] on his thigh which would not heal. He went to a wise physician to phlebotomize him from his arm and he saw black, thick blood. He [therefore] only removed a little [blood] on the first day and similarly on the second and third and fourth days. He then purged him three times with a drug that eliminates black chymes and fed him nutriments that produce good chymes [nourishing foods]. He then returned to the treatment of the boil and it healed. *De Melancholia VI*

60. If you feel that an operation is indicated [lit. if it is proper in your eyes to make an incision], but the patient is soft-hearted [cowardly or frightened] or his relatives [lit. those who surround him] are in doubt, then pretend to palpate or massage the area surrounding the site of the affliction, and amputate at a time when the patient does not recognize it. *Katagenes I*

61. There is no benefit to be derived by removing any liquid which is in the process of being converted to pus [lit. who desires to turn it to pus] because it is being withheld from inside until the complete transformation [to pus] has taken place [i.e., do not incise an area of hyperemic inflammation until pus is visible and the boil comes to a head] of that which is best and most [desirable] to change together.[7]

62. If the nasal bone is broken, bandage the break and it will heal and unite in ten days. However, the maxillary bone and the clavicle reunite in twenty days, the arm in thirty days, and the thigh bone and calf bone [femur and tibia respectively] in forty days. *Comment. Peri Trophes IV*

63. Bones of young people unite earlier than those of children, because children require humors in order to grow and to replace

_____

7. The last phrase is unclear. The entire aphorism is lacking in the Arabic manuscript and the Latin translation.

that which dissolves from the bones. This was pointed out by [the ancient Greek physician] Asklepiades. *Comment. Peri Arthron I*

64. Do not attempt to reduce any broken bone until four or more days have passed, lest you cause the patient great harm. *Comment. Peri Arthron I*

65. At the time of a fracture apply splints [lit. supports] that were immersed in black, astringent wine [alcohol], especially in the summer. If you do this in oil or wax [cerota] in the summer, putrefaction will occur in the limb. *Megatechne III*

66. In a comminuted fracture [lit. break and ulceration] the patient should feel the pressure of the bandage more at the site of the ailment and less at the two ends thereof. For a bandage with which you intend to fatten [swell] the lean limb, leave loose the part above the thin limb but bind the nearby healthy parts [lit. organs] in order to send blood into the lean limb. *Antidotarium III*

67. When you bandage the arm or leg in the case of a fracture, place it in the position that it was in [lit. its usual form or picture] which is customary for the particular patient, because there are some people whose legs are stretched during the day but flexed at night, and there are others [whose legs are] flexed during the day and extend at night. *Antidotarium III*

68. Fractures of the leg require the application of a cast lest [the leg] move and the limb crepitate [lit. make noise] during movement. In an illness that requires a cast, closely reflect whether the damage that might arise from the cast will be greater than its benefit. In such a case, do not do it [do not apply a cast but use other therapeutic means]. *Antidotarium III*

69. First place some cushioning [lit. bandage] under the splints. Begin at the site of the injury and terminate at the uppermost sites in order to hinder the pouring out of humors and thus prevent the development of an abscess. Then apply the splints, and support the splints from above so that they do not slip [lit. become confused]. Begin [this supporting bandaging of the splints] at the site of the injury and terminate below in order to restrain to one side the

blood which has putrefied [hematoma?] in the injured limb. After this second bandaging, apply the tight bandage to fasten and support the whole area, Thus, there are four layers that surround the [fractured] limb: the bandage directly on the wound, the splints, the bandaging on these, and the bindings. *Megatechne III*

70. Place the splints over the thinnest place of the [injured] limb so that the ends will adhere to the thicker parts. Then bind them with a good binding equal [in all areas] so that [the splints] do not fall off. When you change [the bandage], tighten [it]. The gauze should be three or four fingerbreadths wide. *Megatechne III*

End of the fifteen treatise.

# ❧ 8 ❧

# Geriatric Aphorisms

The selections from the *Aphorisms of Moses* in this chapter concern the subject of geriatrics. Of particular interest is Maimonides' dissertation on a regimen of health appropriate for the elderly (chap. 17). As in the preceding chapters, the source, usually from Galen, is given at the conclusion of each aphorism.

Once again, in reading these materials, bear in mind that they were translated into English by a twentieth-century physician with a modern medical outlook. Hence, certain of the interpretations may not coincide with Maimonides' understanding and knowledge of geriatrics.

Chap. 3:3. The temperament during the years of old age and senility is cold and dry. The clear difference which distinguishes between the years of old age and those of senility is the predominance of moist secretions [in the former] versus the overt weakening of all bodily functions [in the latter]. *Peri Marasmou*

Chap. 3:11. It is impossible for the power [of resistance to disease] of one who is in his older years to be very strong. Many physicians have also thought that children do not have strong [resistance] forces, but this assumption is erroneous. *De Phlebotomia VI*

Chap. 4:5. The pulse of a newborn during the neonatal period is very rapid and full [lit. successive]. The pulse of old people is rather slow and weak [lit. hindered]. The other age groups between these two [extremes] have [appropriate] gradations. The pulse is fullest and strongest in the prime years of youth. The fullness and strength [of the pulse] diminish by gradations until, in old age [the pulse] is weakest and smallest. However, from birth until the prime of youth, the pulse increases in fullness and strength by gradations. *De Pulsu XI*

Chap. 6:1. One can prognosticate regarding the stroke called apoplexy. If the "attack" is severe, then the patient will certainly die, but if it is minor [lit. weak], then cure is possible, though difficult. Regarding breathing, the worst situation that can occur following a stroke is the complete irreversible suppression of respiration. Even if respiration proceeds but is labored and heavy, this too is extremely perilous and mostly fatal, but is one degree less [dangerous] than the first case. Should respiration proceed without any difficulty or work, but is irregular without maintaining its rhythm, this too is serious but less so than the previous case. If respiration has any type of rhythm, even though it is [intermittently] irregular, if not labored, then the stroke was a mild one from which cure is possible, if all appropriate [therapy] is instituted. *Comment. Aphorismorum II*

Chap. 9:100. For wasting [emaciation] which resembles old age, and wasting which is secondary to fever, as well as the wasting called *do algashi* [Arabic for coma] which occurs in patients with collapse—in these three instances, milk, barley gruel, and groats cooked in vinegar in the same manner that barley is cooked, are beneficial, in order to distribute them [rapidly and easily] into [all bodily] organs. On the other hand, honey water is only helpful for cold [bodily] constitutions. *De Marasmo*

Chap. 12:3. Do not phlebotomize a youth below age fourteen nor anyone over the age of seventy. Guide yourself not only by the number of years [of age of any particular patient], but by examination of his facial appearance. This is because many people who are only sixty years old cannot tolerate phlebotomy at all, whereas others who are seventy years old can tolerate it well because their blood is plentiful and their strength is great. *De Phlebotomia VI*

Chap. 17:27. The regulation of health in the elderly [geriatrics or gerontology], in general, consists of massage with oil in the morning, after sleep, followed by walking or slow riding. Further, washing in comfortably [warm] water, the drinking of wine, and the consumption of warming and moistening foods [are all part of this regimen]. *Regimen Sanitatis V*

Chap. 17:28. Just as wine is extremely damaging to young people, it is extremely beneficial to the elderly. For them the most salutary wines are those which are particularly warming [in their effect], and markedly diluted, and which have a red or yellowish appearance. This is the one that Hippocrates calls *vinum rucham*. *Regimen Sanitatis V*

Chap. 17:29. Strive to have a weak, elderly person consume some food three times daily, because a weakened body should be nourished in small amounts, at frequent intervals. Those who are strong can be nourished with large meals, at infrequent intervals. *Regimen Sanitatis V*

Chap. 17:30. Bread for the elderly should be bread which is toasted. Milk is not good for all old people; only for those who can digest it well, and in whom no gas [i.e., flatulence] develops below the loins. *Regimen Sanitatis V*

Chap. 17:31. Food for the elderly in the summer should include fresh figs that have already ripened. Be careful to avoid other fruits. In the winter, [give them] dry figs. *Regimen Sanitatis V*

Chap. 17:32. Watery secretions of white bile usually accumulate and become abundant in the bodies of the elderly. Therefore, it is appropriate to promote diuresis in them, daily, not with medications, but with parsley and honey and [some types of] wine. In particular, soften their stools with oil, and give them a confection of prunes cooked in honey to enjoy, prior to meals. *Regimen Sanitatis V*

Chap. 17:33. Prior to any food or beverage consumption, it is proper to give elderly people something that softens their stool, be it sweet wines or softening vegetables which are taken with oil and fish soup. After the meal, they should consume some sharp foods to strengthen the mouth of the stomach. *Regimen Sanitatis VI*

Chap. 17:35. Old age has three gradations. In the first stage of old age, which is relatively short, the [elderly] person is permitted to engage in business activities and carry them out. The second is where the [elderly] person may [also] conduct himself as we have just described, and execute his affairs. During the third stage, the elderly person should act so as to conserve his strength. He cannot tolerate a daily steambath, nor can his body accumulate that which is warming and irritating [i.e., he should not eat sharp, spicy foods]. *Regimen Sanitatis V*

Chap. 17:36. It is impossible to repel or hinder [the advent of] old age. However, the postponement thereof, so that it not hasten [to occur], is possible. This is effected by the elderly being careful with their diet, much bathing, [adequate] sleep, pleasant [but not strenuous] walks, and avoidance of everything that will dry or cool [the body]. *De Marasmo*

Chap. 17:38. I advise that no aloe or hiera picra be given to the elderly. If they suffer from constipation for one or two days, then it suffices to soften their stool with [the roots] of a small bindweed plant, or with oil, or with safflower hearts, together with barley gruel, or with the hearts of dried figs with safflower, in the amount of one shekel [a solid measure] or two [shekels] of the burning of oak [trees]. The latter softens the stool without harm and cleanses the intestines, liquefies that which is in the liver, spleen, both kidneys, the urinary bladder, and the lung. [One should utilize] this laxative once, and another type once, so that nature not become accustomed to one type [of laxative], since then it would become ineffective. *Regimen Sanitatis V*

Chap. 18:11. Elderly people require that their bodies move, because the constitution of their bodies needs warmth. No elderly person should rest and repose without having done some exercise. On the other hand, he does not need to do strenuous exercise, because exertional athletics cools [body] warmth that is weak, and extinguishes it. *Regimen Sanitatis V*

Chap. 20:16. The most valuable and most appropriate bread for someone who does not perform any physical exercise, or for the elderly, is bread which has been well-baked in the oven, and which contains a large quantity of sourdough. However, matza bread [unleavened bread] in all its forms is not appropriate for any type of individual. *De Alimentorum Virtutibus I*

# { 9 }

# Diseases of the Chest

The sixth of Maimonides' ten medical treatises is his *Discourse on Asthma*.[1] The patient for whom this book was written suffered from violent headaches which prevented him from wearing a turban. His symptoms began with a common cold, especially in the rainy season, forcing him to gasp for air until phlegm was expelled. Might a change of climate be beneficial? Maimonides, in thirteen chapters, explains the rules of diet and climate in general, with emphasis on those rules specifically suited for asthmatics. He outlines the recipes of food and drugs and describes the various climates of the Middle East. He states that the dry Egyptian climate is efficacious for sufferers from this disease and warns against the use of powerful remedies.

The last chapter of this work contains concise admonitions and aphorisms which Maimonides considered "useful to any man desirous of preserving his health and ministering to the sick." The chapter begins as follows: "The first thing to consider . . . is the provision of fresh air, clean water and a healthy diet." Fresh air is described in some detail:

> City air is stagnant, turbid, and thick, the natural result of its big buildings, narrow streets, the refuse of its inhabitants. . . . one should at least choose for a residence a wide-open site. . . . living quarters are best located on an

---

1. See above, chap. 2.

upper floor . . . and ample sunshine . . . Toilets should be located as far as possible from living rooms. The air should be kept dry at all times by sweet scents, fumigation, and drying agents. Concern for clean air is the foremost rule in preserving the health of body and soul.

Maimonides' book on asthma is of interest for all physicians who deal with diseases of the chest and provides both medieval and modern concepts of disease causation, symptomatology, and therapy.

The famous *Medical Aphorisms of Moses* (*Pirkei Moshe bi-Refuah*), the most voluminous of Maimonides' medical writings, is replete with references to the anatomy, physiology, and pathology of the heart and lungs and other parts of the chest.[2] A few excerpts dealing with diseases of the chest from this most important work will give the reader the flavor of Maimonidean medical thinking.

In chapter 1, aphorisms 29 and 30, Maimonides describes the process of respiration from the standpoint of the muscles that move air in and out of the lungs.

When the diaphragm stretches the way all muscles are able to undergo tension, meaning its foreshortening and contraction, then inhalation [of air] is facilitated. When it extends from the aforementioned contraction, which occurs at the same time that the abdominal muscles are contracting or at the time of intercostal muscle contraction, then exhalation is facilitated. The diaphragm alone is responsible for the ease of inhalation and exhalation. However, when exhalation becomes difficult, then the intercostal muscles, pectoral muscles, shoulder and neck muscles participate as well.

Maimonides recognizes that respiration continues even during sleep when he says "activities of all muscles cease during sleep. Only the actions of the muscles that move the breast [i.e., chest] continue unimpeded" (chap. 1, aphorism 32).

The relationship and connection of the brain to respiration was poorly understood but described by Maimonides as follows:

This thin brain membrane [i.e., *pie mater*] is adherent to the brain, whereas the thick brain membrane [i.e., *dura mater*] is separated from the thin membrane. There is nothing attached between it and the brain except for the passing blood vessel.

---

2. See above, chap. 4.

The *dura mater* is perforated by a hole like a sieve. This hole is cleansed by the two cycles of respiration. During both, a constant stream of air cleanses, in inspiration and expiration. The bone that protects the brain from the inside and the palate is hollow. Anatomists call it the sieve [i.e., *lamina cribrosa*]. The openings are not straight, as in a sieve, but are rather irregularly placed, as in a sponge, so that cold air, if inhaled, does not enter the interior of the brain directly.

(chap. 1, aphorism 42)

The lesser pulmonary circulation is beautifully depicted by Maimonides.

The right chamber of the two chambers of the heart was created for the benefit of the lung. The lung is the organ of respiration and voice. Every living being [i.e., mammal] inhales air only through its nostrils and mouth. Should the lung die, the right chamber of the two chambers of the heart also dies.

(chap. 1, aphorism 53)

The supreme importance of the heart over the other organs of the body is clearly enunciated by Maimonides.

Should the heart muscle dry out even a trifle, then the strength will rapidly wane. However, one can live many years in such a state. He whose heart muscle completely dries out, however, is in a condition which leads to rapid wasting and weakness, and he will shortly expire. Similar to this [but dangerous] is the wasting which occurs due to drying up of the liver [i.e., cirrhosis]. After this is the wasting which begins when the stomach dries out, and after this is the wasting which begins in organs other than the above.

(chapter 3, aphorism 14)

Aphorisms 32, 33, 34, and 35 of chapter 3 describe the physiology of the heart, lungs, liver, stomach, and spleen.

Although every single organ in the body attracts nourishment to itself, not all have the same attracting force. Therefore, it is important that their nutritional status at a time of sparse blood [flow] be unequal. The power of attraction of the heart is the strongest, followed by the liver. Therefore, the heart never lacks in nourishment even when other bodily organs are most blood-deficient. For this reason, it is not proper for us to fear that when the body appears very thin due to prolonged illness, the heart and liver will have the same nutritional status as the other bodily organs.

The natural tendency that unites humans and other living beings is that the heart attracts that which is beneficial to it and repulses that which could harm it. Its attraction power is stronger and more specific than that of the liver. The repulsion force and attraction power of the liver are stronger and more specific than the attractive force of the intestines and stomach. Should the arteries be working harder than the veins, and should the liver be full and stretched while the stomach is empty and desirous of attracting [nutrition], then the attraction force of the liver is transferred to the usual attractive power of the stomach.

The filtering of food that comes from the stomach to the liver is through boiling and cooking in the blood of the liver, where blood is transformed. There two secretions are produced, the red and the black [biles], which are then attracted to the gallbladder and spleen. The thin-substanced blood travels in the large vessel which sprouts from the convex side of the liver and nourishes the two halves of the body, the upper section and the lower. As long as the blood is in this vessel, it is mixed with many liquids, thin and fluid, and needs them to facilitate its passage through the vessels in the liver, which are many and narrow. Then the blood reaches the main vessel, which lies in close proximity to the right side of the heart; then these secretions are sifted out, the kidneys extracting them and sending them to the urinary bladder.

The liver is nourished by thick red blood. The spleen is nourished by thin black blood, and the lung by blood that is already maximally cooked, light-red and thin, nearly of a gaseous nature.

The medieval medical concept that health represents an equilibrium between the four bodily humors is readily apparent. Coughing and the production of sound or speech are clearly described a little later in chapter 3.

There are five activities [related to respiration] which follow each other in ascending order [of importance]. These are the exhalation of air during breathing, cough unassociated with sputum, cough that is associated with sputum, voice, and speech. Should only one of these five functions be damaged, then take care of the next one and do not look at the preceding one.

Expulsion of air during respiration is mediated through the breast muscles, and the throat muscles participate in coughing unassociated with sputum. During strong coughing, the intercostal muscles come into play. Voice is produced by activity of the larynx and its musculature, and speech is completed by the tongue, which is aided by the teeth, the lips, the nostrils, the upper palate, and the uvula.

Some disorders of the heart mentioned by Maimonides cannot be identified by the modern physician except by speculation. For example, does the following aphorism, "Any type of pulse with more than one irregularity is a direct result of an abnormal constitution [of humors] of the heart which is also irregular" (chap. 4, aphorism 9), refer to an arrhythmia? What afflictions are meant in the following aphorisms?

If the heart muscle itself becomes cool or heated or moist or extremely weak, then the cause is a bad constitution [or mixture of humors] which came to it, causing a weak pulse which signifies that the affliction has settled in the heart itself. However, if the blood or pneuma, which are enclosed within the heart, become heated or cooled, or if the pericardial sac or the lung parenchyma become warm or cool, and should that bad constitution spread to the heart without affecting the heart muscle, then nothing more than a transformation [in the pulse] according to the circumstances will occur, but not as strong as when the illness afflicts the heart action.

If blood or pneuma enclosed by heart muscle or pericardial substance or lung parenchyma are converted to dryness or moisture, then the necessity for a change [in the pulse] from this does not occur, because only warmth and coldness can cause a change in the pulse.

(chap. 4, aphorisms 27–28)

Other illnesses are mentioned by name. For example, pleurisy or empyema: "I have never seen a case of pleurisy that could be saved where the pulse was extremely hard, small, and very accelerated" (chap. 4, aphorism 42). "In pleurisy, first examine the sputum and afterwards do a urinalysis" (chap. 5, aphorism 1).

The cessation of respiration, whether due to cerebral disease, chest muscle disease, or pulmonary disease, is fatal. This was stated by Maimonides eight hundred years ago.

One can prognosticate regarding the stroke called apoplexy. If the "attack" is severe, then he will certainly die, but if it is minor [lit. weak], then cure is possible, though difficult. Regarding breathing, the worst situation that can occur following a stroke is the complete irreversible suppression of respiration. Even if respiration proceeds but is labored and heavy, this too is extremely perilous and mostly fatal, but is one degree less [dangerous] than the first case. If respiration proceeds without any difficulty or work but is irregular without maintaining its rhythm, this too is serious, but less so than the previous case. If respiration has any type of rhythm, even though it is [intermittently] irregular, if not labored, then the stroke was a mild one from which cure is possible if all appropriate [therapy] is instituted.

The cessation of respiration can occur either through weakening of the energy that moves the breast musculature or due to severe cold which overpowers the brain.

(chap. 6, aphorisms 1–2)

Maimonides further states that "sneezing in prolonged illness of pleura and lungs is a favorable sign" (chap. 6, aphorism 4) and "sputum reflects the cooking [metabolism?] in the organs of respi-

ration" (chap. 6, aphorism 30). A lengthy description of diseases of
the lung and pleura begins in the middle of chapter 6:

> In some acute illnesses, bad liquids flow to the lungs. If they are in small
> quantities, then no inflammation will occur and they will be excreted in the
> sputum. The uninformed thinks that such a patient is suffering from pleu-
> risy or pneumonia, which is not the case.
>
> A malignant cough is one whose cause is either catarrh which descends
> from the head or a boil or ulcer or inflammation in a part of the organ of
> respiration. It is due to a collection of viscous sputum in the breast. A
> benign cough is one secondary to a bad lung or laryngitis or bronchitis. This
> benign cough, when very strong and associated with fever, causes the sides
> of the breast and lung [or pleura] to become warmed, thus adding to the
> elevation of the fever and the strength of the thirst. If it is weak but of pro-
> longed duration, then it will cause these organs to attract thin [watery] liq-
> uids, thus diminishing the thirst and the degree of fever.
>
> It has already been clarified that respiratory impairment associated with
> [abnormal] movements of all the breast [pectoral] muscles and intercostal
> muscles has three causes. Either bodily strength has become weakened or
> the respiratory passages are narrowed or heat prevails over the heart and
> lung. If the only reason [for breathing difficulties] is the domination of fever,
> then respirations will be rapid, deep, and cut off, and air will be expelled in
> very warm [short] puffs. If the only reason is bodily weakening, then respi-
> rations will not be rapid or cut off, and the expired air will flow [smoothly]
> without [intermittent short] puffs. During inhalation of air the two nostrils
> will appear as if their two sides, called *alae nasi*, are contracting. This is the
> main sign [of respiratory disturbance] due to bodily weakening. If the only
> reason [for the respiratory embarrassment] is narrowing of the organs of res-
> piration [i.e., bronchospasm], then the breast will be seen to greatly expand
> [obstructive emphysema?]. This expansion will produce rapid and cut-off
> [respirations], but the expiration of air will be without puffs from the
> mouth.
>
> If an abnormal, usual, or unusual constitution [of liquids] occurs in the
> lungs, then a cough will ensue. If this even abnormal liquid is minor and
> warm, then the rhythm of respiration will be altered. If it is strong and
> warm, then a desire to inhale cold air and drink cold fluids will be pro-
> duced. Should it be prolonged, then a fever will develop. However, a cold
> abnormal liquid will produce a craving for warm air and warm drinks, as
> long as it remains minor. Should it become stronger [colder], then the lung
> will continue to be filled with liquids [mucus].
>
> (chap. 6, aphorisms 40–43)

Cyanosis and clubbing of the fingers associated with pulmonary
disease are beautifully depicted: "With an illness affecting the lungs
called *hasal*, namely phthisis [bronchiectasis?], there develops

rounding of the nail as a rainbow. If the tongue becomes dark, this is a sign of a caustic fever" (chap. 6, aphorism 51). The signs and symptoms of pneumonia are remarkably accurately described.

> The basic symptoms of pneumonia, which are never lacking, are as follows: acute fever, sticking [pleuritic] pain in the side, short, rapid breaths, serrated pulse, and cough moistly [associated] with sputum. Occasionally a nonproductive [lit. without sputum] cough occurs which signifies imminent death or a prolonged illness [pulmonary cripple].
>
> (chap. 6, aphorism 54)

Maimonides also recognized that not all pain in the chest is of pulmonary or cardiac origin when he said: "One finds pain radiating between the scapulae in all those diagnosed as having a painful illness in the esophagus [esophagitis]. The reason for this is that the esophagus stretches along the bones of the vertebral column" (chap. 6, aphorism 56).

Further diseases of respiration, the lungs, the chest wall, larynx, and bronchi are depicted in the following several aphorisms:

> An alteration in respiration leading to syncope is due either to a dissolution of the organ of respiration, which represents a quantitative loss, or to a deterioration of the substrate of respiration, and this represents a qualitative loss. Deterioration of the substrate of respiration follows degeneration of air or following damaging poisons or following infections from living beings. Dissolution of life spirits occurs either following disturbed emotions, such as hedonia, and strong pleasures popularly called great happiness and jubilation; or marked fear or anxiety or anger. One usually also includes pain and insomnia among these emotions. I am of the opinion however, that the two latter situations should be separately categorized, because there is no stronger means for dissolution of life spirits than pain and, after that [in importance], insomnia. Life spirit is also dissolved if it is too thin or if its organs are weak and perforated. Life spirit is further dissolved by lack of food and following severe diarrhea. These last two causes also alter organs and liquids. Galen, on the other hand, categorizes them with disturbance of life spirits.
>
> (chap. 7, aphorism 12)

> The causes of impaired respiration that force the patient to lose all the upper chest [lit. breast ] muscles together with the intercostal muscles are one of the following three: either weakening of strength, or narrowing and compression of the respiratory passages causing a choking sensation, or excessive heat in the heart and lung. If all three occur together, the patient will die immediately. If two occur, it is difficult to save [the patient], but if only one occurs, then the patient will either die or be spared.
>
> (chap. 7, aphorism 47)

Laryngitis, hemoptysis (perhaps tuberculosis), and related chest problems, together with certain therapeutic approaches thereto, are mentioned in the following series of aphorisms from chapter 9:

> Synanche [hoarseness] refers to every illness in the throat where the patient suffers a choking sensation during swallowing. The most fatal of these [i.e., diphtheria] is where no inflammation is visible in the throat nor any redness, since the inflammation and swelling are in the esophagus and larynx [epiglottis] or only in their muscles. Sometimes synanche occurs from cold, raw, viscous liquids.
>
> If the laryngopharyngitis is very severe, internal medications alone will not suffice, and one must externally apply compresses and casts poured in hot water. Do not bathe until the time of defervescence of the illness. Nourishment for a patient with laryngopharyngitis consists of egg yolks cooked in the form of the omelette called *chassu* [in Arabic], which should be soft in order to make its transit through the sites of inflammation more rapid and [also] have it act as an ["internal"] compress.
>
> (chap. 9, aphorisms 32–33)

> Medications for [a patient with] hemoptysis are composed of drugs that dry without irritating, drugs that have some viscosity, and astringent drugs. This [is the prescription] if one intends to arrest the hemorrhage from the lung or breast or bronchi or larynx. We mix medications which mildly warm into these drugs, although their action is maximally opposite [what is desired for] this illness. The reason for this is to dilute and lead the astringent medications to the sites where they are needed to act there. If the hemorrhage is from the esophagus or stomach or abdomen or intestines, then there is no need to mix these [mildly warming] medications in. Sometimes one should mix soporific drugs, such as *papaver somniferum*, in the medications for hemoptysis in order to induce sleep. This is greatly beneficial, because [otherwise] the cough would vehemently shake [the patient] and cause him harm and discomfort. Also, through its coolness, it will prevent renewed expectoration of blood and will stop and arrest its flow to the artery within which the hemoptysis is originating. The amelioration of bad liquids at a time when people claim that the taste of their sputum is like the taste of sea water [i.e., salty] requires a prolonged period. Therefore, he who is afflicted with sores of the lung cannot be healed save after a long time, [i.e.,] until the liquids have become localized, and the ulcers and boils [pulmonary tubercles?] have dried up and become hard [encapsulated?] or putrefied [caseous?]. [In the latter instance,] the surrounding areas will decay until the entire lung caseates [and the patient dies].
>
> (chap. 9, aphorisms 37–39)

There are many additional aphorisms dealing with the lungs, heart, and chest and their diseases in the medical writings of Maimonides. I hope that the reader has been stimulated by these excerpts to read further in the works of the giant of medieval Judaism, specifically his *Treatise on Asthma* and his *Medical Aphorisms of Moses*.

# ⸙ 10 ⸙

# The Heart

## The Heart in the Bible

The Hebrew word for "heart" is *lev*. This word occurs 190 times in the Bible. Variations of the word, such as "the heart," "and the heart," "in the heart," "like the heart," "from the heart," "my heart," "in my heart," "from my heart," "our heart," "your heart," etc., are found an additional 388 times. Another Hebrew word for "heart" is *levav*. This word is present 26 times in the Bible, and variants as above occur an additional 223 times. Hence, the word *lev* and its variations are found a total of 827 times in Scripture.

Most often the term for "heart" is used in a figurative sense. For example, the Bible speaks of "circumcising the foreskin of the heart" (i.e., opening the heart) (Deut. 10:16, Jer. 4:4), "heart of the ocean" (Exod. 15:8; Ezek. 27:25–27; Prov. 23:34, 30:19; Ps. 46:3), "heart of heaven" (Deut. 4:11), and "heart of Jerusalem" (Isa. 40:2).

The heart can reflect the emotions of anguish (Jer. 23:9), wisdom (Exod. 31:6), evil (Gen. 8:21) and good (Ezek. 13:22) inclinations, delight (I Kings 8:66), pleasure (Ps. 16:9), praise (Ps. 9:2), warmth (Ps. 39:4), shame (Ps. 69:21), singing (Ps. 84:3), and charity (Exod. 35:22).

Statements are made regarding the heart of a villain (I Sam. 25:36), the heart of a king (Prov. 25:3), the heart of a prince (Jer.

4:9), the heart of a fool (Prov. 12:23), the heart of a widow (Job 29:13), the heart of a man (Prov. 19:21), and the heart of an understanding person (Prov. 14:33).

Various adjectives are used to describe the heart, including "haughty" (Ezek. 31:10), "frightened" (Deut. 28:67), "pure" (Ps. 24:4), "happy" (Prov. 15:13), "fleshy" (Ezek. 11:19), "melting" (Nah. 2:11), "perfect" (I Chron. 28:9), "intelligent" (Prov. 11:29), "broken" (Ps. 51:19), "upright" (Ps. 97:11), "stout" (Ps. 76:6), "trembling" (Deut. 28:65), "listening" (I Kings 3:9), "fat" (Isa. 6:10), "oppressed" (Isa. 57:15), "pained" (Isa. 65:14), and "uncircumcised" (Jer. 9:25).

In Midrash Rabbah (Lev. 4:4), the heart is described as the decision-making organ, as follows:

> Ten things serve the soul: the gullet for food, the windpipe for the voice, the liver for anger, the lungs for drinking, the first stomach to grind the food, the spleen for laughter, the maw for sleep, the gall for jealousy, the reins think out, and the heart decides; and the soul is above them all.

Perhaps the most complete exposition of the heart's functions and activities is found in the Midrash Rabbah commentary on the phrase "I spoke with my own heart" (Eccles. 1:16). It is presented here in its entirety.

> The heart sees, as it is said, "My heart hath seen much." It hears, as it is said, "Give Thy servant therefore a heart that hears" (I Kings 3:9). It speaks, as it is said, "I spoke with my own heart." It walks, as it is said, "Went not my heart?" (II Kings 5:26). It falls, as it is said, "Let no man's heart fail within him" (I Sam. 17:32). It stands, as it is said, "Can thy heart stand?" (Ezek. 22:14). It rejoices, as it is said, "Therefore my heart is glad and my glory rejoiceth" (Ps. 16:9). It cries, as it is said, "Their heart cried unto the Lord" (Lam. 2:18). It is comforted, as it is said, "Bid Jerusalem take heart" (Isa. 40:2). It is troubled, as it is said, "Thy heart shall not be grieved" (Deut. 15:10). It becomes hard, as it is said, "The Lord hardened the heart of Pharaoh" (Exod. 9:12). It grows faint, as it is said, "Let not your heart faint" (Deut. 20:3). It grieves, as it is said, "It grieved Him at His heart" (Gen. 6:6). It fears, as it is said, "For the fear of thy heart" (Deut. 28:67). It can be broken, as it is said, "A broken and contrite heart" (Ps. 51:19). It becomes proud, as it is said, "Thy heart can be lifted up" (Deut. 8:14). It rebels, as it is said, "This people hath a revolting and rebellious heart" (Jer. 5:23). It

invents, as it is said, "Even in the month which he had devised of his own heart" (I Kings 12:33). It cavils, as it is said, "Though I walk in the stubbornness of my heart" (Deut. 29:18). It overflows, as it is said, "My heart overfloweth with a goodly matter" (Ps. 45:2). It devises, as it is said, "There are many devices in a man's heart" (Prov. 14:21). It desires, as it is said, "Thou hast given him his heart's desire" (Ps. 21:3). It goes astray, as it is said, "Let not thy heart decline to her ways" (Prov. 7:25). It lusts, as it is said, "That ye go not about after your own heart" (Num. 15:39). It is refreshed, as it is said, "Stay ye your heart" (Gen. 18:5). It can be stolen, as it is said, "And Jacob stole Laban's heart" (ibid. 31:20). It is humbled, as it is said, "Then perchance their uncircumcised heart be humbled" (Lev. 26:41). It is enticed, as it is said, "He spoke enticingly unto the damsel" (Gen. 34:3). It errs, as it is said, "My heart is bewildered" (Isa. 21:4). It trembles, as it is said, "His heart trembled" (I Sam. 4:13). It is awakened, as it is said, "I sleep, but my heart waketh" (Song of Songs 5:2). It loves, as it is said, "Thou shalt love the Lord thy God with all thy heart" (Deut. 6:5). It hates, as it is said, "Thou shalt not hate thy brother with thy heart" (Lev. 19:17). It envies, as it is said, "Let not thy heart envy sinners" (Prov. 23:17). It is searched, as it is said, "I the Lord search the heart" (Jer. 17:10). It is rent, as it is said, "Rend your heart, and not your garments" (Joel 2:13). It meditates, as it is said, "The meditation of my heart shall be understanding" (Ps. 49:4). It is like a fire, as it is said, "There is in my heart as it were a burning fire" (Jer. 20:9). It is like a stone, as it is said, "I will take away the stony heart out of thy flesh" (Ezek. 36:26). It turns in repentance, as it is said, "That turned to the Lord with all his heart" (II Kings 23:25). It becomes hot, as it is said, "While his heart is hot" (Deut. 19:6). It dies, as it is said, "His heart died within him" (I Sam. 25:37). It melts, as it is said, "The hearts of the people melted" (Josh. 7:5). It takes in words, as it is said, "And these words, which I command thee this day, shall be upon thy heart" (Deut. 6:6). It is susceptible to fear, as it is said, "I will put My fear into their hearts" (Jer. 32:40). It gives thanks, as it is said, "I will give thanks unto the Lord with my whole heart" (Ps. 111:1). It covets, as it is said, "Lust not after her beauty in thy heart" (Prov. 6:25). It becomes hard, as it is said, "He that hardeneth his heart shall fall into evil" (ibid. 28:14). It makes merry, as it is said, "It came to pass when their hearts were merry" (Judg. 16:25). It acts deceitfully, as it is said, "Deceit is in the heart of them that devise evil" (Prov. 12:20). It speaks from out of itself, as it is said, "Now Hannah, she spoke in her heart" (I Sam. 1:13). It loves bribes, as it is said, "But thine eyes and thy heart are not but for thy covetousness" (Jer. 22:17). It writes words, as it is said, "Write them upon the table of thy heart" (Prov. 3:3). It plans, as it is said, "A heart that deviseth wicked thoughts" (ibid. 6:18). It receives commandments, as it is said, "The wise heart will receive commandments" (ibid. 10:8). It acts with pride, as it is said, "The pride of thy heart hath beguiled thee" (Obad. 3). It makes arrangements, as it is said, "The preparations of the heart are man's" (Prov. 16:1). It aggrandizes itself, as it is said, "Will thy heart therefore lift thee up?" (II Chron. 25:19). Hence, "I spoke with my own heart, saying: lo, I have gotten great wisdom."[1]

In the classic verse "Thou shalt love the Lord thy God with all thy heart" (Deut. 6:5), "heart" is interpreted by the rabbis to refer to the desires and passions, i.e., emotions, rather than the intellect.

## The Heart in the Talmud

In the Talmud the Hebrew word *lev* (or its Aramaic equivalent, *libba*) has meanings other than "heart," e.g., "stomach," "chest," "breast," or "mind." The word *lev* is used to denote the stomach, as exemplified by the phrase "all medicines are to be imbibed on an empty stomach [lit. empty heart]" (Gittin 70a). Another illustration is the statement of R. Judah that "he who eats asafetida on an empty stomach [lit. empty heart] will shed his skin" (Hullin 59a). Finally, R. Joseph said that "he who eats sixteen eggs, forty nuts, and seven caperberries, and drinks one quarter of a log of honey in one meal on an empty stomach [lit. empty heart], in the summer months, snaps his heart strings asunder" (Hullin 59a). R. Joseph seems to indicate that such gross overeating puts a strain on the heart. Even the Bible occasionally uses the word "heart" to mean stomach. For example, "and wine maketh glad the heart of man ... and bread sustains man's heart [i.e., his stomach]" (Ps. 104:15).

The word *lev* is also used by the Talmud to refer to the chest or the breast. Mourning for a father or mother in Jewish law includes the tearing of one's garment (Moed Katan 22b) to expose the chest or breast. The expression in the Talmud is that one "rends one's garments up to the heart" (Semahot 9:5, Sanhedrin 68a), meaning that the chest is bared. R. Akiba is said to have kept beating his heart (i.e., chest) until the blood flowed, as a sign of mourning for his deceased colleague R. Eliezer.

The Pentateuchal passage dealing with a suspected adulteress (Num. 5:11–31) is commented upon in the Mishnah as follows: "A priest seizes her garments [at the neck]—if they are torn they are

---

1. Reprinted from the English translation of the Midrash with kind permission from the Soncino Press, Ltd., London.

torn, and if they become unstitched, they are unstitched—until he uncovers her bosom [lit. heart]" (Sotah 1:5).

Elsewhere (Kelim 26:5), the Talmud describes a covering for the heart (i.e., chest) of a child which served either to protect the clothes from becoming soiled (commentary of Moses Maimonides) or to protect the child from being scratched by a rabid cat (commentary of Bertinoro).

The placing of phylacteries (*tefillin*) "on your hearts" (Deut. 11:18, 6:6–9) is interpreted by the Talmud to mean on the left biceps, in apposition to the left chest or breast (Menaḥot 37a). Also of interest is the quotation "set me as a seal upon thy heart" (Song of Songs 8:6). Seals were suspended from the neck with a cord worn by a woman over her heart (i.e., chest or breast).

Finally, the Hebrew word *lev* connotes the mind. The Talmud (Bava Batra 12b) states that before a man eats and drinks he has two hearts (i.e., he cannot make up his mind), but after he eats and drinks he has only one heart, as it says, "A hollow man is two-hearted" (Job 11:12).

## The Anatomy of the Heart and Great Vessels

The Mishnah recognized that "if the heart [of an animal] was pierced as far as the cavity thereof" (Ḥullin 3:1), the animal cannot survive and is declared *terefah* (unfit for ritual slaughtering and consumption). R. Zera raised the question: "Does it mean as far as the small cavity or as far as the large cavity?" (Ḥullin 45b). "Small cavity" apparently means the right part of the heart, and "large cavity" the left part, not a differentiation of atrium and ventricle as we now know it. Moses Maimonides, in his *Mishneh Torah*, reiterates the fatal outcome of a pierced heart, but also describes left and right chambers of the heart as follows:

> If the heart is pierced as far as the chambers thereof, whether as far as the large chamber on the left or the small one on the right, the animal is *terefah*. If only the flesh of the heart is pierced, but the perforation does not penetrate inside the chamber, it is permitted. The aorta, that is, the large artery which leads from the heart to the lung, is like the heart: if it is perforated to the smallest extent into its cavity, it is *terefah*.
>
> (Hilkhot Sheḥitah 6:5)

The code of Jewish law of Joseph Karo states that "the heart has three chambers" (*Shulḥan Arukh,* Yoreh Deah 40:1). It remained for more recent anatomists to correctly describe the four chambers of the mammalian heart. There is also no mention of heart valves in the Talmud and the major commentaries thereon.

The piercing of an animal's heart, and the possible use to which such a "nonviable" animal may be put, is discussed in other parts of the Talmud (Avodah Zarah 29b, Sefer Torah 1:2, Soferim 1:2).

The aorta is also described in the Talmud as follows:

> As to the aorta [lit. the artery of the heart], Rab says that the slightest perfo-
> ration therein [will render the animal *terefah*], and Samuel says [that it is *tere-*
> *fah* only if] the greater portion [of its circumference was severed]. . . .
> Amemar said in the name of R. Naḥman: "There are three main vessels,
> one leads to the heart [aorta], one leads to the lungs [pulmonary artery],
> and one leads to the liver [inferior vena cava?]."
>
> (Ḥullin 45b)

The two carotid arteries are described by Maimonides in his *Commentary on the Mishnah* (Ḥullin 1:1), where he calls them "the pulsating vessels on the side of the neck."

## Symptoms Related to Diseases of the Heart

Disorders of the heart are described in the Talmud under several categories, including "pain of the heart" (*ke'ev lev*), "weakness of the heart" (*ḥulsha de'libba*), "heaviness of the heart" (*yukra de'libba*), "palpitations of the heart" (*pirḥa de'libba*), and "pressure on the heart" (*kirḥa de'libba*). These will be discussed individually.

### Pain of the Heart

The following statement is quoted from the Talmud: "Rather any complaint, but not a complaint of the bowels; any pain, but not heart pain; any ache, but not headache; any evil, but not an evil wife" (Shabbat 11a). Although "heart pain" in this passage may, in fact, refer to organic heart disease, the following citation obviously describes psychological heart pain: "If one draws out his prayer and therefore expects it to be fulfilled, he will in the end suffer heart pain, as it says, 'Hope deferred maketh the heart sick' [Prov.

13:12]" (Berakhot 55a). The expression "heart pain" in Isa. 65:14 also refers to vexation of spirit, and not organic disease.

Therapy for heart pain (perhaps heartburn?) consists of the ingestion (but not inhalation) of black cumin: "One who regularly takes black cumin will not suffer from heart pain. . . . The mother of R. Jeremiah used to take bread for him and stick black cumin on it [so that it would absorb the taste] and then scrape it off [to remove the smell]" (Berakhot 40a). Apparently smelling the aroma of black cumin was thought to be harmful, but eating black cumin was considered to be specific therapy for heart pain.

## Weakness of the Heart

R. Ḥisda and R. Huna sat all day engaged in judgment and their "hearts grew weak" (Shabbat 10a). Perhaps hunger pangs or hypoglycemia is meant here. R. Zera was unable to teach because "his heart felt faint" or weak (Ta'anit 7a). R. Avia had "weakness of the heart" and did not go to hear the lecture of R. Joseph (Berakhot 28b). Therapeutically, the Talmud advises that taking mustard regularly once in thirty days keeps sickness away. Taking it every day, however, is not advisable, because it "weakens the heart" (Berakhot 40a). A final talmudic citation dealing with weakness of the heart is the following:

> Abaye's nurse said: "If a man suffers from weakness of the heart, let him fetch the flesh of the right flank of a male beast, and excrement of cattle cast in the month of Nissan; and if excrement of cattle is not available, let him fetch some willow twigs, and let him roast the flesh on the fire of the twigs, eat it, and after that drink some diluted wine."
>
> (Eruvin 24b)

Preuss, in his classic book, states that the above remedy is evidently an emetic.[2]

## Heaviness of the Heart

Heaviness of the heart is not described in the Talmud, but two remedies for it are enunciated. If *ḥiltit* (probably asafetida, an

---

2. J. Preuss, *Biblical and Talmudic Medicine*, p. 179.

umbelliferous plant used for medicinal purposes) is dissolved in cold or warm water and three gold dinar weights thereof imbibed on three consecutive days, it is therapeutically effective for "heaviness of the heart" (Shabbat 140a). Omitting the last dose may be detrimental to the patient's health (ibid.). The Soncino English version of the Talmud translates *yukra de'libba* in the preceding citation as "asthma," whereas Preuss suggests that it refers to melancholy or depression.[3]

The other remedy for heaviness of the heart is to eat three barley cakes streaked with *hamak* (a Persian sauce of milk) and wash them down with well-diluted wine (Gittin 69b).

## Palpitations of the Heart

The remedy suggested in the Talmud for palpitations of the heart is to take three cakes of wheat, streak them with honey, eat them, and wash them down with strong wine (Gittin 69b).

## Pressure of the Heart

The remedy for pressure of the heart is to consume three eggs' volume of mint, an egg of camon, and an egg of sesame (Gittin 69b). Some commentators suggest that *kirha de'libba* refers to inflammation of the heart rather than pressure of the heart.

Preuss points out that the last three conditions discussed above (*yukra de'libba*, *pirha de'libba*, and *kirha de'libba*) are described in the Talmud among the remedies for stomach ailments.[4] Hence the word *libba* may refer to the stomach or abdomen rather than the heart.

A final talmudic citation dealing with disorders of the heart concerns a certain pious man who groaned or cried out from "pain in his heart" (*goneiah mi-libbo*). When the doctors were consulted, they said that there was no remedy for him unless he sucked hot milk from a goat every morning (Temurah 15b).

It cannot be determined with certainty whether or not any of

---

3. Ibid., p. 179.
4. Ibid., p. 180.

these "heart" ailments in fact refer to organic heart disease in the modern sense. Hence, it is impossible to state whether or not any of the proposed remedies has scientific validity or justification.

## The Heart as a Food

The consumption of heart as a food substance is said to be contraindicated in at least one circumstance:

> Five things make one forget one's studies: eating something from which a mouse or a cat has eaten, eating the heart of a beast, frequent consumption of olives, drinking the remains of water that was used for washing, and washing one's feet one above the other. Others say: he also who puts his clothes under his head . . .
>
> (Horayot 13b)

## The Heart in the Medical Writings of Maimonides

In his most famous and voluminous medical work, the *Medical Aphorisms of Moses*,[5] Maimonides quotes Galen, who states that the right chamber of the heart was created for the benefit of the lung. The lung is the organ of respiration and voice. Should the lung die, the right chamber of the heart also dies. The liver is a right-sided organ, and the heart leans toward the left side. Galen also described various constitutions of the heart. The heart attracts beneficial nourishment to itself and repulses that which is harmful. Death always follows an extreme aggravation of a bad constitution of the heart. If much cold humor comes to the heart at the height of a fever, the patient is near death. If the heart muscle itself becomes cool or heated or moist or extremely weak, the cause is a bad constitution. A bad combination of cardiac humors leads to palpitations of the heart. Sudden heart palpitations can occur in seemingly healthy people, both young and old. All are helped by venesection and a light diet.

The exact diseases or conditions being described are not readily clear in modern terms. However, it is apparent that Galen, Maimonides, and other ancient and medieval physicians described the anatomy, physiology, and pathophysiology of the heart as under-

---

5. See above, chap. 4.

stood in those days. Health was present if the four bodily humors (white bile or phlegm, red bile or blood, black bile, and yellow bile) were qualitatively and quantitatively normal. Dysequilibrium of the humors led to illness.

Maimonides ridicules a statement by Galen that the testicles are of greater benefit to a living being than the heart. If a man's heart is excised, asks Maimonides, can he remain alive and live a good life? Can he engage in sexual intercourse and show his male sexual potential? Obviously not! Maimonides agrees with Aristotle's thesis that the heart sends power to each of the other organs, such as the brain and the liver, so that these organs can perform their special functions.

In his medical treatises on the *Regimen of Health*, Maimonides speaks of extremely bad gases, especially melancholic vapors which enter the heart and the brain and corrupt their humors.[6] He also describes pain in the heart resulting in syncope and severe heart-ache following venesection for indigestion. He lists a variety of re-cipes to strengthen the heart and give it normal rhythm. A special concoction is detailed for palpitations of the heart.

Several key passages in Maimonides' *Medical Aphorisms* as well as his *Regimen of Health* suggest that he may have been alluding to movement of the blood long before William Harvey's revolutionary concept of blood circulation.[7] In fact, Jewish writers and sources earlier than Maimonides may have presaged the circulation of the blood based on biblical and talmudic concepts.[8] The historical development of our knowledge of the circulation and its disorders is described in detail elsewhere.[9]

In his *The Art of Cure: Extracts from Galen*, Maimonides speaks of sickness in the heart, dryness of the heart, and heart disturbances. He states that hectic fever, of necessity, affects the heart adversely.

---

6. See F. Rosner, *Moses Maimonides' Three Treatises on Health.*
7. J. O. Leibowitz, "Harveian Items in Hebrew Medicine."
8. D. Margalith, "The First Anticipations of the Idea of Circulation in Ancient Jewish Sources"; E. Lieber, "A Medieval Hebrew Presage of the Circulation of the Blood."
9. P. S. Roy, "Historical Development of Our Knowledge of the Circulation and Its Disorders."

Leibowitz suggests that Maimonides was alluding to coronary artery disease in his *Medical Aphorisms*.[10]

## Concluding Note

The Hebrew Bible contains the word "heart" or a variant thereof 827 times, mostly in the figurative sense. The Talmud serves as a prime source of preoccupation with the anatomy of the heart (recognition of chambers but not valves) and great vessels, symptoms related to diseases of the heart (pain, weakness, heaviness, palpitations, pressure) and remedies for these disorders, and the contraindication of using heart as a food. Some doubt exists as to whether the Hebrew word *lev* in the Bible and the Aramaic word *libba* in the Talmud always refer to the heart, since the context of some of the citations suggest alternative meanings, such as stomach, chest, or breast. The anatomy and pathophysiology of the heart are described in Moses Maimonides' medical and other writings. A variety of heart ailments are mentioned, as are numerous recipes for remedies to strengthen the heart.

---

10. J. O. Leibowitz, *The History of Coronary Heart Disease*, pp. 46–47.

# ❧ 11 ❧

# Headache

In this chapter I review the topic of headache as found in the writings of Moses Maimonides and other Hebrew sages. Various talmudic pronouncements on headache are also cited. In the *Medical Aphorisms of Moses*, drawing heavily on the works of Galen, Maimonides speaks about the causes of headache as follows:

> Thick viscous humors cause headache. All thick black humors [i.e., black bile] cause headaches if they are retained in the passages of the cavities of the brain [i.e., the cerebral ventricular system]. If this [black humor] prevails and increases in the brain substance itself, black confusion [melancholy or manic depressive psychosis] ensues.[1]

Implicit in this passage is the medieval concept of the four bodily humors: white bile (phlegma), black bile (melancholy), red bile (blood), and yellow bile. Disease was thought to result from a dysequilibrium of these humors with one or more predominating over the others. Thus, an excess of black bile results in melancholy, and an excess of red bile in plethora. With this synopsis as background, one can readily understand Maimonides' citation from Galen's *Megatechne*:

> If white, thick, cold phlegma which has not yet putrefied increases in the brain, a headache develops from deep sleep without arousal. This somnolence is called a coma [lit. sunken and frozen]. If this [phlegma] putrefies

---

1. F. Rosner, *The Medical Aphorisms of Moses Maimonides*, p. 111.

with time, these things develop but with fever, and the illness is then called lethargy.[2]

Elsewhere, Maimonides states that:

Severe headache occurs from heat or cold. On the other hand, headache produced by dryness is mild, whereas moisture causes no [head] pain at all. However, if much moisture is present in the head, a heaviness is produced, not [true] pain, unless the illness called vertigo, otherwise known as scotodinia, ensues therefrom. Headache occurs proportional to the degree of obstruction.[3]

Another very similar aphorism is the following:

Strong headache occurs from [excessive] heat or cold. The headache occurring because of dryness is a mild one, and that due to dampness is not associated with pain at all. Excessive moisture in the head, however, leads not to pain but to a heaviness, unless an obstruction develops, because the headache is commensurate with the degree of obstruction.[4]

Maimonides seems to be describing the patient's inability to excrete "bad" humors or liquids, thus resulting in headache. In addition, heat, cold, and dryness (absence or marked reduction of normal humors or liquids?) can lead to headache.

Again quoting Galen, Maimonides asserts that:

The seat of a headache-producing illness is occasionally in all parts [of the head] outside the skull or in all the parts within the skull. Sometimes it is only in some of these parts, such as in the arteries [lit. pulsating vessels] or veins or select nerves or in the meninges [lit. membranes] or in the scalp. The illness may also be in the brain substance itself. To know the exact location of the illness is most difficult and complicated, and can only be accomplished by one who is greatly experienced and has often seen such cases.[5]

Occipital headaches are one of the sixteen symptoms of phrenesia.[6] Maimonides' description of the symptoms and causes of migraine headaches is as follows:

Some people with the unilateral headache called migraine feel the pain sensation outside the membranes of the brain, whereas others feel the pain into the depths of the head. The pain in sufferers of unilateral headaches only

---

2. Ibid., pp. 369–70.
3. Ibid., p. 151.
4. Ibid., p. 51.
5. Ibid., p. 89.
6. Ibid., pp. 84–85.

extends to the linea mediana, which separates the two halves of the skull. If it is due to biliary humors, the pain is burning. If it is due to an excess of humors [whose vapors ascend to the brain], a sensation of heaviness is also felt. If the heavy sensation is associated with a red appearance and warmth, the excessive humors are sharp. If it is not associated with redness or warmth, the excessive humors are without sharpness.[7]

Several of Maimonides' medical aphorisms recommend a variety of treatments for headaches. The therapy of migraine headaches is described as follows:

> People who suffer from a strong mid-line headache [i.e., migraine] or the like secondary to thick blood or internal coldness are overtly benefited by drinking undiluted wine either after a meal or during the meal. Their pain is alleviated by the warming effect of the wine and its thinning [of the blood]. Also, feed them bread or toast [soaked] in undiluted wine, because the mixing of pure wine with food will positively prevent the ascent of warm gases from it which are harmful at the site of the pain. Thusly, an even [degree of] warmth is produced throughout all parts of the painful organ. Moreover, this nongaseous warmth dissolves mental perturbation by liquefying the humors which have already become viscous and also induces sleep and heals the organs which surround the painful, abscessed organ, widening their pores and eliminating all that pains them. All these things usually occur when the warmth is evenly [distributed].[8]

Further, Maimonides asserts, patients with severe migraine headaches sometimes derive benefit from bloodletting from "the pulsating arteries behind the ears."[9] If they are not benefited by this procedure, it is due to the fact that "the vapors which produce the illness rise to the brain through other pulsating arteries which are not visible on the surface substance, and which rise to the base of the brain." Elsewhere, I have discussed at length the subject of bloodletting as described in the Talmud and other classic Jewish sources.[10]

Maimonides states that headaches, in general, can be alleviated by mild pressure on the head "if the humors that are activating the headache require an even degree of warmth."[11] Again quoting Galen, Maimonides states:

---

7. Ibid., p. 84.
8. Ibid., pp. 146–47.
9. Ibid., pp. 221, 245.
10. F. Rosner, "Bloodletting in Talmudic Times."
11. Rosner, *Medical Aphorisms of Moses Maimonides*, p. 147.

If head-illnesses occur due to a faulty warm constitution, it is proper to bathe often in comfortably-warm sweet water, because this dissolves the sharp vapors that arise in the head and improves the body's disposition to a more favorable one. If the headache is strongly localized, it is most appropriate to massage [the site] in the summertime with oil of roses which is prepared in omphacite oil [oil from unripe grapes].[12]

Maimonides recognized, as did the ancient Greek physicians, that headache can occur secondary to alcoholic intoxication.[13] In another of his medical treatises, Maimonides recommends that wine should not be imbibed when the stomach is full or empty, because, at least in the latter case, it induces headache.[14] The Talmud also describes a sage who, after drinking the prescribed four cups of wine on the night of Passover, had to bind his temples for seven weeks until Pentecost because of severe headache (Nedarim 49b). The binding of the temples may be analogous to the mild pressure recommended by Maimonides, as mentioned above. Maimonides also suggests that people who suffer from headaches should refrain from physical exercise and other activities until the pain begins to diminish.[15] The patient should then become active until the remainder of the pain is dispelled.

As part of an overall regimen of health, Maimonides advises vomiting once or twice a month, provided that the patient does not suffer from frequent headaches.[16] One should be careful about eating fruits rich in moisture, such as melons, peaches, apricots, mulberries, fresh dates, and the like, because they give rise to headaches. These fruits should be eaten when juicy and full of substance.[17] For a mild headache it is prudent not to take any medication, counsels Maimonides.[18] Nature does well without help; a normal, healthy conduct of life is quite sufficient. Moreover, if one makes an error while treating a mild headache, the situation may be aggravated, while the use of medication may

---

12. Ibid., pp. 287–88.
13. Ibid., p. 150.
14. F. Rosner, *Moses Maimonides' Three Treatises on Health*, p. 123.
15. Rosner, *Medical Aphorisms of Moses Maimonides*, p. 150.
16. Rosner, *Moses Maimonides' Three Treatises on Health*, p. 45.
17. S. Muntner, *The Medical Writings of Moses Maimonides, Treatise on Asthma*, pp. 15, 75.
18. Ibid.

make nature lazy and dependent on that medication.[19] Headache secondary to inflammation or "hypersensitivity of the nerve which grows at the mouth of the stomach [vagus nerve?]" should be treated by strict adherence to dietary principles.

> That is, he should daily hasten to ingest some food, before superfluities pour into his stomach. He should then adjust his mode of life toward cooling and moistening [foods]. If bitter liquids pour into the stomach, he should eliminate them by emesis and dissolution of the abdomen [i.e., purgation]. From time to time, he should utilize drugs such as absinthium, oil of roses, or other similar mildly astringent oils.[20]

Maimonides also speaks of headache in his legal code, the *Mishneh Torah*, where he rules that a man who has aches in his head is legally considered to be in good health in regard to the validity of transactions like buying, selling, and giving gifts.[21] Many neurological and psychiatric signs and symptoms other than headache due to an excess of one or more humors are described by Maimonides, including mania, confusion, mental perturbation, vertigo, visual disturbances, seizures, stupor, apoplexy, delirium, somnolence, spasms, paralysis, phobia, melancholy, lethargy, hysteria, hallucinations, dizziness, brain abscess or inflammation, meningitis, aphasia, and amnesia. These topics are beyond the scope of this essay.

## Headache in the Talmud

The Talmud is a collection of rabbinic discussions and commentaries of biblical law compiled during the second through sixth centuries of the common era. It is replete with references to headache. One famous talmudic sage said: "I can tolerate any illness but not an intestinal disease, any pain but not heart pain, any ache but not headache" (Shabbat 11a). The Talmud considers the blowing away of the froth or foam of beverages like beer or mead to be one cause of headache (Hullin 105b). Headache can also be inflicted by divine decree for sins which a person commits. The headache is then cured by repentance and the performance of good deeds

---

19. Rosner, *Maimonides' Three Treatises on Health*, p. 75.
20. Rosner, *Medical Aphorisms of Maimonides*, p. 278.
21. F. Rosner, *Medicine in the Mishneh Torah of Maimonides*, p. 156.

(Shabbat 32a). Elsewhere, the Talmud advises that a person who suffers from headache should engage in the study of Torah (Eruvin 54a) because the words of Torah are "an ornament of grace on your head" (Prov. 1:9).

The Talmud rules that one should not visit patients with intestinal diseases (i.e., diarrhea), eye disorders, or headaches, the first because of embarrassment and the latter two because speech is harmful to them (Nedarim 41a). Perhaps the reason is that patients with headache would rather lie quietly without speaking, because conversation is uncomfortable for them. The Talmud also rules that patients ill with diseases, including those suffering from eye pain or headache, are free from the obligation of living in booths (Heb. *sukkot*) on the holiday of Sukkot (Sukkah 26a).

The Talmud points out that Jabez prayed to God "that Thou wouldst keep me from evil" (I Chron. 4:10), which is interpreted to mean "that I have no headache nor earache nor eye pain" (Temurah 16a). The name of King Ahasuerus (Heb. *aḥashverosh*), associated with the holiday of Purim, is interpreted by one talmudic sage to mean "headache-inducer" (Heb. *ḥash be-rosh*) (Megillah 11a).

The Jerusalem Talmud has at least two references to headache. The first is a remedy to treat headache: rub the head with wine, vinegar, or oil (Jer. Ma'aser Sheini 3:53b). Preuss points out that this remedy was already recommended by physicians in antiquity, such as Celsus and Caelius Aurelianus.[22]

The other reference to headache in the Jerusalem Talmud is to a talmudic sage who only wore the arm phylactery but was not able to wear the phylactery on the head during the summer because his head was heavy from the heat (Jer. Berakhot 2:4c).

## Headache in the Midrash

The homiletical commentary on the Bible known as Midrash Rabbah quotes one of the great rabbis of the Middle Ages who suffered from headache (Genesis Rabbah 34:11). The rabbi lamented, "This

---

22. J. Preuss, *Biblical and Talmudic Medicine*, p. 305.

is what the generation of the Flood did for us," for only since that time have "cold and heat . . . not cease[d]" (Gen. 8:22). Apparently, he felt that extreme cold or heat were associated with headache, a concept later reiterated by Maimonides (see above).

Elsewhere, the Midrash describes the case of a king who reminds his convalescing son, as they pass various stopping places on their return journey from a health resort: "Here we slept, here we cooled ourselves, here you had a headache" (Genesis Rabbah 23:3). The cause of the son's headache and its treatment are not cited. Finally, Preuss quotes another Midrash in which a famous rabbi said that if one of two twin sisters has a headache, the other feels it as well, perhaps a genetic or hereditary form of headache.[23] Although the Midrash is an important homiletical resource, it does not have scriptural infallibility.

## Summary and Conclusion

The present chapter extracts Maimonides' pronouncements dealing with headache. Since most of the statements about headache in his *Medical Aphorisms* were derived from Greco-Roman medical writers, such as Hippocrates and, especially, Galen, Maimonides was merely a compiler, not an innovator, in this area. Some of his ideas about the causes of headaches being related to a dysequilibrium of the bodily humors are clearly medieval in origin. Other statements demonstrate his concern with preventive medicine and the maintenance of a healthy regimen of daily living. Medications should not be used to treat illness, he advised, unless non-medicinal means, such as diet and exercise, are ineffective.

---

23. Ibid., p. 304.

# ⸙ 12 ⸙

# Hemophilia

## Introduction

Classical hemophilia is a hereditary bleeding disorder which occurs almost exclusively in males but is transmitted as a sex-linked recessive gene by the female. The first accurate description of hemophilia in the modern medical literature was that of John Conrad Otto in 1803.[1] In 1820, Nasse formulated the genetic transmission of this disease.[2] The name hemophilia was given by Schoenlein in 1839.[3]

This chapter points out the recognition and description of hemophilia, including its precise genetic transmission, in the fifth-century Talmud. Further medical details are provided by Maimonides in the twelfth century and by subsequent rabbinic codifiers of Jewish law. Nearly all modern textbooks of hematology and blood coagulation cite the pertinent talmudic passage to indicate the amazing knowledge and understanding of the ancient rabbis of Israel of the genetics of this sex-linked bleeding disorder.

---

1. J. C. Otto, "An Account of an Hemorrhagic Disposition Existing in Certain Families."
2. C. F. Nasse, "Von einer erblichen neigung zu todtlichen blutungen."
3. A. Castiglioni, *A History of Medicine*, p. 707.

## The Classic Talmudic Passage on Hemophilia

The Babylonian Talmud states that if a woman circumcises her first child and he dies as a result of exsanguination, and a second one dies similarly, Rabbi Judah the Prince rules that she must not circumcise her third child. Rabban Simeon ben Gamliel, however, rules that she may circumcise the third but not the fourth son (Yevamot 64b). The Talmud continues with a statement made by Rabbi Ḥiyya bar Abba in the name of Rabbi Yoḥanan:

> It once happened with four sisters at Sepphoris that when the first had circumcised her child he died [of exsanguination], when the second [circumcised her child], he died similarly, and when the third [circumcised her child], he also died [of exsanguination]. The fourth sister came before Rabban Simeon ben Gamliel, who told her, "You must not circumcise [the child]." . . . he meant to teach that sisters also establish a presumption.

Rabbi Judah the Prince and Rabbi Simeon ben Gamliel are not arguing about the question of the genetic transmission of a hereditary bleeding disorder. Rather, they differ on a technical point of talmudic law—the number of repetitive events required to establish a pattern and thus remove a subsequent similar event from the category of chance. In general, three repetitive events are necessary to establish a pattern, but in matters of life and death, the view of Rabbi Judah the Prince is upheld that two suffice.

The Talmud later offers an explanation for post–circumcision exsanguination when it states that the members of some families have "loose blood," whereas those of other families have blood which is "held fast," i.e., coagulates.

Another pertinent ruling is found in identical language in two places in the Talmud (Shabbat 134a, Ḥullin 47b), where the following story is related:

> Rabbi Nathan said: I once visited the coastal towns and a woman came before me who had her first son circumcised and he died, and her second son and he died. The third [son] she brought before me.
> I saw that he was red, so I told her to wait until his blood was absorbed.[4] She waited until his blood was absorbed and had him circumcised, and he

---

4. The talmudic commentator Rashi (1040–1105) explains that all the blood was beneath the skin and thus that circumcision might have led to exsanguination.

lived and he was called Nathan the Babylonian after my name. On another occasion, I went to the land of Kaputkia and a woman came before me who had her first son circumcised and he died, and her second son circumcised and he died. The third [son] she brought before me. I saw that he was green, and I examined him and saw no covenant blood in him.[5] I told her to wait until he became full-blooded. She waited and then had him circumcised, and he lived and he was called by the name Nathan the Babylonian after my name.

This talmudic discussion is interpreted by one author to refer to neonatal thrombocytopenic purpura.[6] Another writer asserts that the "red" and "green" probably refer to newborn erythema and neonatal anemia, respectively.[7] Preuss, Krauss, and Ebstein also consider jaundice or anemia to be the greenness here described.[8] Most rabbinic sources, however, discuss this talmudic passage together with the earlier-cited classic talmudic reference to hemophilia.

## Maimonides' Writings on Hemophilia

The medical writings of Moses Maimonides and especially his *Medical Aphorisms* are replete with references to blood and bloodletting. His major pronouncements on hemophilia, however, are found in the *Mishneh Torah*, his famous code of Jewish law. In the tractate dealing with the laws of circumcision, Maimonides states:

An infant found on the eighth day to be excessively yellow should not be circumcised until it develops blood and its complexion becomes like that of other healthy infants. So, too, if it is excessively ruddy as if it were dyed, it should not be circumcised until its blood is absorbed and its complexion becomes like that of other infants—because that is an illness and great care must be taken in such cases. One may only circumcise an infant that is totally free of disease, because danger to life overrides everything else. It is possible to circumcise later, but it is impossible to restore a single departed soul of Israel forever.

---

5. Rashi explains that he was anemic and weak from lack of blood production as yet.
6. D. Ehrlich, "Neonatal Purpura in the Talmud."
7. I. L. Katzenelsohn, *Ha-Talmud ve-Hokhmat ha-Refuah.*
8. J. Preuss, *Biblical and Talmudic Medicine*, p. 245; S. Krauss, *Talmudische Archaeologie*, vol. 1, p. 255; W. Ebstein, *Die Medizin im Neuen Testament und im Talmud*, p. 255.

> If a woman had her first son circumcised and he died as a result of the circumcision, which enfeebled his strength, and she similarly had her second [son] circumcised, and he died as a result of the circumcision—whether [the latter child was] from her first husband or from her second husband—the third son may not be circumcised at the proper time [the eighth day of life]. Rather, one postpones the operation for him until he grows up and his strength is established.

(Hilkhot Milah 1:18)

In his *Kesef Mishneh* commentary on the *Mishneh Torah*, Rabbi Joseph Karo (1488–1575) begins his discussion of Maimonides' rulings by citing the talmudic passage about the woman whose first two sons exsanguinated as a result of circumcision. He states that Rabbi Judah the Prince and Rabban Simeon ben Gamliel differed in many situations about whether two or three repetitive events establish a presumption. He cites Rabbi Isaac Alfasi (1013–1103), the first codifier of talmudic law, who ruled that for danger to life two repetitive events establish a presumption. The hemophilic infants look perfectly healthy. Otherwise, if they appear ill, even the first may not be circumcised until it becomes healthy. Finally, says Karo, the expression "if a woman had her first son circumcised" rather than "if a man . . ." indicates to Maimonides that the third child may not be circumcised even if it is from a second husband.

Rabbi Ezekiel Landau (1737–1793), in his *Responsa Noda bi-Yehudah* (Yoreh Deah 165), questions Maimonides' rule that the circumcision should take place when the child's strength is established. There is no talmudic source for this rule, claims Landau. If the infant's life is in danger from circumcision, it remains so forever. Later codifiers of Jewish law, such as Rabbi Jacob ben Asher (1269–1343), in the *Tur* (Yoreh Deah 263), and Rabbi Joseph Karo, in his *Shulḥan Arukh* (Yoreh Deah 263:2–3), agree with Maimonides. An answer to Landau's question has been provided in the twentieth century by Rabbi Joseph Kapach in his new edition of Maimonides' *Mishneh Torah*. Kapach suggests that Maimonides, Jacob ben Asher, and Karo all relied on the talmudic passage about Rabbi Nathan, where the woman waited until her son became full-blooded and healthy and then had him circumcised, and he lived. Since the infant appeared ill, it could not be circumcised until it became well, at which time circumcision was allowed.

Maimonides may be alluding to the mode of death when he states "enfeebled his strength," i.e., exsanguination. This conclusion may be unwarranted, however, as Maimonides may have lumped together circumcision mortality from numerous causes, such as prematurity and anemia in addition to bleeding disorders. As a physician, he sought to delay circumcision until health was established. Rabbi Joseph Karo in his *Kesef Mishneh* states that the prohibition against further circumcision in an afflicted family was "because there are families in which the blood is loose." Furthermore, whereas the Talmud does not state when circumcision can be performed in an afflicted child (perhaps never, as discussed below), Maimonides specifically sets a time limit; circumcision, he says, may be performed at such time that the child is declared medically fit. Maimonides thus seems to feel that spontaneous remission or perhaps medical therapy can control or even cure hemophilia. Maimonides also recognizes that a woman transmits the disease to all her male offspring even if the latter were conceived from different fathers. A contemporary writer notes that many centuries elapsed between the talmudic pronouncement and Maimonides' classification thereof in the twelfth century.[9]

## Other Codifiers of Jewish Law

After Maimonides' *Mishneh Torah*, the most important code of Jewish law is the sixteenth-century *Shulḥan Arukh*, compiled by Rabbi Joseph Karo. In Yoreh Deah 263:2–3, he states:

> If a woman had her first son circumcised and he died as a result of the circumcision, which enfeebled his strength, and she also had her second [son] circumcised, and he died as a result of the circumcision, then it is established that her children die as a result of circumcision irrespective of whether she had one husband or two. The third [child] should not be circumcised. Rather, one postpones [the operation] for him until his strength is established. The same applies if a man circumcised his first son and then his second, and they [both] died as a result of the circumcision; he should not circumcise his third [son], whether he had them from one woman or two. And the same rule applies if a woman had her son circumcised and he died as a result of the circumcision, and her sister also had her son circumcised; then the other sisters should not have their sons circumcised but wait until they are grown and their strength established.

---

9. T. Mildner, "Eine gewissensfrage an Maimonides."

Karo thus introduces the possibility of hemophilia being transmitted through the male line. He prohibits the circumcision of the third son of a man whose earlier sons, born of different mothers, died as a result of the circumcision. This view is subscribed to by Rabbi Hayyim Joseph David Azulai (1727–1806), who states, in his *Birkei Yosef* (Yoreh Deah 263), that if two sons of a man and woman die as a result of circumcision, and the parents then are divorced and remarry others, the man's sons from his new wife and the woman's sons from her new husband may not be circumcised until they grow up and their health is established. Rabbi Azulai quotes Rabbi Jacob Reischer (ca. 1670–1733) to support this viewpoint. Rabbi Reischer, in his *Shevut Ya'akov* (pt. 2, no. 82), states that if in one family there are three women whose firstborns die as a result of circumcision, then these women should not circumcise their sons until they grow up and become healthy. The same applies to brothers and to a father and son or grandson whose children die as a result of circumcision.

Contrary to the opinions of Rabbis Karo, Azulai, and Reischer that males can occasionally transmit the disease is the viewpoint of Rabbi Moses Isserles (1510–1572), known as Rema. Isserles agrees with the Talmud, Maimonides, and Jacob ben Asher that only females transmit hemophilia, although males are afflicted with it. Isserles specifically states in his gloss on Yoreh Deah 263:2, "There are some who disagree with Karo and consider this [rule] not to apply to a man [with more than one wife] but only to a woman [with two or more husbands]."

Rabbi David ben Samuel Halevi (1586–1667), in his *Turei Zahav* (Yoreh Deah 263:1), and Rabbi Elijah of Vilna (1720–1797), known as the Vilna Gaon, in his *Biyur ha-Gra* (Yoreh Deah 263:4) both explain Isserles in that they mention "because the blood comes from the woman."

Rabbi Solomon Eger (1786–1852), in his *Gilyon Maharsha* commentary on Karo's code (Yoreh Deah 263:4), tries to differentiate a bleeding disorder from other causes of neonatal death after circumcision by observing whether the blood actually clotted at circumcision and deciding if the death could be attributed to other recognized causes of neonatal morbidity. He raises the question of whether it is only true lack of coagulation at circumcision that would preclude the circumcision of subsequent siblings if they appear healthy at birth. Indeed, in the talmudic story, Rabbi Nathan seems to have attempted to differentiate bleeding disorders from other causes of neonatal morbidity by carefully examining the newborn and not to have accepted the blanket dictum that all subsequent children not be circumcised.

## Rabbinic Responsa Literature

The responsa literature represents the formal replies of rabbinic scholars to legal queries addressed to them over the generations. Rabbi Ezekiel Landau's responsum has already been cited earlier in this essay. He was asked about a three-year-old boy whose three brothers died as a result of circumcision. In his responsum Rabbi Landau answered that even the third brother should not have been circumcised. He further states that if it were not for Maimonides, Jacob ben Asher, Karo, and others who say that circumcision should only be postponed, he would recommend that circumcision never be performed on the child under consideration. He quotes the Talmud, Alfasi, and Rabbi Asher ben Yeḥiel, known as Rosh (1250–1327), another codifier of Jewish law—all of whom simply state that "the third [son] should not be circumcised"; the implication is forever. Several talmudic references establish the fact that there occasionally were uncircumcised adult Israelites (Yevamot 8:1, Ḥullin 4b).

According to Zimmels, the questions and statements in the rabbinic responsa indicate that the cause of death of brothers "who died in consequence of circumcision" was not always hemophilia. In many cases the death was due to an illness resulting from the circumcision.[10]

The principle cited in the Talmud that "sisters establish a presumption" was extended by Rabbi A. S. B. Schreiber (1815–1871), in his *Responsa Ketav Sofer* (Yoreh Deah 117), to mother and sister;

---

10. H. J. Zimmels, *Magicians, Theologians and Doctors*, p. 90.

by Rabbi Ḥayyim David Azulai, in *Birkei Yosef* (Yoreh Deah 263:4), to three women of the same family, so that if death occurred in three sons of three women of the same family, no child in the whole family should be circumcised until it has grown up; and by Rabbi J. Boaz, in his *Shiltei ha-Gibborim* (Shabbat, chap. 19), to the male line, so as to include brothers, father, son, and grandson.

Other interesting questions cited by Zimmels include the situation of twins who die following circumcision. Do they count as two sons to establish the repetitive pattern? The question is answered in the affirmative by Rabbi J. S. Nathanson in his *Responsa Sho'el u-Meshiv* (pt. 1, no. 238). Another question concerns a man who was not circumcised because his two brothers died in consequence of circumcision. Should this man don phylacteries on the Sabbath? Rabbi I. Isserlein, in his *Pesakim u-Ketavim* (no. 108), and Rabbi David ibn Zimra, in *Responsa Radvaz* (pt. 6, no. 2334), decided in the negative.

Additional rabbinic responsa dealing with the subject of brothers dying as a consequence of circumcision are cited by Rabbi Abraham Zvi Hirsch Eisenstadt in his *Pitḥei Teshuvah* to *Shulḥan Arukh*, Yoreh Deah 263:1–11. Rabbi Nachum Rabinovitch discusses at length Maimonides' pronouncements cited above about waiting until the infant's strength is established before circumcising it.[11] He concludes that the case of the four sisters probably refers to hereditary hemophilia. This diagnosis can be made even without circumcision, since any wound or cut in such a patient bleeds indefinitely, indicating that the family has "loose blood." Even the first son in such a family should not be circumcised. However, other causes of death following circumcision are also possible.

## Summary

Jakobovits summarizes the talmudic and rabbinic discussions about hemophilia as follows: If a mother loses two sons through weakness from bleeding following their circumcision, it is assumed that her

---

11. N. L. Rabinovitch, *Yad Peshutah* commentary on *Sefer Ahavah* (Jerusalem: Ma'aliyot, 5744 [1984]), pp. 1263–67.

children are predisposed to die from the operation. Hence, her third son must not be circumcised until he grows up and becomes strong. It makes no difference whether or not the brothers have a common father.[12] Karo and others also grant the exemption to brothers who share a common paternity but have different mothers. All rabbinic authorities, however, agree on extending this law to maternal cousins. Thus, if the death of a woman's son due to circumcision is followed by the death of her sister's son, the remaining sisters must defer the operation on their sons until they are adults.

## Conclusion

The sages of the Talmud and subsequent rabbinic authorities had a remarkable knowledge of the genetic transmission of a familial bleeding disorder, probably hemophilia. All recognized that females transmitted the disease, but some thought that males could also do so. It is unclear, however, whether the rabbis were dealing only with hemophilia. Some of the cases they discussed may have involved Vitamin K deficiency, possibly determined by diet in certain families, or other bleeding disorders, such as congenital hypofibrinogenemia or thrombocytopenia. While a recognized bleeder who continued to bleed throughout his life would not be circumcised, some of the rabbis felt that an individual who proved to be healthy should be circumcised. The rabbis who postulated that a male sibling of bleeders who died as a result of circumcision should never be circumcised may have feared the possibility of causing bleeding in a hitherto-undiscovered hemophiliac. They had no way of diagnosing the presence of a covert bleeding tendency except by the sibling history. No rabbi stated that a known hemophiliac should be circumcised. Since many of the rabbis did not understand the true nature of hemophilia and did not discuss the natural course of the disease, they probably lumped hemophilia together with other causes of neonatal mortality precipitated by circumcision.

The observations recorded in the Talmud and by codifiers of Jew-

---

12. I. Jakobovits, *Jewish Medical Ethics*, pp. 198–99.

ish law are incomplete, however. Although families with "loose blood" (i.e., bleeding disorders) were recognized, the question of the circumcision of a child whose maternal uncles died of bleeding after circumcision was not considered. A woman whose brothers bled to death after circumcision could well be a carrier. Only the direct maternal transmission of the disease was recognized, whether demonstrated in siblings or in maternal cousins.

For practical purposes, in our era of hematological sophistication, when anti-hemophilic globulin (factor VIII) assays can establish the diagnosis of hemophilia at or shortly after birth, it is not permitted to circumcise any young child so diagnosed even if he does not have older siblings who exsanguinated after this operation.[13] A positive diagnosis established by the finding of low to absent antihemophilic globulin levels in the plasma of a newborn infant is equivalent in Jewish law to a history of two siblings having died after circumcision. A woman whose brothers bled to death after circumcision cannot have her child circumcised until the coagulation profile of her son is shown to be normal.

With the availability of clotting factor concentrates which can replace the missing or nonfunctional anti-hemophilic factor, it is relatively safe to circumcise an older child or adult. Rabbinic consultation should be obtained, however, in each specific case.

---

13. M. Feinstein, personal communication, Oct. 12, 1966.

# ⚡ 13 ⚡

# Obstetrics

## Pregnancy and Fetal Development

Maimonides concludes the first chapter of the *Medical Aphorisms of Moses* with a description of the physiology of procreation:

> The force in semen which can be found in material within blood is capable of making bones. It is material capable of making nerves and is similar to other materials which make flat-appearing organs. This is called the procreating force, since it gives birth to and generates material not previously present. It is also called the developmental force. The force which gives shape and quality to that material until the bone has reached a certain size and a certain form as other flat-appearing organs is called the structure-forming force. It is the one which has a different origin, namely, intellectual, in addition to its natural origin. The force which causes growth of that small bone and enables the small nerve to grow and mature is called the growth force. The force which nourishes a limb until it grows and is able to eliminate superfluities is called the nutritive force. It has four powers: attraction, retention, expulsion of wastes, and alteration of form. The power of alteration is also called the digestive force. It does not complete its function save through its powers of retention and assimilation.
>
> (aphorism 1:72)

> The procreating and structure-forming forces dominate as long as the fetus is still in the uterus, while the nutritive and growth forces are like servants ministering to them. Following birth, the structure-forming force ceases to exist, and the growth force dominates until the end of adolescence. At the same time, the nutritive force and the alteration power of the procreating force will help it, serve it, and minister to it.
>
> (aphorism 1:73)

149

Later in the same work, Maimonides states that the time for complete formation of the fetus is thirty-five days or forty-five days, and fetal movement is created in twice that many days. Birth occurs in three times the amount of time from the onset of fetal movement (aphorism 16:32).

In Maimonides' Code, chapter 10 of Hilkhot Issurei Bi'ah, the treatise on forbidden intercourse, deals with fetal development and embryology. Confinement, regardless of result, entails ritual uncleanness for the woman (Hil. Issurei Bi'ah 10:1). In an earlier chapter, various forms and shapes of abortuses are cited which also render a woman unclean (ibid. 5:13–15). Forty days after conception, a fetus is said to take human form (ibid. 10:2). Embryological development and fetal sex recognition are described by Maimonides as follows:

> At the beginning of the formation of a human being, the body resembles a lentil; the two eyes are like the two eyeballs of a fly, widely spaced; the two nostrils are like the two eyeballs of a fly, placed close to one another; and the mouth is open like a fine hair. The fetus has no clear-cut hands or feet. After its form has become more clearly defined than this, but before its sex can be determined . . . one takes a chip of wood with a smooth tip and passes it from the top downwards over the place of the genitals. If the chip gets caught, it is certain that the embryo is male. If the place of the genitals looks like a split barley corn, the embryo is female.
>
> (Issurei Bi'ah 10:3)

Teratology and monster births are discussed in detail, including abortuses resembling a domestic or wild animal or a bird, or a snake (Issurei Bi'ah 10:8–10). Esophageal atresia, anencephaly, spina bifida, and other congenital abnormalities are cited by Maimonides as follows:

> If the fetus is born with an obstructed gullet, or if it lacks everything from the navel downwards and is, therefore, shapeless, or if its skull is shapeless, or if its face is covered over so that it is unrecognizable, or if it has two backs and two spines, or if the abortion consists of a head which has no recognizable articulation, or an arm without recognizable lines—a fetus of any of these kinds does not render the mother unclean through childbirth.
>
> (Issurei Bi'ah 10:11).

An expert veterinarian is required to distinguish between an embryo or fetus or placenta and a blood clot discharged from the womb of an animal (Hilkhot Bekhorot 4:10). A human fetus is said to take form forty-one days after conception (ibid. 4:12). This Maimonidean assertion is probably based on the amazing knowledge of embryology and fetal development of the talmudic physician-sage known as Samuel.[1] In Samuel's view, a true embryo, as opposed to a clot shaped like a fetus, had hair on its head (Niddah 25a). He also said that "an aborted sac on which a hair that lay on one side could be seen through the other side" was not a true embryo, because "if it were in fact a fetus, it would not have been so transparent" (ibid.). Samuel further thought that a placenta can be attributed to an embryo as late as ten days after the latter's birth (ibid. 26b). Monster births are also described by Samuel (ibid. 24a). Finally and perhaps most important is Samuel's recognition that the human fetus takes recognizable form forty-one days after conception (ibid. 25b).

A woman is considered pregnant from the time that the fetus becomes discernible, i.e., at three months (Issurei Bi'ah 9:4). An unborn fetus does not have the status of a person, and therefore, if one transfers ownership through a third party to a fetus, the transaction is not valid (Hilkhot Mekhirah 22:10). However, if a man on his deathbed enjoins that a gift be given to his child which is still an embryo in the womb of its mother, the embryo acquires title to it (Hilkhot Zekhiyah u-Matanah 8:5). An unborn fetus is part of the mother. Therefore, someone who sells a pregnant female slave also sells thereby the unborn fetus (Hilkhot Mekhirah 27:7).

A one-day-old baby inherits his mother (Hilkhot Neḥalot 1:13) and need not prove its viability for thirty days. An unborn fetus or embryo does not inherit (ibid. 2:5). Midwives used to deliver babies (ibid. 2:14). A stillbirth is not considered a firstborn in relation to the laws of inheritance (ibid. 2:10). Nor is a child born by cesarean section considered a firstborn in this regard (ibid. 2:11). If a fetus of a pregnant woman extrudes a limb and then withdraws it, the mother is deemed unclean through childbirth (Hilkhot Mishkav Umoshav 3:9).

---

1. See F. Rosner, "Mar Samuel the Physician."

Pregnancy in general is discussed in the *Medical Aphorisms of Moses*. For example, Maimonides states that the discomforts of pregnancy (e.g., morning sickness) and the cessation of menses in the first and second month are not necessarily clear indications of the existence of a pregnancy (aphorism 16:1). An alternative explanation of amenorrhea is the obstruction of menstrual outflow from the mouth of the uterus (ibid.). The result of such a situation is vividly depicted as follows:

> Spasm of the uterus occurs if menstruation is withheld, and the uterus and the vessels leading to it become filled [with blood], and its ligaments tighten, and the uterus is stretched upward, and presses on the diaphragm. Respiration then becomes difficult, and pressure on the stomach causes severe pain.
>
> (aphorism 16:16)

Maimonides seems to be describing pica in pregnancy when he asserts that

> Perverse craving for food occurs to one who has bad superfluities in the folds of the stomach, which penetrate it. This occurs in women with bad liquids at the time of conception. Mostly, they crave sour and pungent things and anything sharp, as well as soot and dust. This occurs in most women during the first three months of pregnancy and afterward subsides in the fourth. This is because these liquids are ejected through vomiting, and the other parts will eventually be digested, since the alimentary intake of the woman is small, because of the occurrence of loss of appetite in these [patients]; also because the fetus then draws out all it can. Then, the filling of the body of the woman diminishes, and the bad liquids therein also decrease.
>
> (aphorism 16:23)

> The illness which occurs due to craving for things originates from alterations in the mouth of the stomach. Indeed, all disorders that develop in women at a time when they have a ravenous appetite or only craving for bad things, arise from a disturbance at the mouth of the stomach.
>
> (aphorism 16:24)

Maimonides ridicules Galen's assertion that male fetuses are mostly conceived by a woman on the right side of the uterus, whereas female fetuses are conceived on the left side. The apparent recognition by Maimonides of the increased blood volume during pregnancy seems to be reflected in the statement that "the pulse is greater, the beat is stronger and also more rapid" (aphorism 16:28).

Returning to Maimonides' Code, he rules that a divorcee or a widow may not remarry or become betrothed without waiting ninety days in order to determine whether or not she is pregnant, so as to be able to distinguish between the seed of the first husband and the seed of the second (Hilkhot Gerushin 11:18). The establishment of the child's true paternity is important because the father is responsible for the child's maintenance, and because the child inherits the father. Maimonides and the sages even extend the ninety-day waiting period to women physically incapable of bearing children, minors, aged women, sterile women, barren women, and women whose husbands are across the sea or in ill health or confined in prison (ibid. 11:20).

The following four women are deemed ritually unclean only from the time they suffer a flow and do not convey uncleanness retroactively; one who is pregnant, one who gives suck, a virgin, and an old woman (Hilkhot Mishkav Umoshav 4:1). A pregnant woman is one whose unborn child is discernible (ibid.). One who gives suck is a woman who nurses throughout twenty-four months after childbirth (ibid.). A virgin is a woman who has never yet suffered a flow. The sages were speaking here of a woman who is virginal as regards blood and not of one who is virginal as regards "virginity." Thus, even if she is married and has suffered a flow of blood by reason of the marital act, or if she bears a child and suffers a flow of blood by reason of childbearing, she is still a "virgin" as regards ritual uncleanness (ibid.). An old woman is one over whom three months pass without her suffering a blood flow near to her time of old age. What does "near to her time of old age" mean? That her companions can call her "old woman" to her face without her feeling resentful (ibid.).

## Abortion and Embryotomy

In Jewish law, a fetus is not regarded as a complete human being until it is born and, hence, may be destroyed to save the mother's life.[2] Both here, in relation to an ox goring a pregnant woman and inducing a miscarriage (Hilkhot Nizkei Mamon 11:3), and later, in relation to a human being who assaults a woman, even unintentionally, causing accidental abortion (Hilkhot Ḥovel u–Mazik 4:1), Maimonides speaks only of the compensation for injury and pain that must be paid to the woman for the premature loss of her fetus. Since the fetus is considered to be an appendage of the mother and belongs jointly to her and her husband, damages must be paid for its premature death. However, the one responsible is not culpable for involuntary homicide, since the unborn fetus is not considered to be a person or full human being. The morality of abortion in Jewish law and the partial-person status of the fetus are discussed elsewhere.[3]

Murder is a capital crime (Hilkhot Roẓe'aḥ u-Shemirat Nefesh 1:1). The preventive killing of a "pursuer" is described by Maimonides as follows: "If one person is pursuing another with the intention of killing him, even if the pursuer is a minor, it is the duty of every Israelite to save the pursued, even at the cost of the pursuer's life" (ibid. 1:6).

The ruling about the pursuer is based on scriptural passages (Lev. 19:16, Deut. 25:11–12) and talmudic discussions (Sanhedrin 72b, 73a) which assert that it is a duty to disable or even take the life of an assailant to protect the life of a fellow human being. Maimonides and others extend the concept of the pursuer to an unborn fetus that is endangering the mother's life. Thus,

> The sages ruled that if a pregnant woman is having difficulty in giving birth, the child inside her may be removed, either by drugs or by surgery, because it is regarded as a pursuer that is trying to kill her. But once its head has appeared, it must not be touched, for we may not set aside one human life to save another, and what is happening is the course of nature.
>
> (Roẓe'aḥ u-Shemirat Nefesh 1:9)

Maimonides is telling us several things. Firstly, an unborn fetus is technically not a human being and hence may (or must) be

---

2. F. Rosner, "The Jewish Attitude Toward Abortion"; I. Jakobovits, "Jewish Views on Abortion"; D. M. Feldman, *Marital Relations, Birth Control and Abortion in Jewish Law,* pp. 251–94.

3. F. Rosner, "The Morality of Abortion."

destroyed to preserve the mother's life. Secondly, once birth begins, the baby is considered to be a human being and cannot be destroyed even to save the mother because one is not allowed to destroy one life to save another, the only exception being the case of a pursuer, as described above. Thirdly, Maimonides permits abortion or embryotomy to save the mother's life not only because the unborn fetus is not a human being, but also because it is equated with a pursuer, whereby the fetus is considered to be pursuing the mother and trying to kill her. Many rabbinic authorities are puzzled by this assertion. They claim that the concept of pursuit is totally inappropriate here because the fetus's endangering the mother's life is an act of God. The child has no willful intention to kill the mother. It is a case of heavenly pursuit. Maimonides himself seems to agree when he states that "what is happening is the course of nature."

A contradictory ruling seems to be emerging. On the one hand, the concept of pursuit is invoked by Maimonides and others to allow therapeutic abortion to save the mother's life. On the other hand, the validity of this argument is dismissed because nature and not the fetus is pursuing the mother. The problem can be resolved as follows: The nonperson status of the fetus prior to birth is not sufficient to warrant destruction of the fetus to preserve the mother's life, since such destruction is a serious moral offense, even if it is not a penal crime. Thus, one must invoke the additional argument of pursuit. After the baby begins to be born, however, the fetus attains the status of a human being, and the "weak" argument of pursuit no longer justifies killing the child even if the mother's life is threatened, since it is a case of heavenly pursuit.

One of the major talmudic sources on abortion (Arakhin 7a) is codified by Maimonides, who states that if a pregnant woman is taken out to be executed following conviction for a capital offense, one does not wait for her to give birth but carries out the sentence promptly (Hil. Sanhedrin 12:4) in accordance with Jewish law, which requires implementation of the sentence on the same day that the verdict of conviction has been rendered.

In the *Medical Aphorisms of Moses*, referred to at the beginning of this chapter, Maimonides cites the physiological cause for abortion according to the medieval concept that disease is caused by a dys-equilibrium of the four bodily humors:

> If a woman is pregnant and aborts after two months, or three or four, then one knows that the cause for this is the white liquids which accumulated in the openings of the arteries that are in the uterus. Depending upon these liquids, the connection between the pulsating vessels and nonpulsating vessels in the uterus and placenta becomes weaker, because [the womb] is unable to tolerate the additional weight of the fetus; rather [the woman] will abort it and easily expel it from herself.
>
> (aphorism 16:27)

He also states that a woman may abort because of exertional activity or because of steambathing, "because a bath softens the body and the nerves" (aphorism 16:30). A woman may also miscarry following excessive anointing of her head with oil because this produces and evokes coughing, and as a result the uterus is shaken up and expels the fetus (ibid.).

Returning to Maimonides' *Mishneh Torah*, he points out that six precepts were given to Adam: the prohibitions of idolatry, blasphemy, murder, adultery, and robbery, and the command to establish courts of justice (Hil. Melakhim 9:1). An additional commandment was given to Noah: the prohibition of eating a limb from a living animal (ibid.). These are known as the seven precepts of the offspring of Noah. Intentional abortion is included in the prohibition of murder, as Maimonides asserts:

> A Noahide who kills a person, even the fetus in its mother's womb, is put to death therefor. So, too, if he kills one suffering from a fatal disease, or ties a man with a rope and places him before a lion, or leaves him to starve to death, he is executed because in each case, he caused the death of the victim . . .
>
> (Hil. Melakhim 9:4)

Abortion in Judaism has already been referred to above and will not be further discussed here except to say that greater stringency applies to a Noahide than to an Israelite in regard to the prohibition of abortion.

Maimonides discusses embryotomy in animals to save the mother's life (Hil. Bekhorot 4:14). Embryotomy in humans to save the mother's life is described in the Talmud (Oholot 7:6) and is the basis for the Jewish attitude toward abortion, where abortion or embryotomy is not only permissible but mandated if the mother's life is at stake. Also described by Maimonides in this treatise are a variety of uterine abnormalities, such as a double uterus (Hil. Bekhorot 4:18) and uterine tears or lacerations (ibid. 4:19).

An abortion conveys ritual uncleanness (Hil. Tumat Met 2:1), as does a placenta (ibid. 25:10). Women are said to bury their abortions in the fields (ibid. 8:3), although abortions are sometimes thrown into cisterns (ibid. 9:2, 9:11). Only an abortus forty days or older conveys uncleanness (ibid. 11:8), a recognition of the fact that an embryo begins to take form forty days after conception. A woman becomes ritually unclean not only after the birth of a healthy child but also if she delivers a dead infant or even a small fetus (ibid. 25:12). Habitual aborters are discussed by Maimonides when he says that "if she miscarries three times in succession, the presumption is that she is prone to miscarry; perchance he is not destined to build a family by her" (Hilkhot Ishut 15:12).

The firstborn son of every Israelite must be redeemed (Hilkhot Bekhorim 11:1) for five silver coins (ibid. 1:6). If a fetus was dismembered in its mother's womb and extracted limb by limb, any baby that is subsequently born is not considered to be the firstborn (ibid. 11:15). A male firstborn child delivered by cesarean section is exempt from redemption (ibid. 11:16). Redemption of a firstborn son occurs on the thirty-first day of life so that the infant proves its viability (ibid. 11:17). Mourning is not observed for an aborted child nor for a newborn infant that does not survive for thirty days (Hil. Evel 1:6).

Furthermore, someone who kills an infant less than thirty days old, even a Down's Syndrome or Tay-Sachs or other physically or mentally handicapped infant, is not put to death, although the offense is morally considered to be infanticide (ibid. 2:6). Killing someone who is dying or even a person in his death throes is murder, and the death penalty is imposed (ibid. 2:7). Killing someone who suffers from a fatal organic disease is not permitted (ibid. 2:7). Mercy killing in Judaism is a topic beyond the scope of this essay, and the interested reader is referred elsewhere for detailed discussion.[4]

## Lactation

The protection of children in Judaism extends even to the unborn fetus and the nursing infant. Thus, a man is not permitted to marry a woman who is pregnant or nursing (Hil. Gerushin 11:25). In the case of a pregnant woman, the objection is that the fetus might be hurt by sexual intercourse, since the second husband, not being the fetus's father, would not be concerned about its welfare and would not take the proper precautions. In the case of a nursing woman, the fear is that the stepfather would not provide the necessary nourishment and medicaments to preserve the wholesomeness of the milk, which might, therefore, spoil and harm the nursing infant (ibid.). The usual lactation period is twenty-four months (ibid. 11:26). Elsewhere in his Code, Maimonides reiterates the twenty-four-month lactation period for a nursing woman (Hil. Issurei Bi'ah 9:4, Hil. Ishut 21:13).

A wife who is nursing her child should work less than usual and consume more than usual of foods and beverages which are beneficial for lactation (Hil. Ishut 21:11). If she gives birth to twins, she may not be compelled to nurse both of them; rather, she should nurse one of them, and the husband should hire a wetnurse for the other (ibid. 21:12). Nursing of a child by a divorcee is also discussed (ibid. 21:16–17).

Finally, in his *Aphorisms*, Maimonides devotes three aphorisms to lactation:

> If a nursing woman's milk is withheld, although not completely withheld, this signifies that an illness will occur in this woman. If it is abundant, it shows that the nature of the breasts is of normal strength in its activity.
> (aphorism 16:35)

> If the milk from a pregnant woman flows out, the fetus is weak and, because of its weakness, cannot attract liquids to itself, and they return to

---

4. F. Rosner, "The Jewish Attitude Toward Euthansia"; I. Jakobovits, *Jewish Medical Ethics*, pp. 119–25.

the breasts, and then milk is formed. If the liquid remains in the breasts, then the fetus is healthier.

(aphorism 16:36)

Mother's milk is the proper nutrition for a newborn infant, because its composition is the same as the blood from which he was created. If the milk ceases, then one should choose [another] suitable milk for him.

(aphorism 16:37)

# ❧ 14 ❧

# Dentistry

This chapter presents a review of dentistry, with a variety of references to the teeth, as found in the Bible and Talmud, as well as a description of the vignettes and authentic statements about dentistry and the teeth in the medical and rabbinic writings of Moses Maimonides.

## Dentistry in the Bible and the Talmud

Julius Preuss's classic text on medicine in the Bible and the Talmud devotes a whole chapter to dentistry.[1] Another book is devoted in its entirety to the history of dentistry in the Talmud.[2] Articles on this subject also appear periodically in the medical literature.[3]

The prophet Jeremiah laments that God broke his teeth with gravel stones (Lam. 3:16). Homiletically, a broken tooth is said to be "like confidence in an unfaithful man in time of trouble" (Prov. 25:19). Esau wept on his encounter with Jacob because his teeth were loose and painful (Genesis Rabbah 78:9). A priest lacking teeth is not fit for Temple service because of his unsightly appearance (Bekhorot 7:6, 44a).

---

1. J. Preuss, *Biblical and Talmudic Medicine*, chap. 7. See also F. Rosner, "Dentistry in the Bible and Talmud."
2. G. Nobel, *Zur Geschichte der Zahnheilkunde in Talmud.*
3. See Asbell, "Review of Hebrew Dentistry."

Vinegar is harmful to the teeth, as is smoke to the eyes (Prov. 10:26). Vinegar loosens healthy teeth but heals a toothache or gum wound; on the other hand, sour fruit juice is efficacious for toothache and does not harm healthy teeth (Shabbat 111a, Bezah 18b). In case of need, one may even use vinegar produced during the Sabbatical year, when fields must lie fallow; such fruits are otherwise permitted only "for nourishment" (Lev. 25:12). Vapors of a bathhouse are also harmful to the teeth (Jer. Avodah Zarah 3:42d). Prolonged fasting causes the teeth to become black (Jer. Shabbat 5:7c, Nazir 52b, Hagigah 22b).

Rabbi Judah the Prince was liberated from a severe toothache when the prophet Elijah touched his tooth (Jer. Ketubbot 12:35a). A special remedy for the teeth is to place a garlic root ground with oil and salt on the side where the tooth aches. A rim of dough should be placed around it, taking care that it not touch the flesh, as it may cause leprosy (Gittin 69a).

Tooth extraction was a serious operation in antiquity. Rav told his son not to have a tooth extracted (Pesahim 113a). The talmudic commentator explains that the extraction of a molar tooth might affect the eyesight. Great emphasis was placed on beautiful teeth. A person who whitens his neighbor's teeth is better than one who gives him milk to drink (Ketubbot 111b). Lovers extol one another by saying that their teeth are like a flock of sheep which has come up from the washing (Song of Songs 4:2, 6:6). Jacob promised his son Judah "teeth whiter than milk" (Gen. 49:12).

Spleen is considered in the Talmud to be good for the teeth, whereas leek is harmful. However, the spleen should be chewed and spit out, because if swallowed, it harms the digestion (Berakhot 44b). Sour grapes set the teeth on edge (Jer. 31:29).

Artificial teeth of silver and gold are described in the Talmud (Shabbat 65a), as is a wooden toothpick (Bezah 33a). A reed should not be used for this purpose because it might injure the gums (Hullin 16b). A gold tooth prepared for a young maiden rendered her beautiful so that she was able to be married (Nedarim 66b). Artificial teeth were prepared by craftsmen (Jer. Shabbat 6:8c). Wood chips or toothpicks were constantly carried between the teeth (Tos.

Shabbat 5:1), perhaps to achieve proper alignment of misaligned teeth. The expression "take the chip out from between your teeth" was often followed by the retort "take the beam out from your eyes" (Arakhin 16b).

Teeth also play an important and specific role in the Jewish legal sphere. The phrase "eye for eye, tooth for tooth" (Exod. 21:24, Lev. 24:20) is not understood literally in Jewish law. Rather, it means that the injured party is entitled to financial compensation. Whereas the Code of Hammurabi interprets "tooth for tooth" literally, so that a man who knocks out the teeth of another man must have his own teeth knocked out, Jewish law rules that if someone knocks out the tooth of his servant, the servant is given his freedom as a substitute for the tooth (Exod. 21:27). This rule applies even if the tooth is already loose but still usable, and also if the tooth was only loosened but became unusable as a result of the blow by the master (Tos. Bava Kamma 9:27). A physician who drills his servant's tooth and causes it to fall out must give his servant his freedom (Bava Kamma 26b).

Various remedies are cited for scurvy of the gums. This ailment is defined as bleeding from the gums if one places anything between the teeth. The cause of this illness is said to be the chill of cold wheat-food and the heat of hot barley-food, as well as the remnant of fish hash and flour. The remedies are leaven water with olive oil and salt, geese fat smeared with a goose quill, and ashes from burned unripe seeds of an olive (Avodah Zarah 28a).

### Dentistry in the Writings of Maimonides

In 1939, Khalifah published an article on dentistry in Maimonides' medical writings.[4] In it he quotes extensively about the treatment of toothache, extraction of teeth, a remedy for the throat, a remedy for the teeth, a remedy for halitosis, remedies for the mouth, remedies for wine odor, and prescriptions to keep the tongue healthy.

---

4. E. S. Khalifah, "Dentistry in the Twelfth Century as Revealed in the Medical Writings of Maimonides."

Khalifah claims to be quoting from Awad Wasif's Arabic edition of Maimonides' *Regimen of Health.*[5] If one examines Wasif's work, published in Cairo in 1908, one notes that the first part of the book is actually part of the *Regimen of Health* of Maimonides. Two prescriptions concern dentistry. Additional quotations by Khalifah on dentistry are not from Maimonides' medical works. These misquotations were perpetuated by Asbell, who quoted Khalifah verbatim in 1943 and again in 1946.[6]

Dentistry and subjects of dental interest are mentioned often in the *Medical Aphorisms of Moses.*[7] In the first chapter, quoting Galen, Maimonides states that nerves do not insert into the cartilage, ligament, or adipose tissue of bone except one organ, the penis. Teeth are the exception among bones because fine nerves are found in their roots.

In the seventh chapter, again quoting Galen, Maimonides states:

The reason which necessitates the tranquilization of pain following the extraction of a painful tooth is that the nerve which attaches to the root of the painful tooth heals through the severance of this connection and attachment to the bone through which this stretching was originally produced. Thus, place is formed therein through which dissolved liquids which have gathered there can exit.

The cause for the breaking of teeth and their corrosion lies in their softening. Therefore, it is important to harden them and strengthen them with astringent medications. The same is true for changes in their appearance to yellow and the like, which occurs due to bad liquids which descend to them. Heal them with remedies which produce an intermediate degree of dryness, and [believe] not, as some physicians think, that the more powerful the drying agent, the more beneficial it is [to the teeth].

In the ninth chapter of his *Medical Aphorisms*, Maimonides points out that a warm cataplasm or compress applied to the teeth, either externally or directly inside the mouth, should be applied before meals on an empty stomach or after a long period following a meal.

In his *Treatise on Poisons and Their Antidotes*, Maimonides discusses

---

5. For further information on the *Regimen of Health*, see above, chap. 1.

6. M. B. Asbell, "A Review of Hebraic Dentistry from Earliest Times Through the Middle Ages," and "Vignettes in Dental History."

7. See above, chap. 4.

the treatment of someone bitten by a poisonous snake or other animal.[8] He recommends that a ligature immediately be tied above the site of the bite to prevent the poison from spreading throughout the body. An incision should be made at the site of the bite and the wound sucked. The person sucking on the wound should spit out all that he sucks. He should first rinse his mouth with olive oil or wine and oil, and should not have any oral illness nor decayed teeth.

In the Arabic version of his *Regimen of Health* quoted by Khalifah, Maimonides cites the following remedy for toothache and tooth extraction.

> The remedy is that the sufferer should take two grains of mountain raisins and wrap them in cotton wool and wet them in water and crush them between two stones and apply to the affected tooth, for it will soothe the pain locally: or take one *qirat* [1/16 of a drachm] of *Colotropis procera* and wrap it in cotton wool and apply to the tooth, for it alleviates pain. He [the sufferer] may also use alkali, tar, cautery, or betel leaves and others. For tooth extraction without using steel [instruments], take pyrethra and leave it [immersed] in vinegar for a month until it becomes soft as dough; then apply it to the [affected] tooth, which should be removed instantly; or take the root of the mulberry, let it solidify in the sun in a glass, and apply it to the tooth, which will drop out immediately.

Another remedy for the teeth is the following:

> Take one ounce of *kabuli* [myrobalan of Kabul] and an ounce of *Phyllanthus embelica*, and half an ounce each of cinnamon bark and coriander, two drachms of Indian nard, and one drachm of mastic. Each is pounded alone and then the whole is crushed together and rubbed against the teeth, then rinse in the bath.

In his famous compilation of biblical and talmudic law, the *Mishneh Torah*, Maimonides describes therapeutic and hygienic rules for the Sabbath.[9] He rules that

> One who has a toothache may take sips of vinegar, but may not spit it out—he must swallow it. One who has a sore throat may not gargle with oil, but may drink it in large quantities, and if this cures his soreness it does not matter. One may not chew mastic or rub his teeth with a medicament on the Sabbath if the purpose is medicinal, but if the intention is to remove mouth odors he may do so.

---

8. F. Rosner, *Moses Maimonides' Treatises on Poisons, Hemorrhoids, and Cohabitation,* p. 39.
9. F. Rosner, *Medicine in the Mishneh Torah of Maimonides,* pp. 160–61.

Maimonides is alluding to the talmudic discussion about the efficacy of vinegar for a toothache (Beẓah 18b, Shabbat 111a). Sipping vinegar or rinsing one's teeth with it is not permitted on the Sabbath, since healing, except in cases of danger, is ordinarily prohibited on the Sabbath, lest the ingredients of the medication be crushed in contravention of the rules governing work. It is permitted, however, to dip food in vinegar and eat it in the usual manner, and if one's toothache is cured in the process, there is no violation of the law.

Also in the laws pertaining to the Sabbath, Maimonides rules that a woman may not go out into a public domain on the Sabbath wearing

> an artificial tooth worn in the mouth to replace a missing tooth, or a gold tooth worn over one of her own teeth that has turned black or red. A silver tooth, however, is permissible, because it is not noticeable. The reason she is forbidden to go out wearing any of these articles is that it might fall off and she would then be tempted to carry it home in her hand, or else she might take it off to show it to her friends.
>
> (Hilkhot Shabbat 19:7)

Maimonides bases his ruling on the talmudic discussion as to whether or not a woman is allowed to go out on the Sabbath with an artificial or gold tooth. Rabbi Judah the Prince permits it, but the sages forbid it (Shabbat 6:5). Rabbi Zera states that this prohibition only applies to a gold tooth, but that all the rabbis agree that a silver tooth is permitted (Shabbat 65a). The talmudic commentator Rashi explains that a gold tooth, being valuable, is likely to be removed by a woman from her mouth and displayed to her friends. Meanwhile, she may carry it on the street, an act forbidden on the Sabbath. Maimonides, in his *Commentary on the Mishnah* (Shabbat 6:5), explains the permissive ruling of Rabbi Judah the Prince in that the gold tooth is covering one of the woman's own diseased teeth; therefore, she will not take it out to show to her friends, because that would uncover her blemish.

## Summary and Conclusion

In ancient times, the art of dentistry was closely related to its mother science, medicine. Ancient and medieval Jewish sources, such as the Bible and Talmud, are replete with references to both dentistry and medicine. Those relating to dentistry are briefly reviewed in this chapter.

The greatest Jewish scholar of the Middle Ages was Moses Maimonides. A few references to dentistry are found in his medical and rabbinic writings. Maimonides is an important figure in the history of dentistry primarily because of his stature and renown as a physician. His medical legacy is found in his ten medical treatises.

# ❧ 15 ❧

# Urology and Urinalysis

In a series of articles, Herzl Kook describes genitourinary items in the writings of Maimonides as seen by a modern urologist.[1] Kook points out that Maimonides describes two kidneys from which distilled urine passes through the "two vessels" (ureters) in the "reservoir" (urinary bladder) where it is kept until the sphincter relaxes and the urine is excreted through the urethra. He also describes the testicles, the scrotum, the penis and the uterus. Maimonides quotes Galen, who wrote that a man whose right testicle is larger than the left has male children whereas a man with a large left testicle has female offspring. The same applies to a woman's breasts.

Maimonides accurately describes the symptoms of lower urinary tract obstruction, including hesitancy, a narrow stream, dripping, and urinary retention. He distinguishes between urinary retention in the elderly and anuria, which is a condition where "no urine reaches the reservoir because the kidneys cease to function." He also describes renal colic and kidney stones as well as renal abscesses for which he advises early surgery to evacuate the pus. He usually advocates conservative management of genitourinary ailments. He

---

1. H. Kook, "Genito-Urological Items in the Scripts of Rambam," *Koroth* 4:5–7 (Dec. 1967): 448–451; idem, "Genitourinary Items in the Writings of Maimonides," op. cit. 6:3–4 (Feb. 1973): 216–221; idem, "Maimonides the Physician as Seen by a Modern Urologist," op. cit. 6:7–8 (June 1974): 489–496; idem, "Maimonides as Seen by a Modern Urologist," *International Surgery* 61 (Aug. 1976): 390–392.

was quite knowledgeable in the anatomy and pathophysiology of the urinary tract, as the remainder of this chapter will demonstrate.

In his major medical work entitled *The Medical Aphorisms of Moses,*[2] Maimonides quotes Galen, who states that the right kidney is somewhat higher than the left, and that the urinary bladder receives vessels to nourish it and has a tube (urethra) to remove wastes. The bladder is said to be a type of muscle. Although the membranes of the kidneys contain small nerves, the bladder receives a large nerve so that its sensation is finer and stronger. The penis, the genitals, and the uterus have an abundance of nerves necessary for sensation during cohabitation.

Regarding illnesses, Maimonides speaks of bladder stones, renal calculi, and abscesses. Thick chymes are said to cause pain in the kidneys (nephritis?). Kidney disease is present if the patient micturates rusty, thin urine. Diuretics should not be given when bleeding occurs from the kidneys or bladder. The seat of the illness called diabetes is in the kidneys and bladder, according to Galen. Maimonides himself asserts that this disease is due to the prevailing heat which spreads over the kidneys. The word "diabetes" in Hebrew letters is present in the original Arabic manuscript of Maimonides' *Medical Aphorisms* as well as in the medieval Hebrew translations. Maimonides must have taken it directly from the Greek.

The Greeks used the word "diabetes" to refer to a disease characterized either by excessive passage of urine or by the passage of sweet urine. Maimonides discusses both polyuria and glycosuria in his *Medical Aphorisms.* For example, in chapter 6, he quotes Galen as follows:

> Individuals with sweet white humors are very somnolent [hyperglycemia or ketoacidosis?]. Those with an excess of sour white humor are hungry [hypoglycemia?]. If an excess of salted white humor prevails, they are extremely thirsty. When the white liquid is neutralized, the thirst disappears.

2. F. Rosner, *The Medical Aphorisms of Moses Maimonides,* Maimonides Research Institute, (Haifa, 1989).

Later, in chapters 8 and 24, Maimonides again quotes Galen, who said that diabetes is rare and that he had only seen two cases of this disease. Maimonides, however, claims that in the warm climate of Egypt, he saw twenty patients with diabetes and postulates that the sweet waters of the Nile river may play a role in the causation of the disease.

In his *Commentary on the Aphorisms of Hippocrates*,[3] Maimonides quotes Hippocrates' statement that diseases of the bladder and kidneys in the elderly are difficult to heal. He also speaks of patients who discharge copious amounts of thick white urine (pyuria?) or who urinate blood or pus. Fleshy substances or hairlike substances (filaria?) in the urine are said to come from the kidneys or the bladder. Maimonides also describes urinary sediments resembling "pistachio hearts." Fat in the urine, he asserts, is evidence of the dissolution of the kidney. Strangury occurs because of weakness of the bladder or sharpness of the urine. The former is due to a bad constitution or an inflammation which develops there. Sharpness of the urine occurs because of the admixture of stinging humor. An inflammation in the uterus or rectum damages the bladder because of its proximity. A tear in the bladder or kidneys, according to Maimonides, is not always fatal.

In describing urine in various diseases, Maimonides states:

> Most patients with fever have thin urine at the beginning of the illness. The closer they get to the end, the thicker the consistency of the urine. . . . Sometimes the urine resembles lime and is sparse at the beginning of the illness. The reason for the sparseness is that it traverses the kidneys with difficulty. When the major part of the bad humor has been evacuated and the remainder thereof cooked, the patient urinates thinner urine and in large amounts. . . . Transparent urine is the furthest away from being cooked, and it indicates that the illness will be protracted. . . . Urine is turbid only if the heat of the fever acts on the thick substances in, and the copious amounts of, the urine; or if it acts on the substances alone. If the heat is extraordinarily great, gases are produced so that the urine becomes thick and turbid like wax or pitch or cinnabar resin. The thick gases and the heat rapidly ascend to the head, and headache is produced. Sometimes it occurs during the micturition of the turbid urine; at other times it occurs earlier, and at yet other times it occurs later.

---

3. F. Rosner, *Maimonides' Commentary on the Aphorisms of Hippocrates,* Maimonides Research Institute, (Haifa, 1987).

In his *The Art of Cure*,[4] Maimonides states that the kidneys are not as important as the liver and stomach but more important than other organs. Stones form in the kidneys when the latter contain a coarse, viscous humor that was warmed and burned. Wounds in the bladder or kidneys are treated with honey and other substances which make the urine flow. If a patient with continuous fever and putrefaction of humors excretes ripe material in his urine, the fever will resolve completely in eleven days. Hectic fever and consumption may follow a sickness in the uterus or the kidneys. To cure such illnesses, it is necessary to empty the putrefying wastes by stimulating urine flow and bowel emptying. Catheters or tubes to collect urine from the bladder are described. Some kidney sicknesses are treated by bloodletting. Diuretics should be avoided for "hot tumors" of the bladder, penis, or kidneys. One who eats coarse foods forms stones in his kidneys.

In his three treatises on the regimen of health,[5] Maimonides states that it is not proper to exercise until one has cleansed oneself from superfluities, that is to say urine and feces. He also says that wine is not only nourishing and rapidly digested but a good diuretic. People who drink cold water upon leaving the bath may develop chilled kidneys.

In his legal code, the *Mishneh Torah*, Maimonides states that if one interrupts urination or defecation, one may develop very serious and dangerous illnesses (Hilkhot Tefillin 4:20). He does not specify the nature of these illnesses, but the talmudic assertion upon which his statement is based is more explicit: "Withholding feces brings on dropsy, and keeping back urine brings on jaundice" (Berakhot 25a). Elsewhere in the *Mishneh Torah*, Maimonides describes defects and diseases in animals which render them *terefah* (nonkosher) (Hilkhot Sheḥitah 8:26). For example, if a kidney is exceedingly small, or if it is

> afflicted with disease—that is, if its flesh is like dead flesh which has putre-
> fied after several days, so that if one grasps it at one end it disintegrates and

---

4. See U. Barzel, *Moses Maimonides' "The Art of Cure"*.
5. See Rosner, *Moses Maimonides' Three Treatises on Health.*

falls to the ground—and if this disease has progressed as far as the white matter inside the kidney, the animal is *terefah*. Likewise, if secretion—even if not malodorous—or turbid or malodorous liquid is found in the kidney, it is *terefah*; if clear liquid is found in it, the animal is permitted.

An exceedingly small kidney probably represents end-stage renal disease from chronic nephritis. The other disorders may represent benign and malignant tumors or cysts, renal abscesses, or other diseases. One cannot be certain.

In his *Treatise on Asthma*,[6] Maimonides again speaks of pain in the kidneys, stones in the kidneys, and urinary retention. He states that drinking radish juice cleanses the kidneys and bladder, and that diuresis should not be induced in healthy people but only in patients with certain illnesses.

Returning to Maimonides' major medical work, his *Medical Aphorisms*, the entire fifth chapter is devoted to the examination of urine in health and in disease. Maimonides seems to be alluding to hemoglobinuria when he states that "black urinary sediments signify either fiery heat or extreme cold. . . . every urine which turns black is extremely malignant. I have never seen anyone who urinated black urine who survived." The final aphorism in the chapter is a concise outline by Maimonides of Galen's views on the four basic types of urine.

The reader must bear in mind the medieval concept of disease production. Disease was thought to be due to a disruption of the normal equilibrium between the four bodily humors: blood, phlegm or white bile, choler or yellow bile, and melancholy or black bile. These humors were supposed to represent various combinations of the four basic elements that compose the human organism: fire, air, earth, and water. Each of the latter had two qualities: fire warms and dries, air warms and moistens, earth cools and dries, and water cools and moistens. In blood these elements are equally distributed; in phlegm water predominates; in yellow bile fire predominates; and in black bile earth predominates. Every human being is born with a unique combination or mixture of

---

6. For further information on this work, see above, chap. 2.

these elements. Any change or disruption in this equilibrium was thought to result in ill health.

I present below an English translation of chapter 5 of Maimonides' *Medical Aphorisms*. Each aphorism concludes with a citation of the source upon which it is based, mostly works by Galen. Words in brackets are my own additions to clarify the meaning of certain terms.[7] I hope that this translation will provide the reader with additional insight into medieval medicine and the medical genius of Moses Maimonides.

The Fifth Treatise contains aphorisms pertaining to the examination of the urine.

1. It is obligatory to perform tests and to examine the urine during any fever because fevers are sicknesses in arteries. Therefore, in pleuritis first examine the sputum and afterwards examine the urine, because pleuritis is not ordinarily one of the fever-producing illnesses. Similarly, if there is a disease in the abdomen accompanied by fever, first examine the stool and then look at the urine. If there is no fever, only examine the stools. *De Crisibus VI*

2. The most propitious of the sediments that settle in the urine of patients with fever due to sepsis are those which arise from the humor which already has been putrefied by the arteries which contained it. From this, evenly distributed white sediments develop in the urine without detestable odors. *De Febribus I*

3. If the particles of the urinary sediment are all equal in appearance and in substance, it signifies the dominance of nature over the illness and its rule over it. Urine in which foam accumulates is caused by a cold humor and therefore shows the chronicity of the illness. *Comment. Aphorismorum VII*

4. The most favorable urine in ill people, and the one which most closely resembles the urine of healthy individuals and the maximally "cooked" urine in very healthy people, is urine which is even in thickness and whose yellowness leans to a tinge of redness

---

7. The term "cooking" which recurs throughout this chapter is translated literally from the original and probably refers to body humor metabolism with resultant formation of urine that has different qualities, as described in the text.

to deepen the yellow color because some moisture of blood and red bile become mixed into it. *De Crisibus I*

5. The most propitious type of urine has a good appearance and contains white turbidity which is smooth and even. If it settles to the bottom of a vessel, it is the best. If [it settles] in the middle, it is less favorable than the first. If it floats on top, it is less favorable than the second. These three types indicate the [degree of] cooking. Of the other types of urine, some show the opposite of cooking, and some herald a catastrophe. *De Crisibus I*

6. The evenness of sediments and their settling down set forth two conditions. One is that sediments should not be dispersed and diffuse but remain compact, and the second is that they should remain so at all times. Sometimes the urine is clear at a certain time but at another time it contains settlings and sediment. In such a case, the observed sediment is not one of the favorable ones, since it indicates that cooking was not completed. *De Crisibus I*

7. The most favorable urines are those of patients whose urine, when excreted, shows completely favorable sediments which are fully cooked, because this signifies that nature has already triumphed over the illness and has begun to excrete the illness-producing humors. After this in propitiousness is a urine which is micturated turbid but which settles out favorable sediments after standing awhile, since this signifies that nature has commenced the activity of cooking and will soon complete this activity. After this second type in propitiousness is a urine which is micturated thick but then clears and in which no sediment forms at all. This signifies that the cooking time is far off, even though nature has initiated efforts in this direction. *De Crisibus I*

8. A sediment always occurs in the urine of those ill with a fever which has developed from complete rest and relaxation and in those who increase their food intake at the end of the illness. However, in those who develop fever from work and toil, the illness often terminates without any sediment at all developing in the urine. They rapidly complete the cooking with the appearance of a white, flat, and even turbidity in the upper part of the urine or suspended in the middle. *De Crisibus I*

9. If illnesses occur secondary to favorable humors, urinary sediments are plentiful. If these [illnesses], however, originate from red humors, no sediments at all form or only very few. *Comment. Prognostikon II*

10. The most unfavorable of all urines in sick people is the thin, clear one which resembles well water and is clear and translucent. It is the furthest possible from being cooked. Somewhat less dangerous is the urine which is excreted thin and clear but a short time later becomes cloudy, since this signifies that nature, although behind in its task, will soon perform it. Less favorable than the second is the urine which is micturated cloudy and remains cloudy, because this shows that nature is as yet undecided and, although attempting to cook [the urine], has not yet clarified the matter. *De Crisibus I*

11. Among kidney ailments is one in which the patient micturates rusty, thin urine similar to the early excretion of a sick liver, and this one is slightly more bloody than the other. *De Locis Affectis VI*

12. If the urine is of an oily bile type, it is a sign of the dissolution of the fat from the heat of the fever. If the urine is actually fatty, and its appearance and consistency are that of oil, it is a bad [sign] and leads to death by dissolving flesh, because the heat which melts the flesh is more dangerous than the heat which [only] dissolves oil. *Comment. Epidemiarum III*

13. Urine resembling water that is micturated repeatedly, as occurs in people with the illness diabetes, is the most unfavorable of all uncooked urines and occurs because of the death of two powers: the natural power of metabolism, and the retention power. *De Crisibus I*

14. Black urinary sediments signify either fiery heat or extreme cold. They occur in association with what resembles the death of the natural powers. Ashen-appearing sediments, however, only occur secondary to cold. *De Crisibus I*

15. Every urine which turns black is extremely malignant. I have never seen anyone who urinated black urine and survived. Black sediments [in otherwise clear urine] signify a less dangerous situa-

tion. A black cloud suspended in the middle of the urine is even less dangerous than black sediments. A black cloud floating on top of the urine is even less dangerous than one suspended in the middle. *De Crisibus I*

16. If a cloud or black sediments, either black in appearance or which actually contain particles resembling groat kernels or beaten-out plates, floats on top of white urine which is thin as water, these are fatal signs. The same is true of a foul-smelling urine or fatty urine which is called oily, all of which are fatal. These [types of] urines indicate that the patient has in his nature a serious life-threatening situation. *De Morborum Temporibus VI*

17. Every appearance of urine except white, dark yellow, or red is a sign of [imminent] death. The same [is true] of what is excreted in the urine, except for sediments which settle or suspended turbidity or a favorable cloud floating on top of the urine. All three [occurring simultaneously] are a bad sign or an indication of death. *De Crisibus I*

18. If the illness is of long duration and [healing] activity is delayed, and the patient micturates thin urine for a prolonged period, the crisis usually ends with the excretion of an abscess. But if thick urine is excreted, favorable sediments develop which settle [in the urine] and begin to slowly cook the illness. No crisis occurs during the excretion of the abscess. *De Crisibus III*

19. If the urine contains particles resembling peeled barley flakes or lentil kernels, this shows that [the illness] comes from the liver. If the particles resemble flesh, it signifies they originated in the kidneys. If they resemble beaten-out plates, it shows that they come from the urinary bladder. Particles which resemble groat kernels in size and hardness and are not white indicate the melting of flesh and nerves. Black particles signify the dissolving of splenic fat. Urine which resembles donkey urine indicates an excessive accumulation of raw humors called chyme. *Comment. Epidemiarum VI, 5*

20. Moses says: The implication in the words of Galen in his [book] *On Crises* is that the most favorable of all urines of sick patients is the one in which favorable sediments are seen. This is called the first type because nature has already completed its activity

and has cooked the illness–producing material. The next in order of propitiousness is the urine which is micturated cloudy but after being excreted becomes clear through the settling of favorable sediments, since this signifies that nature has already commenced its work and will soon complete its task. This is the second type of urine. After this in propitiousness is that which is nearly cloudy and then becomes clear but where the sediments do not settle, since this demonstrates that nature has already begun its work but is not even close to the time of cooking. This is the third type. After this in propitiousness is one which is micturated turbid and remains turbid, since this one is further away from being cooked than the previous one. This is the fourth type. Following this is the one which is urinated clear and thin and later becomes turbid, because this indicates that nature has not yet begun its activity but will shortly do so. The most unfavorable of all is urine which is micturated thin and remains very thin, since this shows the complete absence of cooking, not at the present time nor in the near future.

End of the fifth treatise.

# ❧ 16 ❧

# Circumcision

## Introduction

The controversy in the medical and lay literatures about routine circumcision for the newborn will not be discussed here, since a religious commandment or rite does not lend itself to a consideration of pros and cons.[1] To Jews, the practice of circumcision requires no medical or social justification.[2] Hertz has summarized the matter succinctly as follows:

> Circumcision is the abiding symbol of the consecration of the Children of Abraham to the God of Abraham. As the sacred rite of the Covenant, it is of fundamental importance for the religious existence of Israel. Unbounded has been the devotion with which it has been kept. Jewish men and women have in all ages been ready to lay down their lives in its observance. The Maccabean martyrs died for it. . . . So vitally significant has loyalty to this rite proved itself, that even an excommunicated semi-apostate like Benedict Spinoza (1632–1677) declared: "Such great importance do I attach to the sign of the Covenant, that I am persuaded it is sufficient by itself to maintain the separate existence of the nation forever."[3]

Historically, circumcision is not exclusively a rite of the Jews. Ishmael, Abraham's first son, was circumcised at thirteen years of age, and the practice remains to this day an integral part of Islam,

---

1. See E. Wallerstein, *Circumcision*.
2. See F. Rosner, "Circumcision."
3. Quoted in J. H. Hertz, *The Authorised Daily Prayer Book* (New York: Bloch, 1959), pp. 1024–25.

although the Koran makes no mention of it. In the last treatise of his *Mishneh Torah*, Maimonides asserts that the practice of circumcision is a commandment given only to Abraham and his descendants, as it is said: "Thou and thy seed after thee" (Gen. 17:9). The descendants of Ishmael are excluded, as it is said: "For in Isaac shall seed be called to thee" (ibid. 21:14). Esau was also excluded because Isaac said to Jacob: "And [God] give thee the blessing of Abraham, to thee and to thy seed" (ibid. 28:4), implying that only those who adhere to His religion and His righteous path are considered seed of Abraham, and they (i.e., Jews) are, therefore, obligated to practice circumcision (Hilkhot Melakhim 10:7).

Throughout history, periods of persecution against the Jews during which circumcision was forbidden under penalty of death have not been uncommon. The first such prohibition was enacted under Antiochus Epiphanes (175–153 B.C.E.), son of Antiochus the Great (I Macc. 1:48). Many mothers who had their sons circumcised suffered martyrdom (II Macc. 6:10). Operations to reconstruct the prepuce surgically, either voluntarily or under coercion, were also practiced. Maimonides mentions the case of a circumcised male whose prepuce had been drawn forward to cover up the corona (Heb. *mashuk*). Such a man must be recircumcised (Hilkhot Terumot 7:10).

In the Hellenistic period, Jews who wanted to participate nude in the Greek games in the gymnasia attempted to make their circumcision unrecognizable by methodically pulling the foreskin to the front. According to Josephus (*Antiquities*, bk. 12, chap. 5:1), these epispastics (from Greek *epispastikos*, "to draw in") covered the circumcision of their penis, so that even when they were naked, they could not be distinguished from Greeks. Some authors believe that they "underwent painful operations to obliterate the signs of circumcision [epispasm]."[4] In the course of the persecutions that preceded the Judean revolt led by Bar Koziba against Rome in 132 C.E., many Jews became epispastics by forcibly drawing their prepuces forward. After the liberation, many were recircumcised with-

---

4. L. V. Snowman, s.v. "Circumcision," *Encyclopaedia Judaica*, vol. 5, cols. 567–75.

out any harm occurring to their health or procreative ability, thus contradicting the assertion of R. Judah that to recircumcise an epispastic is dangerous (Yevamot 72a). Elsewhere, the Talmud states that Achan was an epispastic, based on the biblical passage in Joshua 7:11 (Sanhedrin 44a). The rabbinic exegetical work entitled Midrash Tanḥuma, in its commentary on the Book of Genesis, implies that Esau was also an epispastic. In his classic work on biblical and talmudic medicine, Preuss cites several additional references to epispastics in ancient Hebrew writings.[5] In the *Mishneh Torah*, Maimonides rules that epispastic priests may eat of heave offerings (Hilkhot Terumot 7:10).

**Procedures of Ritual Circumcision**

The child is brought from the mother by the godmother and handed to the godfather, who in turn hands it to the *mohel* (ritual circumciser). The baby is momentarily placed on the chair of Elijah, after which it is placed on a pillow on the knees of the *sandak* (holder). The *mohel* thoroughly cleanses his hands with a disinfectant solution and performs the three major acts of the circumcision: *milah*, or the excision of the prepuce; *peri'ah*, or the severance of the internal mucosa of the prepuce and its retraction over the glans; and *meẓiẓah*, or the sucking of blood from the wound. According to Maimonides' Code, this is done to remove the blood from the distant parts of the wound (Hilkhot Milah 2:2).

The procedure is as follows: the prepuce is protracted anteriorly and adhesions to the glans released with a blunt probe. The shield is applied, the ritual blessings are recited, and the foreskin is excised by applying a knife to the outer surface of the shield. The glans is protected below the shield, thus militating against accidental cuts into the glans or shaft of the penis. The shield is removed, and the prepuce is retracted over the glans. The final act of sucking of the blood from the wound is usually performed with a glass or rubber tube or the inverted barrel of a hypodermic syringe or a similar suitable object, whereby one end of this object is opposed to the

---

5. J. Preuss, *Biblical and Talmudic Medicine*, pp. 240–48.

wound and the other end in the mouth of the operator. Dressings consist of vaseline gauze, oxidized cellulose (Oxycel), absorbable gelatin (Gelfoam), or similar material in addition to plain or antiseptic gauze. Most operators use a shield of some kind as described, although some still circumcise free-hand. This is not recommended, since the danger exists of accidentally cutting into the glans.

After the circumcision, the child is handed to an honored guest and a benediction is recited by the *mohel* or rabbi or honored guest praising God for having established a covenant with His people Israel. The child is then named and a prayer recited for its welfare. The infant is given a few drops of wine to drink from the goblet over which the benediction was recited. The ceremony is followed by a festive meal at which special hymns are sung.

## Reason for Ritual Circumcision

In his *Guide of the Perplexed*, Maimonides provides us with a lengthy discourse in which he explains the reasons for circumcision as follows:

> With regard to circumcision, one of the reasons for it is, in my opinion, the wish to bring about a decrease in sexual intercourse and a weakening of the organ in question, so that this activity be diminished and the organ be in as quiet a state as possible. It has been thought that circumcision perfects what is defective congenitally. This gave the possibility to everyone to raise an objection and to say: How can natural things be defective so that they need to be perfected from outside, all the more because we know how useful the foreskin is for that member? In fact this commandment has not been prescribed with a view to perfecting what is defective congenitally, but to perfecting what is defective morally. The bodily pain caused to that member is the real purpose of circumcision. None of the activities necessary for the preservation of the individual is harmed thereby, nor is procreation rendered impossible, but violent concupiscence and lust that goes beyond what is needed are diminished. The fact that circumcision weakens the faculty of sexual excitement and sometimes perhaps diminishes the pleasure is indubitable. For if at birth this member has been made to bleed and has had its covering taken away from it, it must indubitably be weakened. The Sages, may their memory be blessed, have explicitly stated: It is hard for a woman with whom an uncircumcised man has had sexual intercourse to separate from him (Gen. Rabbah 80). In my opinion, this is the strongest of the reasons for circumcision. Who first began to perform this act, if not Abraham,

who was celebrated for his chastity—as has been mentioned by the Sages (Tractate Bava Batra 16a), may their memory be blessed, with reference to his dictum: "Behold now, I know that thou art a fair woman to look upon" (Gen. 12:11).

According to me, circumcision has another very important meaning, namely, that all people professing this opinion—that is, those who believe in the unity of God—should have a bodily sign uniting them so that one who does not belong to them should not be able to claim that he was one of them, while being a stranger. For he would do this in order to profit by them or to deceive the people who profess this religion. Now a man does not perform this act upon himself or upon a son of his unless it be in consequence of a genuine belief. For it is not like an incision in the leg or a burn in the arm, but is a very, very hard thing.

It is also well known what degree of mutual love and mutual help exists between people who all bear the same sign, which forms for them a sort of covenant and alliance. Circumcision is a covenant made by Abraham our Father with a view to the belief in the unity of God. Thus everyone who is circumcised joins Abraham's covenant. This covenant imposes the obligation to believe in the unity of God: "To be a God unto thee and to thy seed after thee" (Gen. 17:7). This also is a strong reason, as strong as the first, which may be adduced to account for circumcision: perhaps it is even stronger than the first.[6]

Maimonides continues by saying that circumcision leads to perfection and perpetuation of this law only if the act is performed during childhood. Three reasons are offered: lest the child grow up and not perform it, because a child has less pain from circumcision than an adult, and because the parents' attachment to the child is not as strong during infancy as during childhood.

Maimonides concludes by asserting that circumcision is performed on the eighth day because living beings are very weak and exceedingly tender when they are born, as if they were still in the womb, until seven days have passed. This concept is also applicable to animals, as stated in Scripture: "seven days shall it be with its dam" (Exod. 22:29). Similarly with man, he is circumcised after seven days have passed. Maimonides could not have been familiar with, but seems to be alluding to, what is today recognized as hepatic immaturity during the first few days of life.

Circumcision on day eight avoids the bleeding that might occur

---

6. Maimonides, *Guide of the Perplexed*, pp. 609–11.

due to clotting-factor deficiencies during the first week of life and also allows the bilirubin-conjugating system to mature.

## Laws Pertaining to Circumcision

Maimonides discusses the subject of circumcision at great length in the *Mishneh Torah*. He states that the duty to circumcise a child is incumbent upon the father (Hil. Milah 1:1). If a male infant is born without a foreskin, it is required that a drop of blood be drawn from the membrum when the infant is eight days old (ibid. 1:7). Hermaphrodites who have both male and female organs, babies born with two foreskins, and babies delivered by cesarean section are all circumcised on the eighth day (ibid.). If there is a bright leprosy spot on the foreskin, it is removed with the foreskin. Although the cutting off of a leprous plague spot is prohibited, the affirmative precept of circumcision overrides the prohibition (ibid. 1:9).

Circumcision of infants born prematurely after seven or eight months of pregnancy is also discussed by Maimonides (ibid. 1:13). A sick infant is not circumcised until it is well. Seven days must elapse after complete recovery from a generalized illness, such as fever due to sepsis, before the circumcision can be performed (ibid. 1:16). Localized disorders, such as an eye infection, do not require the seven-day waiting period, and circumcision can be carried out promptly after the baby recovers (ibid.). Maimonides rules that circumcision must be postponed if an infant is found on the eighth day to be "excessively yellow, until the blood has become normal and the baby's complexion has returned to be like that of other healthy infants" (ibid. 1:17). Other codifiers of Jewish law omit the term "excessively." The degree of jaundice for which circumcision must be postponed is not further defined by Maimonides. Mild physiological jaundice is not an absolute contraindication to circumcision from a medical standpoint, since the hazard is minimal. However, Jewish law requires postponement of this procedure until clinical jaundice has receded.

Maimonides adds that "if an infant is excessively ruddy, presenting the appearance of one who has been dyed red, it is not circumcised until the blood has been absorbed and the baby's complexion returns to be like that of other infants, this redness being a disease. In these cases, great caution must be exercised" (Hil. Milah 1:17). Maimonides may be describing erythema neonatorum in a normal newborn or neonatal polycythemia perhaps due to maternal-to-fetal or twin-to-twin transfusion in utero. Twin-to-twin transfusion has been suggested by one writer to be the cause of the ruddy complexion of Esau when he was born to Rebecca (Gen. 25:24–26).[7]

Amazing is the recognition of the genetic transmission of hemophilia in the Talmud (Yevamot 64b) and subsequent rabbinic writings. The talmudic decree of Rabbi Judah that the sibling of two brothers who died of bleeding after circumcision may not be circumcised is codified by all rabbinic authorities of the last ten centuries.[8] Modern rabbinic opinion extends this ruling to any child, even the firstborn, in whom a diagnosis of hemophilia can be established. Maimonides' discussion of the subject is as follows:

> If a woman had her first son circumcised and he died as a result of the circumcision, which enfeebled his strength, and she similarly had her second son circumcised, and he died as a result of the circumcision—whether the latter child was from her first husband or from her second husband—the third son may not be circumcised at the proper time, on the eighth day of life. Rather, the operation is postponed until he grows up and his strength is established. One may only circumcise a child who is totally free of disease, because danger to life overrides every other consideration. It is possible to circumcise later than the proper time, but it is impossible to restore a single departed soul of Israel forever.
>
> (Hil. Milah 1:18)

Maimonides may have been alluding to death by exsanguination when he stated: "enfeebled his strength." This conclusion may be unwarranted, however, as Maimonides may have lumped together circumcision mortality from numerous causes, such as prematurity and anemia, in addition to bleeding disorders. As a physician, he sought to delay circumcision until health was established.

Rabbi Joseph Karo (1488–1575), in his *Kesef Mishneh* commentary on the preceding passage from Maimonides' Code, states that

---

7. P. Lanzkowsky, "Twin-to-Twin Transfusion."
8. F. Rosner, "Hemophilia in the Talmud and Rabbinic Writings."

the prohibition against further circumcision in an afflicted family is "because there are families in which the blood is weak [lit. loose]." Furthermore, whereas the Talmud does not state when circumcision can be performed in an afflicted child, Maimonides specifically sets a time limit; circumcision may be performed at such time as the child is declared medically fit. Maimonides thus seems to feel that spontaneous remission or perhaps medical therapy can control or even cure hemophilia. Maimonides also recognized that a woman transmits the disease to all her male offspring even if the latter were conceived from different fathers.

The conclusion to be drawn from the above discussion is that the sages of the Talmud in the second century and subsequent rabbinic authorities, including Maimonides, had a remarkable knowledge of the genetic transmission of a familial bleeding disorder, probably hemophilia. All recognized that females transmit the disease, but some thought that males can also do so. It is unclear, however, whether Maimonides and other rabbis were dealing only with hemophiliacs. Vitamin K deficiency, possibly determined by diet in certain families, or other bleeding disorders, such as congenital hypofibrinogenemia, may have been involved in some cases. Furthermore, the observations recorded in the Talmud, by Maimonides, and by other codifiers of Jewish law are incomplete. Although families with "loose blood" (i.e., bleeding disorders) were recognized, the question of the circumcision of a child whose maternal uncles died of bleeding after circumcision is not considered. A woman whose brothers bled to death after circumcision could well be a carrier. Only the direct maternal transmission of the disease was recognized, whether demonstrated in siblings or maternal cousins.[9]

Maimonides continues his presentation of the laws pertaining to circumcision by describing the procedure as follows:

> The entire foreskin which covers the glans is cut, so that the whole of the glans is exposed. Then the thin layer of skin beneath the foreskin is divided with the nail and turned back, till the flesh of the glans is completely

---

9. For additional discussion, see above, chap. 12.

exposed. The wound is then sucked till the blood has been drawn from parts remote from the surface thus obviating danger to the child. After this has been done, a plaster, bandage, or similar dressing is applied.

(Hil. Milah 2:2)

He is thus describing the three major parts of ritual circumcision: excision of the prepuce, tearing or cutting of the internal mucosa of the prepuce and its retraction over the glans, and the sucking of blood from the wound. The latter act, as cited above, is usually performed with a glass or rubber tube or the inverted barrel of a hypodermic syringe or similar suitable object, whereby one end is opposed to the wound and the other end in the mouth of the ritual circumciser. The nature of the "danger to the child" if the sucking from the wound is omitted is not further specified by Maimonides or other rabbinic writers.

The drugs used for the dressing are also not specified, but an emulsion of wine and oil may be used for this purpose, and cummin seed may be used as a styptic (ibid. 2:7). The baby may be bathed in warm water following the circumcision; either the whole body or just the genital area, in accordance with local custom (ibid.).

For additional source material and bibliographical citations on the biblical and talmudic writings about circumcision, the reader is referred to Preuss's classic book.

# Hygiene and
# Preventive Medicine

# ⚹ 17 ⚹

# Preventive Medicine

## Introduction

An old English proverb states that "an apple a day keeps the doctor away." The task of physicians has always been to promote health by preventing illness and curing it. Prevention is obviously better than cure. It is often much more difficult to keep people well than to cure them of illnesses. Prevention of disease is the goal of every physician. Preventive care is becoming the linchpin of modern medicine.

The famous medical historian Fielding Ha. Garrison states that "The ancient Hebrews were, in fact, the founders of prophylaxis."[1] The Jewish view of the practice of medicine emphasizes prevention over treatment. Evidence to support this thesis is found in the Bible in the following quotation:

> And he said: if thou wilt diligently hearken to the voice of the Lord thy God, and wilt do that which is right in His eyes, and will give ear to His commandments and keep all His statues, I will put none of the diseases upon thee, which I have put upon the Egyptians, for I am the Lord that healeth thee.
>
> (Exod. 15:26)

The Talmud, reflecting on this passage, asks: if God promises "I will put none of the diseases upon thee," what need is there for a

---

1. M. B. Strauss, *Familiar Medical Quotations* (Boston: Little, Brown, 1968), p. 452.

cure? (Sanhedrin 101a). Rabbi Yoḥanan answers that the verse means that if the Jews diligently hearken to the voice of the Lord, He will not bring diseases upon them. The implication is that Jews can prevent illness by obeying the word of God. The same interpretation can be offered to explain the verse "And the Lord will put none of the evil diseases of Egypt . . . upon thee" (Deut. 7:15). But if the Jews fail to obey the laws of the Torah and are divinely stricken with illness, God promises that "I am the Lord that healeth thee." The Torah thus clearly emphasizes prevention over treatment of disease.

Rashi, the famous medieval exegete, explains "I am the Lord that healeth thee" to mean that God teaches the laws of the Torah in order to save man from these diseases. Rashi uses the analogy of a physician who tells his patient not to eat such-and-such a food lest it bring him into danger from disease. So too is it stated, continues Rashi, obedience to God "will be health to thy body and marrow to thy bones" (Prov. 3:8). In a similar vein, the extratalmudic collection of biblical interpretation known as the Mechilta asserts that the words of Torah are life as well as health, as it is written: "For they are life unto those that find them and health to all their flesh" (Prov. 4:22). Other commentators (*Siftei Ḥakhamin* and Rabbi Samson Raphael Hirsch, among others) extend this thought by propounding that the Divine Law restores health, and certainly prevents illness from occurring, thus serving as preventive medicine against all physical and social evil.

Numerous writings of Moses Maimonides provide further emphasis and proof for the goal of preventing rather than treating illness. This chapter examines some of them.

### Maimonides' *Mishneh Torah*

Hilkhot De'ot, a treatise of Maimonides' legal code, the *Mishneh Torah*, is devoted to moral dispositions or human traits or temperaments.[2] Particularly interesting is its fourth chapter, which deals with a variety of hygienic and medical prescriptions for healthy liv-

---

2. See F. Rosner, *Medicine in the Mishneh Torah of Maimonides.*

ing and for the prevention of illness. Among the many subjects discussed are normal bodily excretory functions, recommended times for eating, amounts and types of food to be consumed, beverage imbibition, exercise, sleep habits, cathartics, climatic and weather effects on eating habits, detrimental and beneficial foods, fruits, meats, vegetables, bathing, bloodletting, sexual intercourse, and domicile. The following are excerpts from this most important chapter, which repeatedly emphasizes prevention over treatment:

> Since when the body is healthy and sound one treads in the ways of the Lord, it being impossible to understand or know anything of the knowledge of the Creator when one is sick, it is obligatory upon man to avoid things which are detrimental to the body and to acclimatize himself to things which heal and fortify it. These are as follows: A person should never eat except when he is hungry nor drink unless he is thirsty. He should not postpone his eliminations for even a single moment; rather, every time that micturition or defecation becomes necessary, he should respond thereto immediately.
>
> A person should not eat until his stomach is replete but should diminish his intake by approximately one-fourth of satiation. One should not drink water during meals save a little and mixed with wine. When the food commences to be digested in the intestines, one may drink as much water as one finds necessary. However, even after the food has been digested, one should not imbibe water excessively. One should not eat until one has examined oneself carefully lest it be necessary to excrete wastes. A person should not eat until he has walked prior to the meal so that his body begins to become warmed, or he should perform a physical task or tire himself by some other form of exertion. The rule in this matter is that one should exert one's body and fatigue it every day in the morning until one's body begins to warm. Then one rests a little until one's soul has settled, and then one may eat. If one washes with warm water after the exercise, so much the better. After this, one should wait a little and then eat.
>
> When a person eats, he should always be sitting in his place or reclining on the left side. He should not walk or ride or exercise or agitate his body ... until the food is digested in his intestines. Anyone who walks immediately after his meal or who fatigues himself brings upon himself serious and grave illnesses.
>
> The day and night consist of twenty-four hours. It is sufficient for a person to sleep one-third thereof, which is eight hours. ...
>
> Things which purge the intestines, such as grapes, figs, mulberries, peas, melons, various types of cucumbers, and types of gourds, should be eaten before the meal. One should not mix them with the food but should wait until they have passed out of the upper abdomen and then one may eat one's meal. Things which bind the intestines [i.e., constipate], such as pomegran-

ates, quinces, apples, and small pears, should be consumed immediately after the meal, but one should not eat excessively thereof. . . . .

In the warm summer months, one should eat cooling foods, not use seasoning to excess, and consume vinegar. In the rainy winter months, one should eat warming foods, abundantly spice the food, and eat a little mustard and asafetida. In this manner one should prepare food in cold climates and warm climates, in each and every place that which is best suited thereto.

Some foods are extremely detrimental, and it is proper for man never to eat them, such as large salted old fish, old salted cheese, truffles, mushrooms, old salted meat, wine must, and a cooked dish which has been kept until it acquires a foul odor. Likewise, any food whose odor is bad or excessively bitter is like a fatal poison unto the body. Other foods are also detrimental but are not as injurious as the aforementioned ones. Therefore, of these one should eat only a little and only after intervals of many days. . . . Anyone who lives a sedentary life and does not exercise or who postpones his excretions or whose intestines are constipated, even if he eats good foods and takes care of himself according to proper medical principles—all his days will be painful ones and his strength will wane. Excessive eating is like a deadly poison to the body of any man, and it is a principal cause of all illnesses. Most diseases that man is afflicted with are due to bad foods or because he fills his abdomen and eats excesssively even of wholesome foods.

Maimonides continues with prescriptions for the correct time and manner of bathing, bloodletting, and sexual intercourse. Many of these rules and regulations are based upon discussions in the Talmud. Maimonides codifies these rules in the *Mishneh Torah* to indicate that they are not optional but mandatory. Prevention of illness and a healthy life-style are obligations upon Jews in order to enable them to serve the Lord. One who is ill cannot serve the Lord properly or fulfill the precepts of the Torah. Maimonides concludes chapter 4 of Hilkhot De'ot as follows:

I guarantee anyone who conducts himself according to the directions we have laid down that he will not be afflicted with illness all the days of his life until he ages greatly and expires. He will not require a physician, and his body will be complete and remain healthy all his life unless his body was defective from the beginning of his creation, or unless he became accustomed to one of the bad habits from the onset of his youth, or unless the plague of pestilence or the plague of drought comes into the world.

Maimonides cites exceptions to the goal of preventing rather than treating illness. Genetic diseases and certain epidemic diseases cannot be prevented. For this reason, the final paragraph in Maimonides' chapter on the regimen of health states that a person should not reside in a city that does not have a physician. A similar pronouncement is found in the Talmud (Sanhedrin 17b).

Another axiom in Judaism is the obligation to avoid or, if possible, prevent danger to life. The Torah tells us not to intentionally place ourselves in danger when it states, "Take heed to thyself, and take care of thy life" (Deut. 4:9) and "take good care of your lives" (Deut. 4:15). The avoidance of danger is exemplified throughout the Bible, Talmud, and Codes of Jewish Law in the positive commandment to make a parapet for one's roof so that no one will fall therefrom and be injured or killed (Deut. 22:8). In his *Mishneh Torah*, Maimonides cites the commandment to make a parapet and then enumerates a variety of prohibitions, all based upon the consideration of being harmful to life:

> It makes no difference whether it be one's roof or anything else that is dangerous and might possibly be a stumbling block to someone and cause his death. For example, if one has a well or a pit, with or without water, in his yard, the owner is obliged to build an enclosing wall ten handbreadths high, or else to put a cover over it lest someone fall into it and be killed. Similarly, regarding any obstacle which is dangerous to life, there is a positive commandment to remove it and to beware of it, and to be particularly careful in this matter, for Scripture says, "Take heed unto thyself and take care of thy life." If one does not remove dangerous obstacles and allows them to remain, he disregards a positive commandment and transgresses the prohibition: "that thou bring not blood" (Deut. 22:8).
>
> Many things are forbidden by the sages because they are dangerous to life. If one disregards any of these and says, "If I want to put myself in danger, what concern is it to others?" or "I am not particular about such things," disciplinary flogging is inflicted upon him.
>
> The following are the acts prohibited: One may not put his mouth to a flowing pipe of water and drink from it, or drink at night from a river or pond, lest he swallow a leech while unable to see. Nor may one drink water that has been left uncovered, lest he drink from it after a snake or other poisonous reptile has drunk from it, and die. . . .
>
> One should not put small change or *denar* into his mouth lest they carry the dried saliva of someone who suffers from an infectious skin disease or leprosy, or lest they carry perspiration, since all human perspiration is poisonous except that coming from the face.
>
> Similarly, one should not put the palm of his hand under his arm, for his hand might possibly have touched a leper or some harmful substance, since the hands are constantly in motion. Nor should one put a dish of food

under his seat even during a meal, lest something harmful fall into it without his noticing it.

Similarly, one should not stick a knife into a citron or a radish lest someone fall on the point and be killed. Similarly, one should not walk near a leaning wall or over an unsteady bridge or enter a ruin or pass through any other such dangerous place.

(Hilkhot Roẓe'aḥ 11:1 ff.)

This quotation from Maimonides certainly emphasizes the point that placing one's health or life into possible danger is absolutely prohibited. Prevention of danger and thereby the preservation of life and health are biblical mandates.

The precept of making a parapet is used by Maimonides in his *Responsum on Longevity* to prove that the duration of human life is not necessarily predetermined.[3] King Hezekiah was seriously ill, supplicated to the Lord, and was granted an extension of fifteen years to his life, as recorded in the Bible and Talmud (Isa. 38:1–20, Berakhot 10a). Maimonides first discusses and provides medical proof that the human lifespan is not predetermined. After presenting all the physiologic information, he concludes that if a person is careful concerning the causes of premature accidental death and the causes leading to "disequilibrium of innate body heat," he will more readily attain his natural life's end. The next large body of evidence to support Maimonides' contention that lifespan is not predetermined is gleaned from biblical and rabbinic writings. Among these is the biblical injunction to build a parapet for one's roof to prevent anyone from falling therefrom. This proves, says Maimonides, that the adoption of precautionary measures can prevent accidents and premature death.

As further proof that prevention of danger is a laudatory goal, the *Responsum on Longevity* cites the laws concerning the establishment of cities of refuge for accidental manslayers (Num. 35:11–12, Deut. 19:5–6). If the manslayer was predetermined to die at the hands of the avenger of blood, no purpose would be served by the cities of refuge. Therefore, concludes Maimonides, they serve to protect the

---

3. See F. Rosner, "Moses Maimonides' Responsum on Longevity," reprinted in chap. 20 of this volume.

accidental manslayer against harm, thus preventing his premature death. He then cites several other biblical proofs, the last of which is the verse "that your days may be prolonged, and the days of your children" (Deut. 11:21). This proves that those who obey the commandments of the Torah can retard the end of their lives and thus protect themselves and prevent premature death.

Some of the earlier-cited prohibitions against endangering one's life and the mandates to prevent illness and danger to life are also found in most of the later Codes of Jewish law, including Rabbi Joseph Karo's *Shulḥan Arukh.* The latter devotes an entire chapter, Ḥoshen Mishpat 427, to "the positive commandment of removing any object or obstacle which constitutes a danger to life." Elsewhere, Karo reiterates the prohibitions against drinking water left uncovered, putting money in one's mouth, putting one's hand on a loaf of bread under the armpit, and leaving a knife in a fruit (Yoreh Deah 116). He further states that two people should not drink from the same cup, and that it is dangerous to eat meat after fish unless a certain interval has passed (Oraḥ Ḥayyim 170:16).

Rabbi Moses Isserles, known as Rema, in his glosses on Karo's Code, concludes that

> one should avoid all things that might lead to a danger because danger to life is stricter than a prohibition. One should be more concerned about a possible danger to life than a possible prohibition. Therefore, the sages prohibited walking in a dangerous place, such as near a leaning wall [for fear of a collapse], or alone at night [for fear of robbers]. They also prohibited drinking water from rivers at night . . . because these things may lead to danger . . . and he who is concerned with his health [lit. watches his soul] avoids them. And it is prohibited to rely on a miracle or to put one's life in danger by any of the aforementioned or the like
>
> (Yoreh Deah 116:5)

Rema thus prohibits relying on miracles when one's health is at stake.

The danger and, therefore, prohibition of drinking from uncovered water or wine, codified by Maimonides and others as described above, is based upon the Talmud, which states that it is prohibited to drink from wine, water, or milk that was left uncovered because a snake may have drunk from it and discharged poison into it (Terumot 8:4). How long must these liquids remain uncovered to become forbidden? As long as it would take a snake to come forth from a place nearby and drink (Ḥullin 10a, 49b). All other liquids are permitted, since a snake has no liking for them. For example, uncovered beer in vats and barrels is allowed, because it is assumed that serpents do not drink beer. Some say that it is permitted because the bitter taste of the hops counteracts any venom that might be in the beer, so that it is harmful only to sick people (Avodah Zarah 31b).

The law forbidding the use of liquids left uncovered does not apply to new wine during the first three days of fermentation, because during this period it repels snakes (Ta'anit 30a, Sanhedrin 70a). Fully matured (i.e., fermented) wine and beer are permitted, for if venom were present, the wine or beer would not have fermented (Avodah Zarah 31b). Uncovered water, if filtered through a strainer, is permitted, since the venom of a serpent is like a fungus which floats on the surface and remains where it is (Sukkah 50a). There is a lengthy discussion in the Talmud as to whether or not diluted wine (the usual proportion is two parts water to one part pure wine) becomes forbidden through being left uncovered, as a snake may or may not drink it (Avodah Zarah 30b).

For baking purposes, it is permitted to use water that was left uncovered, because snake poison is destroyed by fire. For this reason, Mar Samuel only drank warmed water. In general, boiled water was permissible even after it cooled. It was thought that a snake does not drink this type of water and, therefore, does not discharge its poison therein (Jer. Terumot 8:45).

Many of the statements in the Bible and Talmud concerning snakes and serpents have primarily homiletical connotations. Perhaps because of this, only a few of the statements have any scientific validity. The danger of drinking from uncovered water or wine is extremely remote and essentially nonexistent. Snakes do not discharge venom into fluids from which they drink. They inject their victims with poison to kill them in order to eat them or to fight off an enemy, such as man. Only if a snake has recently discharged venom and still has a few drops of fresh, moist venom on its fangs could it possibly exude poison into a fluid from which it drinks. Even then there is no danger to a human being who imbibes the same fluid, since snake poison is not absorbed through the intestinal tract of man if taken in orally. Only for someone who had ulcerations in his mouth or stomach would the remote possibility of absorbing some of the poison exist. Hence, the fears of the sages concerning the drinking of uncovered water or wine were unfounded, but they illustrate the Jewish philosophy of avoiding danger and preventing illness.

In addition to prohibiting the intentional endangerment of one's health or life, Jewish law disallows wounding oneself without fatal intent. The Talmud quotes Rabbi Eleazar ha-Kappar Beribbi, who maintains that a man is not permitted to injure himself (Bava Kamma 91b). He derives this point from the scriptural phrase "And make an atonement for him, for that he sinned regarding the soul" (Num. 6:11), which refers to a Nazarite who is called a sinner because he deprived himself of wine. Certainly, says Rabbi Eleazar ha-Kappar, a person who deprives himself of health by injuring himself is considered a sinner. The prohibition against intentionally wounding oneself is codified by both Maimonides and Karo (Hilhot Ḥovel u-Mazik 5:1; Ḥoshen Mishpat 420:31 and Oraḥ Ḥayyim 571).

Elsewhere in the *Mishneh Torah* (Melakhim 6:10), Maimonides states that he who smashes household goods or destroys articles of food, with destructive intent, transgresses the commandment "Thou shalt not destroy" (Deut. 20:19). The sages deduce from this biblical phrase a prohibition against the wanton destruction of anything useful to man (Shabbat 140b). Rabbi Solomon Luria extends the prohibition to the willful destruction of one's own body (*Yam Shel Shelomoh*, Bava Kamma 8:59). An example of this is described in the Talmud, where a footstool was broken up for Rabbah, whereupon Abayye said to him: "But are you not infringing on 'Thou shalt not destroy'?" He retorted: "'Thou shalt not destroy' in respect of my own body is more important to me" (Shabbat 129a).

Thus it is clear from the numerous references to preventive medicine and the avoidance of danger in the legal writings of Maimonides that he considered such practices to be mandatory in Jewish law. Maimonides presents ample evidence to support the adage "An ounce of prevention is worth a pound of cure." Much more evidence is found in Maimonides' medical writings, some of which are cited below.

### The Treatise on Asthma

Maimonides wrote the *Treatise on Asthma* at the request of a member of the Egyptian royal family.[4] In the introduction, he states that "it seems best to write general chapters which might prove useful to all people for the preservation of health and the prevention of illness."

The final chapter of the treatise deals with "advice to help all people preserve their health and avoid illness." Maimonides advises that one must first pay attention to the improvement of the air, then to the amelioration of the water one drinks, and then to the improvement of one's diet. He emphasizes important ecological and environmental factors in the preservation of health, as follows:

> The relationship between the air of cities and its streets and the air of open fields and deserts is comparable to the relationship between thick turbid water and clear, light water. This means that cities, because of their buildings, the narrowness of their streets, the refuse and waste of their inhabitants, their corpses and animal carcasses, and the putrefaction of their foods, provoke stagnation of the air, which becomes turbid and thick. . . . if you cannot find a way to escape from this, having grown up in cities and become accustomed thereto, at least choose a city with wide horizons, preferably in a northeasterly direction. . . . if that is not possible, at least try to live on the outskirts of the city. . . . living quarters should be on an upper floor with large rooms so that the north wind can traverse them and the sun can shine in. . . . pay attention to locate toilets as far removed as possible from the living quarters . . . strive to improve the air and dry it with aromatic, scented substances and fumigations. . . . this is the regimen for preserving the health of body and soul.

Maimonides quotes the famous Persian physician Rhazes (850–923 C.E.), who said that if the illness is stronger than the patient, medicine is not beneficial; if the patient can overpower the illness,

---

4. For further details, see above, chap. 2.

there is no need for a physician; but if they are equal, the physician is needed to reinforce the strength of the patient to help him overcome the illness. This is the credo known to all physicians as *primum non nocere*, "first do no harm." Maimonides also quotes Hippocrates, who said that a physician should have two goals: to benefit the patient and not to harm him. Maimonides himself asserts that those who can manage without a physician are greater than those who need one. Maimonides' preventive approach to illness and to the practice of medicine is thus obvious throughout the *Treatise on Asthma*.

## The Treatise on Hemorrhoids

The *Treatise on Hemorrhoids*, as Maimonides explains in the introduction, was written for a nobleman, probably a member of the sultan's family.[5] Maimonides' whole approach to the problem bespeaks a modern medical trend. The following is part of the introduction to the treatise:

There was a youth, [descended] from knowledgeable, intelligent, and comprehending forebears, from a prominent and renowned family, distinguished and charitable and of great means, in whom the affliction of hemorrhoids occurred at the mouth of the rectum, who interested me in his problem and placed the task [of healing them] upon me. These irritated him on some occasions, and he treated them in the customary therapeutic manner until the pain subsided and the prolapsed rectum [lit. excesses that protruded] became reduced and returned to normal. Because this [illness] recurred many times, he considered having them extirpated in order to uproot this malady from its source so that it would not return again. I informed him of the danger inherent in this, in that it was not clear whether these hemorrhoids [lit. additions] were of the variety which should be excised or not, since there are people in whom they have once been [surgically] extirpated and in whom other hemorrhoids develop. This is because the causes which gave rise to the original ones remained and, therefore, new ones developed.

Here Maimonides provides an insight into the etiology of disease in general, in that he regards operative excision of hemorroids with

---

5. For further details and the full text, see F. Rosner, *Maimonides' Treatises on Poisons, Hemorrhoids, and Cohabition*, pp. 117–52.

skepticism, because surgery does not remove the underlying causes which produced the hemorrhoids in the first place.

## The Regimen of Health

The *Regimen of Health* was written at the request of Sultan al-Malik al-Afdal, the eldest son of Saladin the Great. The sultan was a frivolous, pleasure-seeking man of thirty, subject to fits of melancholy or depression due to excessive indulgence in wine and women, and to his warlike adventures against his own relatives and in the Crusades. He complained to his physician of constipation, dejection, bad thoughts, and indigestion. Maimonides answered his royal patient in four chapters.[6] The first is a brief abstract on diet taken mostly from Hippocrates and Galen. The second chapter deals with advice on hygiene, diet, and drugs in the absence of a physician. The third, extremely important chapter contains Maimonides' concept of "a healthy mind in a healthy body," one of the earliest descriptions of psychosomatic medicine. He indicates that physical well-being is dependent on mental well-being, and vice-versa. The final chapter summarizes Maimonides' prescriptions relating to climate, domicile, occupation, bathing, sex, wine-drinking, diet, and respiratory infections.

There follows the first part of the section on psychosomatic medicine where Maimonides writes that to preserve physical health one must have mental well-being, and vice-versa.

> It is known to my Master, may God prolong his days, that emotional experiences produce marked changes in the body which are apparent and manifest to all. I will prove this to you in that you may see a man of robust build whose voice is strong and pleasant, and whose face shines. When news suddenly reaches him that causes him great anxiety, his facial expression falls and loses its glitter. The color of his countenance changes, his posture droops, and his voice becomes hoarse and weak. Even if he tries with all his might to raise his voice, he cannot. His strength weakens, and sometimes he trembles from his great weakness. His pulse becomes small and weak, his eyes change, and his eyelids become too heavy to move. The surface of his body cools and he loses his appetite. The cause of all these symptoms is the

---

6. For further details and the full text, see F. Rosner, *Maimonides' Three Treatises on Health*, pp. 1–116.

lowering and entrance of the natural [body] heat and the blood into the depths of the body.

The opposite of this is when you see a man of weak body with an altered countenance and a soft voice. When news reaches him that causes him great rejoicing, you see that his body strengthens and his voice becomes raised. His face brightens, his movements become faster, his pulse becomes stronger and larger, the surface of his body warms, and rejoicing and happiness become apparent in his face and his eyelids. These matters are extremely clear, cannot be hidden, and do not require close observation to be recognized. The cause of all these symptoms is the movement of the natural heat and the blood to the surface of the body

Similarly, the situations of hopeful and fearful people and of those who expect security and tranquility are known; so, too, the emotional reactions of the desperate and the successful are manifest. Sometimes a desperate person may be so disheartened by his misfortune that he cannot see because of the diminution of his visual power and its gloominess. On the other hand, the light in the eyes of a successful person markedly increases to the point that the light of the day has increased and grown. This matter is clear. It is not necessary to elaborate thereon.

Because of this, physicians have instructed that one must pay attention to and constantly consider emotional activities. One should maintain them in equilibrium during health as well as during any illness, and not let any other regimen take precedence over them in any wise. The physician should regard every sick person as having a constricted heart and the healthy person as having a broad psyche, and therefore he should remove from him the emotional activities which lead to anxiety. Thereby the health of the healthy is preserved.

## Maimonides' Medical Aphorisms

The preventive-medicine approach and the interrelationship between physical and mental health are also described in Maimonides' *Medical Aphorisms*.[7] In the seventh chapter of this work, Maimonides asserts that fasting, insomnia, anxiety, severe pain, and the like weaken bodily strength. Most people are said to faint following severe emotional strain. This occurs most frequently in the ill, the elderly, and the weak. Many individuals faint following anxiety or happiness or anger. Other times, they break out in profuse perspiration.

Maimonides' understanding of the dependence of physical health on the psyche or mental health is again apparent.

---

7. For further details on this work, see above, chap. 4.

## The Treatise on Poisons

The *Treatise on Poisons* is one of Maimonides' most interesting and popular works because it is very scientific and modern in its approach and was, therefore, used as a textbook of toxicology throughout the Middle Ages.[8]

The first section of the book deals with snake and dog bites and with scorpion, bee, wasp, and spider stings. The first chapter concerns the conduct of the victim in general to prevent the dissemination of the poison.

> When someone is bitten, immediate care should be taken to tie the spot above the wound as fast as possible to prevent the poison from spreading throughout the body; in the meantime, another person should make cuts with a black lancet directly above the wound, suck vigorously with his mouth, and spit out. Before doing that, it is advisable to disinfect the mouth with olive oil, or with spirit in oil. . . . Care should be taken that the sucking person has no wound in his mouth or rotten teeth. . . . should there be no man available to do the sucking, cupping-glasses should be applied, with or without fire; the heated ones have a much better effect because they combine the advantages of sucking and cauterizing at the same time. . . . Then apply the great theriac. . . . Apply some medicine to the wound that will draw the poison out of the body.

This is the same method used to treat snakebites today. Maimonides was far ahead of his contemporaries on this matter. He also discusses at length the prevention of both accidental and intentional poisoning.

> Be careful about foods with altered tastes and about various types of bad odors and about everything whose nature is not known. Also be careful about colored foods which we commonly use, such as thick soups like the Egyptian ones, and foods to which lemons have been added or whose appearance is altered, such as foods containing sumac or pomegranate juice or foods cooked in fishbrine or foods in which an apparently sour or styptic or extremely sweet taste predominates or foods which have a bad odor, such as those prepared with vinegar or those containing onions or those cooked with garlic. Only eat these types of foods if they were prepared by a reliable person about whom you have not the slightest doubt, because the cunning of those who wish to do harm by poisoning is only accomplished through foods in which the taste or the odor or the appearance of the poison is assimilated.

---

8. For further details, see above, chap. 3. For the full text, see Rosner, *Maimonides' Treatises on Poisons, Hemorrhoids, and Cohabitation*, pp. 19–115.

He also cautions against drinking water that was left uncovered lest a poisonous creature discharged poison in it. This topic was discussed in some detail earlier in this chapter.

## Discussion

It is apparent from his legal and medical writings that Maimonides fully subscribed to the Jewish concept of prevention rather than treatment of disease. He championed this cause because someone who is ill cannot serve the Lord properly. Judaism is guided by the axioms of the supreme sanctity of human life and the dignity of man created in the image of God.

In Judaism, the preservation of human life is a divine commandment. If it is a matter of saving a life, all religious laws are automatically suspended, the only exceptions being the prohibitions against idolatry, murder, and forbidden sexual relations such as incest or adultery. The value of human life is infinite and beyond measure. The bodies and souls of human beings are gifts from God. Man does not possess absolute title over his life or body. He is like a steward charged with preserving and dignifying that life. It is therefore required that we follow a regimen of life, as described by Maimonides, that will maintain our health. Man must eat, drink, and sustain himself, and seek healing when he is ill. Asceticism and self-affliction are foreign to Judaism. Even fasting is not allowed except as prescribed for religious purposes.

The maintenance of health requires Jews to avoid harmful foods and activities and to prevent danger wherever possible. This principle is exemplified by the precept of building a parapet on one's roof. One must be concerned about ecological and environmental factors, such as clean air and sunshine, which may impact upon one's health. One must observe the rules of personal hygiene, such as washing the hands before eating. Diet, exercise, sex, and bodily functions must all be tended to as outlined by Maimonides.

If, in spite of all the above, a person becomes ill, healing from a human physician is mandated in the Torah and does not constitute lack of faith in the true Divine Healer. On the contrary, it is forbidden to rely on miracles or on Providence alone. One must do whatever one can to preserve health and maintain life. Physicians, too, according to Maimonides, are mandated with Divine license to heal the sick. These and other general principles of Jewish medical ethics are discussed in greater detail elsewhere.[9]

As a physician, Moses Maimonides tried to prevent illness by prescribing healthy regimens of living. His attitude toward the practice of medicine came from his deep religious background, which made him view the preservation of health and life as a Divine commandment.

---

9. See F. Rosner, *Modern Medicine and Jewish Ethics.*

# ⸙ 18 ⸙

# Human Temperaments and a Regimen of Health

## Introduction

Hilkhot De'ot ("Moral Dispositions"), the second treatise of the *Sefer ha-Mada* ("Book of Knowledge") section of Maimonides' *Mishneh Torah*, deals with human traits or temperaments and ethical tendencies. Particularly interesting is chapter 4, which deals with a variety of hygienic and medical prescriptions for healthy living and for the prevention of illness.[1] Among the many subjects discussed are normal bodily excretory functions, recommended times for eating, amounts and types of food to be consumed, beverage imbibition, exercise, sleep habits, cathartics, climatic and weather effects on eating habits, detrimental and beneficial foods, fruits, meats, vegetables, bathing, bloodletting, sexual intercourse, and domicile.

The other chapters of this treatise are just as interesting and deal with recommended moral traits and ethical standards of practice for which a person should strive. Hilkhot De'ot is of such importance that it is presented in its entirety further on in this chapter, translated and fully annotated.

---

1. See F. Rosner, "The Hygienic Principles of Moses Maimonides."

205

Maimonides also discusses ethical conduct and personal hygiene, as well as sanitation, and environmental health hazards, in other treatises of the *Mishneh Torah*. Among other things, he says that good character and ethical conduct are essential traits of a human being who hopes to fulfill the divine precepts. Thus, one should be scrupulous in conduct, gentle in conversation, pleasant, affable, and courteous toward fellow human beings; moreover, it is necessary to conduct one's business affairs with integrity and honesty, and to devote oneself to the study of Torah (Hilkhot Yesodei ha-Torah 5:11). In another place he writes that every Jew is obligated to study Torah, whether poor or rich, in good health or ailing, young or very old and feeble (Hilkhot Talmud Torah 1:8). It is desirable to become well versed in the Torah prior to marriage, he adds, but if the sexual drive or physical desires are so overpowering as to preoccupy the mind, one should marry and then study Torah (ibid. 1:5).

Eating, says Maimonides, should not be a purely biological function, as it is in animals. Rather, a person should eat in order to be able to study Torah and serve the Lord (ibid. 3:6). One should not derive profit from the study or teaching of Torah but should maintain oneself by the labor of one's hands (ibid. 3:11). Hence, many of the great sages of Israel were woodcutters and water-drawers (ibid. 1:9), and some of the most illustrious of the talmudic sages were physicians. Included among them are Mar Samuel, R. Ammi, and R. Nathan.[2]

Prior to ministering in the Temple, Maimonides writes, the priests had to cleanse their hands and feet (Hilkhot Bet ha-Beḥirah 5:1). Before reciting the Shema, one should wash his hands in water (Hilkhot Keriat Shema 3:1). If water is unavailable, they should be wiped with earth (ibid.). The Shema is not to be recited in a bathhouse or a latrine, even if there is no odor there (ibid. 3:2). Not only the recitation of the Shema, but anything that appertains to sacred things, may not be uttered in a bathhouse or latrine (ibid.

---

2. F. Rosner, *Medicine in the Bible and the Talmud*, pp. 151–70.

3:4). It is also forbidden to recite the Shema when facing human, dog, or swine excrement, or any other filth that emits an odor as foul as these (ibid. 3:6). Nor should the Shema be recited in the presence of a naked person or if the worshipper himself is bare (ibid. 3:16–17).

The treatise on forbidden foods concludes with a number of rules relating to personal hygiene and sanitation, as follows:

> The sages have forbidden the consumption of food and drink of the kind that is revolting to most people, such as food and drink contaminated with vomit, excrement, or putrid secretion, and the like. They have also forbidden eating and drinking out of filthy utensils which offend against one's natural fastidiousness, such as utensils used in the privy, the glass vessels used by barber-surgeons for bloodletting, and the like.
>
> Similarly, the sages forbade eating with grimy and dirty hands, or upon a soiled tablecloth, since all these things are included in the verse "ye shall not make yourselves abominable" (Lev. 11:43). He who eats such revolting foods is liable to the flogging prescribed for disobedience
>
> It is likewise forbidden to delay the normal evacuation of one's large or small orifices, and he who does so is counted among those who make themselves abominable, not to speak of the grave illnesses which he may thereby bring upon himself, thus endangering his life. Man should, on the contrary, accustom himself to bowel movements at regular times, so that he will not make himself offensive in the presence of people nor render himself abominable.
>
> Indeed, he who is painstaking in these things gains exceeding sanctity and purity for his person, and purges his soul for the sake of the Holy One, blessed be He, as it is said, "Ye shall therefore sanctify yourselves and be holy, for I am holy" (Lev. 11:44).
>
> (Hilkhot Ma'akhalot Asurot 17:29–32)

Environmental hazards seem to be described when Maimonides asserts that carcasses, graves, and tanneries must be kept fifty cubits from a town (Hilkhot Shekhenim 10:3). A tannery may be set up only on the east side of the town, because the east wind is mild and reduces the unpleasantness of the odors produced by the tanning of the hides (ibid. 10:4). It is not clear whether the odor is harmful to health or just a nuisance. Discomfort from smoke, the smell of a privy, dust, and the like, and shaking of the ground, are grounds for the aggrieved party to sue his neighbor to compel him to move the damage-causing item to a proper distance (ibid. 11:4).

Environmental health factors are also discussed in Maimonides' *Treatise on Asthma*.[3] In the last chapter, he gives concise admonitions and aphorisms useful to anyone desirous of preserving his health and ministering to the sick. The chapter begins as follows:

> The first thing to consider. . . is the provision of fresh air, clean water, and a healthy diet. . . . city air is stagnant, turbid, and thick, the natural result of its big buildings, narrow streets, and refuse of its inhabitants. . . . one should at least choose for a residence a wide open site. . . . living quarters are best located on an upper floor. . . and ample sunshine. . . . toilets should be located as far as possible from living rooms. The air should be kept dry at all times by sweet scents, fumigation, and drying agents. Concern for clean air is the foremost rule in preserving the health of body and soul.

Maimonides wrote two separate medical treatises on personal hygiene and health at the behest of Sultan al-Malik al-Afdal, eldest son of Saladin the Great. These treatises are briefly described in the introductory chapter of this book and are available in English for the interested reader.[4]

There follows an unabridged, fully annotated English translation of Hilkhot De'ot from Maimonides' *Mishneh Torah*. Material in brackets has been added to help clarify the meaning of the text.

## Laws of Moral Dispositions (Hilkhot De'ot)

These comprise eleven commandments, five positive and six negative. Specifically they are:

1. to imitate His ways
2. to cleave to those that know Him
3. to love neighbors
4. to love proselytes
5. not to hate brothers
6. to admonish
7. not to put anyone to shame [lit. not to whiten faces]
8. not to oppress the unfortunate
9. not to bear tales

---

3. For further details on this work, see above, chap. 2.

4. See H. L. Gordon, *Moses ben Maimon: The Preservation of Youth*; A. Bar Sela, H. E. Hoff, and E. Faris, *Moses Maimonides' Two Treatises on the Regimen of Health*; J. O. Leibowitz and S. Marcus, *On the Causes of Symptoms*; F. Rosner and S. Muntner, *The Medical Writings of Moses Maimonides: Treatise on Hemorrhoids and Maimonides' Answers to Queries*; F. Rosner, *Moses Maimonides' Three Treatises on Health*.

10. not to avenge
11. not to bear a grudge

The explanation of these commandments follows in these chapters.

## Chapter One[5]

1. Every human being is endowed with many temperaments [or: tendencies, moral dispositions, ethical qualities], and each is different from the other and very far apart from it. There is one type of man who is quick-tempered and always angry, and there is another type of man whose mind is at ease and who is not angry at all; and if he does become angry, he is only mildly vexed once in many years. And there is another type of man who is excessively arrogant [lit. of elevated heart]; and one who is extremely humble [lit. of low spirit]. And there is one who is a sensualist, whose soul's desires can never be satisfied; and there is one whose heart is extremely pure and does not even long for the few things which the body needs. And there is one who is so greedy [lit. wide souled] that his soul would not be satisfied with all the money in the world, as the matter is stated: "He that loveth silver shall not be satisfied with silver" [Eccles. 5:9]. And there is one who is frugal [lit. abbreviates his soul], so that he is content with even a very small amount which is insufficient for him; and he does not pursue the attainment of all his needs. And there is one who tortures himself through starvation and hoarding; he does not consume a penny's worth of his own without great anguish. And there is one who intentionally squanders all his money. The other temperaments can be similarly viewed: such as the jovial and the melancholic, the miserly and the generous, the cruel and the merciful, the soft-hearted and the stout-hearted, and the like.

2. Between each human temperament and its counterpart at the opposite extreme, there are intermediate temperaments each dis-

---

5. Maimonides' theory on mental and physical therapy is holistic rather than dualistic, requiring parallel treatment of body and soul, which form a single psychosomatic unit. This chapter is in the nature of a supplement to Maimonides' *Regimen Sanitatis*, in which he recommends the reading of ethical literature as a means of achieving mental equilibrium.

tinct from the other. Of all the temperaments, there are some with which man is innately endowed from the beginning of his creation in accordance with the nature of his body. And there are some temperaments toward which a man's nature is disposed and which he acquires more rapidly than other temperaments. And there are some which are not innate in man from the beginning of his creation but which he learns from others, or towards which he leans according to the thoughts which enter his heart, or because he has heard that a certain temperament is good for him and it is appropriate that he adopt it and conduct himself according to it until it becomes ingrained in his heart.

3. To follow either extreme of each and every temperament is not the right path, and it is not proper to follow such a course or learn it for oneself. If you find your nature inclined toward one of them or predisposed toward one of them, or if you have already acquired one of them and are accustomed thereto, you should reverse yourself to good and follow the path of good people, and that is the proper path.

4. The proper path is the middle [or intermediate] tendency of each of the temperaments with which man is endowed. It is the temperament which is equidistant from the two extremes and is not closer to one extreme than the other. Therefore, the early sages instructed that a man should constantly reevaluate his temperaments [cf. Sotah 5b] and weigh them and direct them to the middle path, in order that his body be perfect. How is this to be done? Do not be an angry person, easily enraged, nor like a dead person, who cannot feel. Rather, steer the middle course. Become ired only over something serious over which it is proper to become angered in order that such a thing not be done again. Similarly, do not lust for things save those which the body needs and without which it is impossible to live, as the matter is stated: "The righteous eats to the satisfaction of his soul" [Prov. 13:25]. Likewise, do not toil in your occupation save to acquire that which is necessary for your sustenance at the moment, as the matter is stated: "The little that the righteous has is better [than the wealth of the wicked]" [Ps. 37:16]. Do not be stingy [lit. tight-fisted] to excess, and do not squander

your money. Rather, give charity according to your means and lend appropriately to one who requires it. Do not be too jovial and frivolous nor too sad and mournful; rather, be pleasantly happy all the days of your life, with a cordial countenance. The same applies to the other temperaments. And this path is the path of the sages. Every man whose temperaments are intermediate and follow the middle path is called a wise man.

5. And he who is extremely strict with himself and deviates slightly from the intermediate temperament to one side or the other is called a righteous man [Shabbat 121b]. How is this done? He who removes himself from haughtiness of an extreme degree and becomes excessively humble is called a righteous person, and this is the characteristic of righteousness. If you only remove yourself to the intermediate degree and become humble, you are called a wise man, and this is the characteristic of wisdom. Similarly with all the other temperaments. And the righteous men of old used to direct their temperaments from intermediate degrees toward the two extremes. There is a temperament which they directed to the last extreme and another temperament which they directed to the first extreme, but this is beyond the line of mere duty.[6] And we are commanded to follow these intermediate paths, and these are the good and proper paths, as it is written: "And thou shalt walk in His ways" [Deut. 28:9].

6. The sages taught the following explanation for this commandment [Sifri on Ekev, Shabbat 133b; cf. *Guide* 1:94]: "Just as He is called Gracious, so you too should be gracious; just as He is called Merciful, so you too should be merciful; just as He is called Holy, so you too should be holy." And in this manner did the prophets call the Almighty with all these attributes, Long-suffering, Abundant in Kindness, Righteous and Just, Perfect, Strong and Powerful, and the like, in order to tell us that these are good and just paths, and that a person is obligated to conduct himself by them and to emulate Him as much as he can.

7. How can you accustom yourself to these temperaments so that

---

6. Some manuscripts begin section 6 here.

they become ingrained in you? Practice again and again[7] the actions that you perform according to these intermediate temperaments and repeat them constantly until these acts become easy for you and until they are no longer a burden on you. And then these temperaments will become ingrained in your soul. And it is because the Creator is called by these names, and they represent the intermediate path which we are obligated to follow, that this path is called the Path of God. And this is what our forefather Abraham taught his sons, as it is written: "For I know him, that he will command [his children and his household after him, that they shall keep the way of the Lord]" [Gen. 18:19]. He who treads in this path brings goodness and blessing upon himself, as it is written: "In order that the Lord bring upon Abraham that which He spoke concerning him" [ibid.].

## Chapter Two

1. To those who have sicknesses of the body, bitter tastes sweet, and sweet tastes bitter. Among the sick are those who long and yearn for foods which are not fit to be eaten, such as dust and coal, and who detest good nutriments, such as bread and meat, all according to the severity of the illness. Similarly, people whose souls are sick lust for and love bad temperaments and despise the proper path and are lazy to walk therein, and it is extremely burdensome on them according to the severity of their ailment.[8] Likewise, Isaiah says of such people: "Woe to those who state that evil is good and good is evil, that put darkness into light and light into darkness, who consider bitter sweet and sweet bitter" [Isa. 5:20]. And concerning them it is stated: "Who forsake the just paths to walk in the paths of darkness" [Prov. 2:13]. And what is the remedy for sickness of the soul? Let them [i.e., those afflicted with illnesses of the soul] go to the sages, who are healers of the soul, and they [the physician-sages] will heal their ailment through temperaments

---

7. Cf. Maimonides, *Commentary on the Mishnah*, Avot 3:19.
8. Cf. Maimonides' *Eight Chapters*, chap. 3.

which they will teach them until they revert to the proper path.[9] And those who recognize their bad temperaments yet do not go to the sages to be healed—of them Solomon said: "Wisdom and discipline fools despise" [Prov. 1:7].

2. And how do you cure them? We tell the one who is easily angered to conduct himself in such a manner that if he is smitten and cursed, he will not feel anything. And he is to follow this path for a long time until the anger is uprooted from his heart. And if he is haughty, he should accustom himself to extreme disgrace and sit below everyone and clothe himself with shabby rags which put to shame those who wear them, and do similar things until the haughtiness is uprooted from him and he reverts to the middle path, which is the proper way. And when he returns to the middle path, he should adhere to it all the days of his life. In this manner should he treat all the temperaments. And if he is far toward one extreme, he should move himself toward the other extreme and conduct himself therein for a long time until he reverts to the proper path. And this is the intermediate measure of each and every temperament.

3. And there are temperaments concerning which man is forbidden to conduct himself to the intermediate degree. Rather, he should distance himself from one extreme to the other extreme. One example is haughtiness, in that it is not good for a person to be only humble. Rather he should be humble in spirit, and his spirit should be lowly to the extreme. And therefore it is stated of Moses our teacher "exceedingly meek" [Num. 12:3], and it is not stated "meek" alone. And therefore the sages commanded us: "Be exceedingly, exceedingly humble-spirited" [Avot 4:4]. And they further stated [Sotah 4b] that whoever is haughty denies a fundamental principle of Judaism, as it is said: "And thy heart will be on high and thou wilt forget the Lord thy God" [Deut. 8:14]. And

---

9. As in Jerusalem Talmud, Ta'anit 1:1, regarding the talebearer who was asked to consult R. Hanina, the psychiatrist. And this is what the latter advised: "Apply yourself to the study of the Law, as it says, 'A wholesome tongue is a tree of life' (Prov. 15:4) and the tree of life is nothing but the Law."

ner stated: "In excommunication shall be he who is
:ven only a little" [Sotah 5a]. The same applies to anger. It
is an extremely bad temperament, and it is proper for man to distance himself from it to the opposite extreme. And he should teach
himself not to become angered [cf. Ta'anit 4a] even over something
for which anger would be appropriate. And if he wishes to instill
fear in his children and the members of his household or in the
community, if he is its leader, and he wishes to be angry at them so
that they revert to good, then he should show himself to be angry
in front of them in order to chastise them, but his own mind
should be at peace with itself, just like a man who simulates anger
at a time when anger is called for but in reality is not angry [cf.
Shabbat 105b].

The sages of old stated: "He who becomes angry is as if he wor-
ships idols" [Zohar, Bereshit 2:26].[10] And they also stated that "he
who becomes angry, if he is a wise man, his wisdom departs from
him, and if he is a prophet, his prophecy leaves him" [Pesaḥim
66b]. The life of the angry is no real life [Pesaḥim 113b]. Therefore,
they commanded us to remain far from anger until we are able to
so conduct ourselves that we do not become irritated even by
things which arouse anger, and this is the good path. And the path
of the righteous is that they are humble and do not humiliate others, they hear their scorn but do not reply, they perform the will of
God out of love and rejoice in affliction [Yoma 23a, Gittin 36b,
Shabbat 88b]. Concerning them Scripture says: "And they that love
Him are like the rising of the sun in its might" [Judg. 5:31].

4. A person should forever indulge in silence and not speak
except for a matter of wisdom[11] or in matters which are required
for the sustenance of his body. It was said of Rav, disciple of our
holy teacher [Rabbi Judah the Prince], that he did not speak idle

---

10. R. Ḥayyim Heller notes that this passage, appearing in the Responsa of Rashbash,
no. 370, was copied from Nedarim 22a, which is probably the original version. In the traditional Talmud, the passage reads: "An angry man is a slave to all the torments of hell."

11. "All idle talk is bad, except that bearing on matters of study" (Jer. Berakhot 9:5).

talk all the days of his life.[12] And such is the talk of most people. Even in regard to necessities of the body, you should not multiply words. And concerning this did the sages command and state: "He who multiplies words brings sin" [Avot 1:17]. And they also stated: "I have found nothing better for the body than silence" [ibid.]. So, too, in words of Torah and words of wisdom, a person's words should be few but their content full of meaning. And this is what the sages commanded and said: "Forever should a man teach his pupils in a concise manner" [Pesaḥim 3b]. However, if the words are many and the content little, this is folly, and concerning this it is stated: "For the dream cometh because of much discussion, and the voice of a fool because of many words" [Eccles. 5:2].

5. "The safeguard of wisdom is silence" [Avot 3:13]. Therefore, do not be hasty to reply, and do not speak much. And teach your pupils calmly and gently, without shouting and without lengthy talk. This is what Solomon stated: "The words of the wise, [spoken] quietly, are heard" [Eccles. 9:17].

6. It is forbidden to conduct yourself to use words of flattery and seduction. And you should not speak one word and have another in your heart;[13] rather, the internal should be as the external, and the matter in your heart should be that which one enunciates with the mouth.[14] And it is forbidden to deceive people [lit. steal the minds of people], even a Gentile. How? Do not sell to a Gentile the meat of an animal which is *nevelah* [not slaughtered according to ritual rules] as if it were meat of a ritually slaughtered animal.[15] And do not sell the shoe of a dead beast as if it were the shoe of a ritually

---

12. In Yoma 19b, Rabbah says, "Engaging in idle talk is a sin," etc. The same is related in Sukkah 28:1 about R. Yoḥanan ben Zakkai. In the Gaonic Responsa, at the end of *Naharot Dameshek*, this is one of the ten modes of pious conduct attributed to Rav. Maimonides mentions Rav in this connection in his *Commentary to the Mishnah* (Avot 1:17).

13. Cf. Pesaḥim 113b, "The following three incur the hatred of God—he who speaks one way with his mouth and another way in his heart," etc.

14. Cf. Yoma 72b, "Any learned man who puts on a false appearance is to be viewed with suspicion," i.e., is not a learned man.

15. The latter is more expensive.

slaughtered animal [Ḥullin 94a]. And do not urge your friend to eat with you if you know that your friend will not eat. And do not shower him with gifts if you know that your friend will not accept them [ibid.]. And do not open barrels which you need to open to sell them in order to flatter your friend so that he thinks you opened them in his honor. And similarly all other deceptions [ibid.]. And even one word of flattery or deceit is prohibited. Rather, you must have truthful lips and an upright spirit and a pure heart free from all travail and mischief [ibid.].

7. Do not be frivolous and jestful nor melancholic and mournful. Rather, be cheerful. Thus did the sages state: "Frivolity and light-headedness accustom a person to lewdness" [Avot 3:13]. And they commanded that we should not be licentious in frivolity nor sad and mournful, but should receive everyone with a cheerful counte-nance [Avot 1:15]. And similarly we should not be overly lustful [lit. have a wide soul] [Avot 5:19], hastening to become rich, nor melancholic and idle from work.[16] Rather we should be contented [lit. with a good eye], work a little for a livelihood [Avot 4:10], and engage in the study of Torah. And we should rejoice in that small amount which is our portion [Avot 4:1]. And we should not be quarrelsome or jealous or lustful or seekers of honor. Thus did the sages state: "Jealousy, lust, and the seeking of honor remove a man from the world" [Avot 4:28]. The general rule is to follow an inter-mediate path in each and every temperament until all your temper-aments are precisely in the middle [between the two extremes]. And this is what Solomon said: "Balance the track of your feet, and all your paths will be exact" [Prov. 4:26].

## Chapter Three

1. If perchance someone says, "Since jealousy, lust, and the pur-suit of honor, and the like, are all evil ways and remove a person from the world, I will separate myself from them to the utmost and will distance myself to the opposite extreme," so that he eats no meat and drinks no wine and does not marry and does not live in a

16. Cf. Avot de-Rabbi Nathan 11, "Idleness kills a man."

fine home and does not wear handsome clothes, but sackcloth and coarse wool and the like, as do the idolatrous priests—this too is an evil path, and following it is prohibited. And he who walks in this path is called a sinner. For it is said concerning a Nazarite: "And he [the priest] shall make an atonement for him because he has sinned against the soul" [Num. 6:11]. The sages said: "Since the Nazarite, who only separated himself from wine, needs atonement, one who abstains from each and every thing certainly requires atonement" [Ta'anit 11a]. Therefore, the sages commanded us to only abstain from those things which the Torah specifically deprives us of. And do not prohibit for yourself, through vows and oaths, those things which are permissible. Thus did the sages state: "Is not that which the Torah forbids sufficient for you that you prohibit for yourselves additional things?" [Jer. Nedarim 9:1]. Included in this general chastisement are those who constantly fast; they are not following a good path. And the sages prohibited a person from afflicting himself through fasting.[17] And concerning all these things and similar matters did Solomon admonish, saying: "Do not be excessively righteous or excessively wise; why destroy yourself?" [Eccles. 7:16].

2. We are required to direct our hearts and all our deeds to knowing the Lord, blessed be He, alone. And our sitting down and getting up and our conversation should all be directed to the attainment of this goal. How is this done? When engaged in business or performing work for wages, do not intend solely to accumulate wealth; rather, do these things in order to obtain the things which your body requires: food, drink, a house to live in, and marriage to a woman. Similarly, when you eat and drink and cohabit, do not intend to do these things solely to obtain gratification therefrom to the point that you find that you only eat and drink that which is sweet to the palate and cohabit for the pleasure thereof. Rather, set your heart to eat and drink only to maintain the health of your body and limbs. Therefore, do not consume all that the palate lusts for, like a dog or an ass, but eat things that are beneficial to

---

17. Said Samuel: "A man who deprives himself of food is a sinner" (Ta'anit 11a).

the body, whether they are bitter or sweet; and do not eat things which are harmful to the body even though they may be sweet to the palate. How is this done? If your flesh is hot [either from fever or because your bodily humors are hot], do not eat meat or honey, and do not drink wine, as the matter was stated by Solomon in proverbial form: "The eating of much honey is not good" [Prov. 25:27]. And drink chickory juice [Mishnah Kilayim 1:2] even though it is bitter, so that you eat and drink solely for medicinal purposes in order to become healthy and remain healthy, since it is impossible for man to live save with food and drink. Similarly, when you cohabit, do not cohabit except to maintain the health of your body and to preserve your race [lit. seed]. Therefore, do not cohabit whenever you have the lust but at such times that you know that you require to emit seed, such as for medical reasons or to preserve your race.

3. Conducting yourself according to medical rules but setting your heart solely on the health of your entire body and limbs, and on having children who will perform your work and will toil for your benefit—this is not a good path to follow. Rather, set your heart on your body's being healthy and strong in order that your soul will be upright to know the Lord. For it is impossible to understand and comprehend the sciences [lit. wisdoms] if you are hungry and ailing or if one of your limbs is aching. And set your heart on having a son who might become a sage and great man in Israel. He who treads in this path all the days of his life is worshipping the Lord constantly, even at times when he conducts his business and even when engaged in sexual intercourse, because his thought in all that he does is to obtain his necessities to the point that his body is healthy to serve the Lord. And even when he sleeps, if he sleeps with the intent of resting his mind and reposing his body so as to fend off illness, since he would not be able to serve the Lord if he is sick, then his sleep is considered service to the Lord, blessed be He. And concerning this matter the sages commanded and said: "And all your deeds should be for the sake of

Heaven" [Avot 2:12].[18] And this is also what Solomon, in his wisdom, said: "In all thy ways, know Him,[19] and He will make your paths straight" [Prov. 3:6].

## Chapter Four

1. Since one treads in the ways of the Lord when the body is healthy and sound, because it is impossible to understand or know anything of the knowledge of the Creator when one is sick, it is obligatory to avoid things which are detrimental to the body and acclimatize yourself to things which heal and fortify it. These are as follows: Never eat except when you are hungry [Berakhot 62b] nor drink unless you are thirsty. Do not postpone your eliminations for even a single moment [Makkot 16b];[20] rather, every time that micturition or defecation becomes necessary, respond thereto immediately.

2. Do not eat until your stomach is replete [Gittin 70a], but diminish your intake by approximately one-fourth of satiation [ibid.]. Do not drink water during meals save a little and mixed with wine [Berakhot 42b].[21] When the food commences to be digested in the intestines, you may drink as much water as you find necessary. However, even after the food has been digested, do not imbibe water excessively.[22] Do not eat until you have examined yourself carefully lest it be necessary to excrete wastes.[23] Do not eat

---

18. Of Hillel it was said [Betzah 16a] that everything he did was for the sake of God, and anytime he went to the baths he used to say to his followers: "I am going to fulfill God's precept" (Vayikra Rabbah 34). See what Maimonides wrote on this in his *Eight Chapters*, chap. 5.

19. Cf. Berakhot 63a, "'In all thy ways acknowledge Him': on these few words depends the entire Torah."

20. Cf. Hilkhot Ma'akhalot Assurot 17;31, "Withholding one's bodily functions comes under the heading of 'You shall not make yourselves abominable' [Lev. 11:43]. Besides, it gives rise to bad diseases and endangers life." Also, "More people die from intestinal disorders than from hunger" (Shabbat 33a).

21. Rashi comments that they used to drink but little during a meal.

22. "Anybody who takes in more drink than food undermines his health" (Niddah 24b).

23. "He who requires easing himself and still goes on eating is like a furnace stoked on top of its ashes, which is the beginning of a bad odor" (Shabbat 82a).

you have walked [Berakhot 23b] prior to the meal so that body begins to become warmed, or perform a physical task or tire yourself by some other form of exertion. The rule in this matter is that you should exert your body and fatigue it every day in the morning until it begins to warm.[24] Then rest a little until your soul has settled, and then you may eat. If you wash with warm water after the exercise, so much the better. After this, wait a little and then eat.

3. When you eat, alway sit in your place [Gittin 70a] or recline on the left side [Berakhot 46b, Pesahim 108a]. Do not walk or ride or exercise or agitate your body, and do not promenade, until the food is digested in your intestines. Anyone who promenades immediately after his meal or who fatigues himself brings on serious and grave illnesses [Shabbat 129b, Ta'anit 10b].

4. The day and night consist of twenty-four hours. It is sufficient to sleep one-third thereof, which is eight hours.[25] These should be at the end of the night,[26] so that from the beginning of your sleep until the rising of the sun will be eight hours. Thus, you will arise from your bed before the sun rises.

5. Do not sleep on your face or on your back but on your side [Berakhot 13b, Niddah 14a]; at the beginning of the night, on the left side, and at the end of the night on the right side. Further, do not go to sleep shortly after eating, but wait approximately three or four hours after a meal. Do not sleep during the day.[27]

6. Things which purge the intestines, such as grapes, figs, mulberries, peas, melons, various types of cucumbers, and types of gourds, should be eaten before the meal [Ketubbot 10b]. Do not mix them with the food, but wait until they have passed out of the upper abdomen and then eat your meal. Things which bind the

---

24. "There are three kinds of perspiration which do the body good, among them that which comes from work" (Avot de-Rabbi Nathan 41). "Work is valuable, because a man gets warmed up by it" (Gittin 16b).

25. The Sephardi *Ma'asei Roke'ah* contains an unspecified quotation from the sages to the effect that it is good to sleep seven hours a day.

26. "Sleeping at dawn is like tempering the iron," i.e., improving it (Berakhot 62b).

27. David is reported to have had the habit of taking a short nap during the day, some sixty respirations in all (Sukkah 26b).

intestines [i.e., constipate], such as pomegranates, quinces, apples, and small pears [Kilayim 1:4], should be consumed immediately after the meal, but do not eat excessively thereof.

7. If you wish to eat fowl meat and cattle meat together, first consume the poultry meat. Likewise, if you desire eggs and poultry meat, eat the eggs first. If you desire the meat of small cattle [e.g., lambs] as well as large cattle [e.g., cows], first consume the meat of the small. Always begin with something light and then proceed to the heavier food.

8. In the warm [summer] months, eat cooling foods, do not use seasoning to excess, and consume vinegar.[28] In the rainy [winter] months, eat warming foods [Eruvin 56a], abundantly spice the food, and eat a little mustard[29] and asafetida. In this manner prepare food in cold climates and warm climates, in each and every place that which is best suited thereto.

9. Some foods are extremely detrimental, and it is proper never to eat them, such as large salted old fish, old salted cheese, truffles, mushrooms, old salted meat [Bava Batra 74b], wine must,[30] and a cooked dish which has been kept until it acquires a foul odor. Likewise, any food whose odor is bad or excessively bitter is like a fatal poison unto the body. Other foods are also detrimental but are not as injurious as the aforementioned ones. Therefore, of these eat only a little and only after intervals of many days. Do not accustom yourself to make a meal of them or to eat them regularly with your meals. Examples of this type of food are large fish, cheese, and milk that is kept for twenty-four hours after milking [Pesaḥim 42a]. The meat of large oxen [Avodah Zarah 29a] and large he-goats, beans, lentils, peas [Kilayim 1:1], barley bread, unleavened bread [Kiddushin 62a], cabbage,[31] leeks, onions [Kiddushin 62a], garlic, mustard, and radishes—all these are detrimental foods. Do not partake

---

28. Ruth 2:14 says, "Dip thy morsel in the vinegar," to which Shabbat 111b comments: "It appears that vinegar is good on a hot day."

29. Regarding mustard Berakhot 40a says: "Mustard taken once in thirty days frees the house from disease. It should not be taken every day because it weakens the heart."

30. Which means at least forty days after leaving the vat (Eduyyot 6a).

31. Boiled cabbage has a curative effect (Avodah Zarah 29a).

of them except a very small amount, and only during the rainy [winter] season. However, during the warm [summer] months, do not eat thereof at all. Beans and lentils alone should not be eaten either in the warm months or in the rainy season. Cucumbers may be consumed during the warm [summer] season.[32]

10. There are other foods which are also detrimental, but not as much as the aforementioned ones. They are water fowl, small young pigeons, dates, bread toasted[33] in oil or kneaded with oil, fine meal that was completely sifted so that not a trace of bran remains [see Pesaḥim 2:7], gravy, and brine of salted fish [Nedarim 51b]. Do not consume these foods excessively. A person who is wise and can control his inclinations and not yield to his appetite, and who does not eat any of the aforementioned [detrimental foods] unless he needs them as a medicine, is indeed a strong man.

11. Always abstain from fruits of trees and do not consume them excessively even when they are dried, and needless to say when they are fresh. Indeed, before they are completely ripe they are like swords to the body. Likewise, carob-pods [locust beans] are always injurious. All sour fruits are detrimental, and do not eat therefrom save a little, and only in the warm season and in warm climates. Figs,[34] grapes, and almonds, however, are always good whether fresh or dried, and you may eat therefrom as much as you require. Do not eat them constantly even though they are better than all other fruits of trees.

12. Honey and wine are bad for children but salutary for the elderly, especially in the rainy season. In the warm months eat two-thirds of what you eat in the rainy months.

13. Always strive to have your intestines relaxed [see Ketubbot 10b] all the days of your life, and your bowel function should approximate diarrhea. This is a fundamental principle in medicine,

---

32. "When cucumbers are soft, patients eat them with their bread; when dry they are extremely harmful" (Nedarim 49a).

33. See Rashi on Lev. 23:14.

34. "The fig is good for consumption, nice to look at, and beneficial to the intellect" (Midrash Kohelet 5:10).

namely, whenever the stool is withheld or is extruded with difficulty, grave illnesses result. How can you heal your intestines if they
are slightly constipated? A young boy should eat salty foods, cooked
and spiced with olive oil, fish brine, and salt, without bread, every
morning; or should drink the liquid of boiled spinach or cabbage
in olive oil and fish brine and salt. An old man should drink honey
mixed with warm water in the morning and wait approximately
four hours, and then should eat his meal. He should do this for one
day, or three or four days if necessary, until his intestines soften [and
move freely].

14. Another major principle of bodily health, physicians state, is
that as long as a person labors and becomes greatly fatigued and
does not satiate himself and keeps his bowels soft, no illness will
befall him and his strength will be fortified even if he eats detrimental foods.

15. Anyone who lives a sedentary life and does not exercise or
who postpones his excretions or whose intestines are constipated,
even if he eats good foods and takes care of himself according to
proper medical principles—all his days will be painful and his
strength will wane. Excessive eating is like a deadly poison to the
body and is a principal cause of all illness.[35] Most diseases that man
is afflicted with are due to bad foods or because he fills his abdomen and eats excessively, even of good [i.e., wholesome] foods.
This is what Solomon in his wisdom stated: "Whoso keepeth his
mouth and his tongue keepeth his soul from trouble" [Prov. 21:23];
that is to say, he who guards his mouth from consuming detrimental food or satiation, and his tongue from speaking except when
necessary [will remain healthy].

16. The correct manner of bathing is to enter the bathhouse and
bathe every seven days. Do not enter the bath immediately after
eating or when you are hungry, but when the food begins to be
digested. Wash your entire body with hot water that does not scald
the body; the head alone may be washed with water hot enough to
scald the body. Then wash your body with lukewarm water, and

---

35. "He who stuffs himself with food is sure to contract many diseases" (Berakhot 32a).

then with tepid water, and so on until you wash with cold water.[36] Do not pour either lukewarm or cold water over your head. In the rainy season, do not bathe in cold water. Do not bathe until you perspire and your entire body becomes supple, and do not remain too long in the bath; as soon as you perspire and your body becomes supple, rinse your body and leave the bath. Examine yourself prior to entering the bath and after leaving it, lest excretion of wastes be necessary. Similarly, always examine yourself before meals and after meals, before sexual intercourse and after sexual intercourse, before and after you exercise and exert yourself, and before and after you go to sleep. The total number of circumstances is thus ten.

17. When you leave the bath, put your clothes on and cover your head in the outer chamber so that you will not be caught in a cold draft. Even in the summer be careful in this regard. After you leave, wait until you are composed, your body rested, and the warmth [from the bath] dissipated, and then eat. Sleeping a little after leaving the bath before you eat is excellent. Do not drink cold water upon leaving the bath[37] and certainly not while in the bath. If you are thirsty upon leaving the bath and cannot restrain yourself from drinking, mix water in wine or in honey [Shabbat 140a] and then drink it. If, in the winter, you anoint yourself with oil in the bath after the rinsing, this is beneficial.

18. Do not accustom yourself to constant bloodletting.[38] Do not phlebotomize yourself except if there is extraordinary need. Do not let blood either in the sunny [summer] months or in the rainy [winter] season; rather, a little in the month of Nissan [approximately April, i.e., spring] and a little in the month of Tishri [approximately October, i.e., autumn]. After fifty years of age, do

---

36. A man taking a hot bath and not following it up with cold water is like iron which has been kept in the fire without being immersed in cold water afterwards, which, Rashi explains, makes for much stronger iron (Shabbat 41a).

37. A warm drink is advisable; "A man taking a hot bath and refraining from having a warm drink is like a furnace which has been stoked from without, not from within, and is therefore of no use" (Shabbat 41a).

38. According to the sages, bloodletting is among the eight things to be applied with moderation (Gittin 70a).

not phlebotomize yourself at all [Shabbat 129b]. Do not be bled and take a bath the same day [Gittin 70a], nor be bled and then undertake a journey, nor be bled on the day you return from a journey. On the day of phlebotomy, eat and drink less than you are accustomed to, and rest on the day of phlebotomy [Gittin 70a] and do not fatigue or exert yourself or promenade [Shabbat 129a].

19. Effusion of semen represents the strength of the body and its life, and the light of the eyes. Whenever semen is emitted to excess, the body is consumed, its strength terminates, and its life perishes. This is what Solomon in his wisdom stated: "Give not thy strength unto women" [Prov. 31:3]. He who immerses himself in sexual intercourse will be assailed by premature aging [Shabbat 152a]. His strength will wane, his eyes will weaken, and a bad odor will emit from his mouth and his armpits. The hair of his head, his eyebrows, and his eyelashes will fall out, and the hair of his beard and armpits and the hair of his legs will increase excessively. His teeth will fall out, and many maladies other than these will afflict him. Wise physicians have stated that one in a thousand dies from other illnesses and the remaining nine hundred and ninety-nine from excessive sexual intercourse. Therefore, be cautious in this matter if you wish to live wholesomely. Do not cohabit unless your body is healthy and very strong and you experience many involuntary erections, and when you divert your thoughts to another thing, the erection persists, and when you sense a heaviness from your loins down, as if the testicular cords were being tightened, and your flesh were warm. A person in this state requires coitus, and it is therapeutic for him to have sexual intercourse.

Do not cohabit when you are satiated nor when you are hungry but after the food is digested in your intestines [Nedarim 20b]. Examine whether need for excretion [of urine or feces] exists before coitus and after coitus. Do not have sexual intercourse standing or sitting, or in a bathhouse, or on the day when you take a bath, or on the day of phlebotomy, or on the day you set out on a journey or return from a journey, or on the day preceding or following such occurrences [all these in Gittin 70a].

20. I guarantee that anyone who conducts himself according to

the directions we have laid down will not be afflicted with illness all the days of his life until he ages greatly and expires. He will not require a physician, and his body will be complete and remain healthy all his life, unless his body was defective from the beginning of his creation, or unless he has become habituated to one of the bad practices from the onset of his youth, or unless the plague of pestilence or the plague of drought comes into the world.

21. All these helpful rules which we have presented should be followed only by healthy individuals. For the ill and for those in whom an organ is ailing or who have been habituated to a bad practice for many years– for each of these there are different directions and rules to follow according to the nature of the illness, as is expounded in the book on medicines: "A change in your living habits is the beginning of illness" [Ketubbot 110b, Bava Batra 152a].

22. Wherever there is no physician, neither the healthy nor the sick should deviate from the rules that we have prescribed in this chapter, because each and every one of them [if observed correctly] will produce a salutary outcome.

23. No disciple of a sage [Sanhedrin 17b] should reside in a city that does not possess the ten following things: a physician [or: circumciser], a surgeon [or: phlebotomist], a bathhouse, a lavatory, a water supply, such as a river or well, a synagogue, a schoolteacher, a scribe, a charity treasurer, and a court of law with authority to punish with lashes and imprisonment.

## Chapter Five

1. Just as a wise man is recognized by his wisdom and temperaments, whereby he is distinguished from the remainder of the people, so too should he be recognized by his deeds: his eating and his drinking and his cohabitation and his elimination of excrement and his speech[39] and his walk and his dress and his conducting his affairs and his engaging in business. And all these deeds should be per-

---

39. Me'ilah 17b says: "I see you are a learned man from the way you hold your mouth."

formed exceedingly befittingly and properly. How is this done? A wise man should not be a glutton but should eat food which is proper for the health of his body. And he should not partake there-from large amounts. And he should not seek to fill his stomach as do those who stuff themselves with food and beverage until their abdomens swell. Of the latter, it is explicitly stated in Scripture: *And I will spread dung on your faces* [the dung of your holidays] [Mal. 2:3]. The sages stated: "These are the people who eat and drink and make all the days of their lives as holidays" [Shabbat 151b]. And they are the ones who say *eat and drink, for tomorrow we die* [Isa. 22:13]. And this is the method of eating of the wicked, and these [festive] tables are those which Scripture shamed by saying: *For all tables are full of filthy vomit without a clean place* [Isa. 28:9]. But a wise man does not eat save a single dish or two, and partakes thereof in order to sustain life, and this is sufficient for him. This is what Solomon stated: "The righteous eats to satisfy his soul" [Prov. 13:25].

2. When the wise man eats the little which is proper for him, he should not eat it save in his house and at his table. And he should not eat in a store [or: restaurant] or in the marketplace [see Jer. Ma'aserot 3:2, Kiddushin 40b], except for extreme necessity, in order not to be disgraced before the public. And he should not eat with ignorant people [Berakhot 43b] or at tables filled with filthy vomit. And he should not eat his meals frequently in all kinds of places even in the company of wise men [Pesaḥim 49a]. And he should not eat at feasts where there are large gatherings. And it is not proper for him to partake of the food of others except for a meal in connection with a religious ceremony, such as an engagement or marriage feast, and then only if it is a wise man who is marrying the daughter of a wise man. The righteous and pious men of old did not partake of meals that were not their own.[40]

3. When a wise man drinks wine, he does not drink save to

---

40. In Ḥullin 7b R. Pinḥas ben Ya'ir is reported to have never partaken of food not his own once he came of age.

moisten the food in his intestines [Ketubbot 8b]. Anyone who becomes intoxicated is considered a sinner[41] and contemptible, and loses his wisdom. And if he becomes intoxicated in the presence of ignorant people, he is considered to have profaned the name of God. It is forbidden to drink wine at noon [Avot 3:6], even only a little, unless it is part of a meal, because drinking which is part of a meal does not intoxicate [Jer. Pesahim 37:74], and we are not warned to avoid wine save that after the meal.

4. Although a man's wife is always permitted to him, it is proper for a wise man to conduct himself with sanctity [Shevuot 18b]. He should not be with his wife like a rooster [Berakhot 22a]. Rather he should cohabit only on Friday nights [Ketubbot 62b] if he has the vigor. And when he converses with her, he should not converse at the beginning of the night, when he is satiated and his stomach is replete; and not at the end of the night, when he is hungry. Rather, he should cohabit in the middle of the night, when the food is digested in his intestines [Nedarim 20b]. And he should not indulge excessively in frivolity [lit. lightheadedness], nor should he profane his mouth with vulgar talk even if only between him and her. For it is stated in Scripture [or: tradition]: "And He relates to man what his discourse is" [Amos 4:13], which our sages interpreted to mean: "Even for light discourse between a man and his wife he will in the future be called to judgment" [Hagigah 5b]. Husband and wife should not be intoxicated [Nedarim 20a], lazy, or melancholic;[42] neither of them. And she should not be sleeping, and he should not coerce her if she is unwilling [Eruvin 100b]. Rather, sexual intercourse should be carried out with the consent of both and while both are happy. He should converse and jest a little with her [Berakhot 72a] in order to put her at ease [Hagigah 5b], and he should then cohabit modestly [Niddah 17b] and not impudently, and he should separate immediately afterward [Nedarim 20b].

---

41. "Drunkenness leads to sin: Do not drink and you will not sin" (Berakhot 29b).

42. "A man should make his wife good-humored in preparation for a good deed" (Pesahim 72b).

5. He who follows this conduct not only sanctifies his soul and purifies himself and perfects his temperaments, but if he has children, they will be pleasant and modest and inclined toward wisdom and piety [Nedarim 20b]. And he who follows the conduct of the remainder of the people, who walk in darkness, will have children just like those of the remainder of the people.

6. Extreme modesty is what the wise accustom themselves to [Berakhot 72a, Tamid 72b]. They should not disgrace themselves or uncover their heads [Kiddushin 30a] or bodies. Even when you enter the lavatory, be modest and do not bare yourself [lit. reveal your clothes] until you sit down [Tamid 27b], and do not wipe yourself with your right hand [Berakhot 62a–b], and remove yourself far from every person [Horayot 13b], and enter a room within a room or a cave within a cave [Berakhot 62a–b] in order to empty your bowels [i.e., in complete privacy]. If you move your bowels behind a fence, distance yourself so that your friend will be unable to hear you if you should sneeze. And if you move your bowels in an open plain, distance yourself so that your friend will not be able to see you bare. And do not talk while moving your bowels, even if there is great need. And in the same modest manner that you conduct yourself during the day in the bathroom, so conduct yourself at night. And train yourself to empty your bowels only in the morning and evening in order not to require distancing yourself.[43]

7. A wise man, when speaking, does not shout or scream, as do animals and beasts. And he does not raise his voice excessively. Rather, his speech with all people is calm [Yoma 86a]. And when he speaks calmly, he is careful not to overdo it lest his speech appear like that of the haughty.[44] Greet everyone first [Avot 4:15, Berakhot 17a] so that their spirit is pleased with you. And judge everyone with the scale of merit [Avot 1:6]. Speak praiseworthy things of

---

43. Because few people are out in the fields at these times (Berakhot 62a).
44. Cf. Derekh Eretz, chap. 2, "Those who pout like pigeons and walk about on their fingertips," concerning whom it says in Psalms 36:12, "Let not the foot of arrogance come against me."

your fellow man[45] and not at all blameworthy things [Nedarim 81a]. Love peace and seek peace [Avot 1:12]. If you see that your words are beneficial and will be heeded, say them, but if not, be silent [Yevamot 65b]. How? Do not appease your friend when he is angry [Avot 4:18], and do not question him about a vow at the time the vow is being made [ibid.], but wait until your friend's mind is cooled and quiescent. And do not offer condolences to a friend while the deceased still remains before him, because mourners are upset until after the burial. And similarly in like matters. And do not show yourself to your friend in the moment of his disgrace but keep your eyes off him. And do not change your word, nor add to nor subtract therefrom, and do not speak save words of wisdom or charity and the like. And do not converse with a woman on the street, even if she is your own wife or sister or daughter [Berakhot 43b, Yoma 86a, Kiddushin 70b, Yevamot 65a].

8. A wise man does not walk with a proud posture and out-stretched neck, as it is written: "And they walk with outstretched necks and wanton eyes" [Isa. 3:16]. And do not walk slowly, bringing heel to toe, as do women and haughty people, as it is written: "Walking and mincing as they go and making a tinkling with their feet" [ibid.]. And do not run about in the street, as is the custom of lunatics, or bend over double like a hunchback, but only gaze downwards as one would do when standing in prayer.[46] And do not walk on the street like a man occupied with his affairs. From a person's gait you can determine whether he is wise and knowledgeable or idiotic and foolish. And similarly did Solomon, in his wisdom, state: "And also when a fool walketh by the way, his understanding faileth him and he saith to everyone that he is a fool" [Eccles. 10:3], meaning that he proclaims to all concerning himself that he is a fool.

9. The clothing of a wise man should be pleasant and clean, and

---

45. "Our masters of old used to praise their colleagues and pupils" (Gittin 67a, Kiddushin 29b and 70a).

46. "A man in prayer should keep his eyes down and his heart uplifted" (Yevamot 105b).

it is forbidden for a stain or grease spot or the like to be found on his clothing [Shabbat 114a]. And he should not wear kingly robes, such as clothing of gold and purple [Shabbat 145a], that all would look at, or clothing of the poor, which disgraces its wearers, but pleasant intermediate clothes. And his flesh should not be seen beneath his garments [Bava Batra 57b], as with the extremely thin [i.e., transparent] linen clothing made in Egypt. And his clothes should not drag on the ground as the clothing of the haughty but only up to the heel. And his sleeves should be up to the tips of his fingers.[47] And he should not let his fringed garment trail,[48] because it appears arrogant, save only on the Sabbath if he has no other to change into. And he should not wear patched shoes in the summertime with patch upon patch, but in the wintertime [lit. days of rain, or rainy season] it is permitted if he is poor. He should not go out on the streets perfumed or with perfumed garments, nor should he place perfume in his hair. However, if he anoints his body with perfume in order to eliminate a bad odor, it is permissible. And likewise, he should not go out at night alone unless he has an appointed time to go out to his studies [all in Berakhot 43b]. All these rules are to avoid suspicion [of wrongdoing] [Hullin 91b, Pesahim 112a, Berakhot 45b].

10. A wise man manages his affairs judiciously. He eats, drinks, and nourishes his household according to his wealth and success, and does not overburden himself more than necessary. The sages commanded [Hullin 84a] that proper conduct means that a person should not eat meat regularly save when he desires it, as it is written: "Because thy soul desireth to eat flesh" [Deut. 12:20]. It is sufficient for a healthy person to eat meat from Friday night to Friday night.[49] And if you are rich enough to eat meat every day, you may

47. "Said Michal, the daughter of Saul, to David: 'My father's was a better family than yours. They never allowed their wrist or ankle to show behind their garments'" (Yalkut Shimoni, II Samuel 143). See also Jer. Bezah 5:2.

48. "Rich men walk about with their outer garments sweeping the ground because they do not mind getting them spoiled, but a learned man must not do it lest he be regarded as a vulgar person, except on a Sabbath if he has no other suit of clothes" (Shabbat 113a).

49. Once weekly on Friday nights.

do so. And the sages commanded [Hullin 84a], saying: "Always eat less than what your wealth can afford, dress within your means, and honor your wife and children with more than you can afford."[50]

11. The way of the sensible is to first select a permanent vocation which will provide a livelihood, and afterwards to purchase a home, and then to marry, as it is written: "And who is the man that hath planted a vineyard and hath not redeemed it? Who is the man that hath built a new house and hath not dedicated it? And who is the man that hath betrothed a woman and hath not taken her?" [Deut. 20:5–7].[51] But a fool begins by marrying; then, if he can afford to, he purchases a house, and after that, at the end of his days, he turns to seeking a vocation or receives his livelihood from charity. And so is it stated in the verses "A wife shalt thou betroth, a house shalt thou build, a vineyard shalt thou plant" [Deut. 28:30], meaning that all your actions will be reversed in order that your ways not be successful. And in the blessings it is stated: "And David acted wisely in all his ways, and the Lord was with him" [I Sam. 18:14].

12. And it is prohibited to declare all your property ownerless or to bequeath it all for holy purposes and then become a burden on society [Arakhin 28a]. And you should not sell a field and buy a house with the proceeds [*Torat Kohanim*, Behar; Gittin 52a], or sell a house and buy chattels or engage in business with the money from the house. However, you may sell chattels and buy a field. The general rule in this matter is to strive for success in regard to your property and exchange the perishable for the durable [Ketubbot 79a]. And your intention should not be to enjoy a little for a moment or to derive pleasure and thereby incur a great loss.[52]

13. A wise man's business dealings should be conducted with truth and in good faith [Yoma 86a]. He should say nay for a nay and yea for a yea. He should be scrupulous with himself in his accounts, honest and benevolent [cf. Megillah 28a] with others when he buys from them, and should not exact from them more

---

50. On which the ancients remarked: "His wife and children depend on him, and he in turn depends on God Almighty."

51. The actual biblical text has "house" before "vineyard."

52. "The best way to lose a fortune is to wear linen and use glassware" (Bava Mezia 29b).

than required. He should pay the money for his purchase promptly [Yoma 86a] and not become a guarantor for others or act as a trustee [cf. Eccles. 11:7] or accept a power of attorney. In matters of buying and selling, he should obligate himself even where the Torah does not make it obligatory upon him, standing fast to his words and not changing them. If others are found obligated to him in judgment, he should delay and forgive them, lend them [money without interest], and be gracious unto them. And he should not go into his friend's vocation [i.e., encroach upon his business] [Sanhedrin 81a]. And throughout his life he should never oppress anyone.[53] The general principle in this matter is to be among the pursued and not among the pursuers, among the humiliated but not the humiliators. And of him who does all these things and the like [Yoma 86a] does Scripture state [Isa. 49:3]: "And he said unto me, thou art My servant, Israel, in whom I will be glorified" [Gittin 52b, Yoma 86a, Sanhedrin 81b, Shevuot 31a, Bava Kamma 93a].

## Chapter Six

1. It is natural to be influenced by friends and neighbors in regard to temperament and conduct, and to follow the customs of the people of one's country. Therefore, it is advisable to attach yourself to the righteous and sit constantly in the presence of the wise in order to learn from their conduct [Avot 1:7]. And distance yourself from the wicked who walk in darkness, in order not to learn from their conduct. This is what Solomon stated: "He that walketh with the wise shall be wise, but the companion of fools shall smart for it" [Prov. 13:20]. And it also states: "Happy is the man that hath not walked in the counsel of the wicked" [Ps. 1:1]. And similarly, if you live in a country whose practices are evil and whose inhabitants do not follow the right path, move to a place whose inhabitants are righteous and conduct themselves in the paths of goodness. And if all the countries that you personally know or hear reports about

---

53. Especially by cheating (Mekhilta, Mishpatim). Bava Meẓia 59b says: "The gates of heaven are all closed except those through which complaints against cheating are voiced, because the heart of the cheated is aching and his eyes well up with tears." (Rashi: God sees to their anguish and takes up their cause.)

conduct themselves in a path that is not good, as in our own time,
or if you cannot go to a country whose customs are good because
of military operations or illness, then live alone, by yourself, as the
matter is stated: "Let him live alone and be silent" [Lam. 3:28]. And
if the people are evil and sinners who do not permit you to live in
the country unless you mingle among them and conduct yourself
according to their evil practices, then go to caves, thickets, or
deserts and do not conduct yourself in the way of the sinners, as it
is written: "Oh, that I were in the wilderness [Berakhot 35b] in a
lodging place of wayfaring men" [Jer. 9:1].

2. It is a positive commandment to cleave to the wise and their
disciples in order to learn from their deeds [Ketubbot 111b], as it is
written: "And unto Him shalt thou cleave" [Deut. 10:20]. Is it possible to cleave to the Shekhinah? Rather, this is what the sages
stated in their interpretation of this commandment: cleave unto the
wise and their disciples. Therefore, endeavor to take the daughter
of a scholar as a wife and to give your daughter in marriage to a
scholar. Eat and drink with wise men [Berakhot 64a], handle the
business of scholars,[54] and associate with them in all types of rela-
tionships, as it is written [Deut. 11:22]: "And to cleave unto Him"
[Sifri, Ekev 49]. Similarly did the sages command, saying: "And sit
amidst the dust of their feet, and thirstily drink their words" [Avot
1:4, Pesaḥim 49a, Bava Batra 126a, Shabbat 63a].

3. It is a commandment upon every person to love each and
every Israelite as himself, as it is stated: "And thou shalt love thy
neighbor as thyself" [Lev. 19:18]. Therefore, speak in praise of your
neighbor and be careful with his money, just as you are careful with
your own money [Avot 2:10–12] and desire your own honor. He
who glorifies himself by disgracing his friend does not have a share
in the world-to-come [Jer. Ḥagigah 2:1].

4. Love for the proselyte [Bava Meẓia 59b] who came and
entered under the wings of the Shekhinah comprises two positive
commandments: one because he is included among neighbors
[whom we must love, as mentioned above] and one because he is a

---

54. "So they can sit and study" (Rashi in Ketubbot 111b).

proselyte, and the Torah has stated: "And ye shalt love the stranger" [Deut. 10:19]. God commanded us concerning the love of the stranger just as He commanded us concerning the love of His name, as it is stated: "And thou shalt love the Lord thy God" [Deut. 6:5, 11:1].

5. Whoever entertains hatred in his heart against any fellow Israelite transgresses a negative precept, as it is stated: "Thou shalt not hate thy brother in thy heart" [Lev. 19:17], but flogging is not meted out as punishment for this prohibition because there is no act involved in it [Makkot 16a], and the Torah did not admonish save regarding hatred within the heart. However, he who smites his fellow or disgraces him—even though it is not permitted—has not transgressed the precept of "Thou shalt not hate" [Arakhin 16b].

6. When someone sins against you, you should not hate the sinner and remain silent, as it is stated concerning the wicked: "And Absalom spoke unto Amnon neither good nor evil, for Absalom hated Amnon" [II Sam. 13:22]. Rather, it is incumbent upon you to inform him and say to him: "Why did you do such and such to me? And why did you sin against me in that particular matter?" as it is stated: "And thou shalt surely rebuke thy neighbor" [Lev. 19:17]. And if the sinner repents and asks forgiveness, you must forgive. And do not be cruel in forgiving, as it is stated: "And Abraham prayed unto God" [Gen. 20:17].[55]

7. If you see that your fellow has sinned or walked in a path that is not good, you are obliged to bring him back to good, and to inform him that he is sinning against himself with his evil deeds, as it is stated: "And thou shalt surely rebuke thy neighbor" [Lev. 19:17]. He who rebukes his fellow, whether for matters between the two of them or for matters between the sinner and God, must rebuke him in private [lit. between themselves; cf. Arakhin 16b], and speak to him calmly and with a soft tongue, and inform him that he is only rebuking him for his own good, to bring him to the life of the world-to-come. If the sinner accepts the rebuke, it is

---

55. Although Abimelech sinned against him, Abraham nevertheless forgave him and even prayed for him (Bava Kamma 92a).

well, but if not, he should be rebuked a second and third time. And similarly you are always obligated to rebuke the sinner till he smites you and says: "I will not listen." Whoever is in a position to prevent a sin and does not do so is responsible for that sin, since he was able to prevent it from being committed.[56]

8. In rebuking your fellow, do not begin so harshly as to shame him, as it is stated: "And thou shalt not bear sin because of him" [Lev. 19:17]. Thus did the sages explain: "I might have thought that you must rebuke him till his face changes color. [Not so!] Therefore, it is said: 'And thou shalt not bear sin because of him,' from which we deduce that it is prohibited to shame an Israelite [even in private] and certainly in public" [Arakhin 16b]. While he who shames his fellow man is not flogged, it is still a grievous sin. Thus did the sages state: "He who shames [lit. whitens the face of] his fellow in public does not have a share in the world-to-come" [Avot 3:11, Bava Meẓia 59a]. Therefore, be careful not to shame your friend in public, whether he be young [Bava Kamma 86a] or old. And do not call him by a name of which he is ashamed, nor relate in his presence something of which he is ashamed. When do all these rules apply? Only in matters between man and man. But in heavenly matters, if he does not repent privately, then he is publicly shamed, and his sin is proclaimed, and he is disgraced and humiliated and cursed until he repents and returns to good, as did all the prophets in Israel [Yoma 86b].

9. If the person against whom someone sinned does not wish to rebuke him or to speak aught to him, because the sinner is very common or of unsound mind, but forgives him in his heart and neither bears animosity against him nor rebukes him—this is the quality of the pious.[57] The Torah only objects to the harboring of animosity.

---

56. Thus it was said of the pious people who failed to exhort their fellows before the destruction of the First Temple: "They should have suffered humiliation and assault, as it says, 'I gave my back to the smiters and my cheeks to them that plucked off the hair' [Isa. 50:6]." See also Shabbat 54b, Berakhot 31b.

57. "Mar Zutra, every night before going to bed, used to say: 'May God forgive all those who wronged me today'" (Megillah 28a).

10. We are obligated to be careful concerning widows and orphans, because their souls are extremely depressed and their spirits low even when they are wealthy. This holds even for the widow and orphans of a king, as it is stated: "Ye shall not afflict any widow or fatherless child" [Exod. 22:21]. How should we conduct ourselves toward them? Always speak softly to them and treat them with respect. And do not pain their bodies with physical labor or their hearts with harsh words. And care for their money more than your own.[58] Whoever annoys them or angers them or pains their hearts or subjugates them or causes them loss of money, violates a negative commandment,[59] and even more so he who smites them or curses them. And the punishment for this negative commandment, even though it does not incur flogging, is explicit in the Torah: "And My wrath shall wax hot, and I will slay you with the sword" [Exod. 22:23]. He who spoke and thus created the world made a covenant with them that whenever they cry out because of violence, they will be answered; as it is stated: "For if they cry at all unto Me, I will surely hear their cry" [Exod. 22:22]. When is all this applicable? Only when someone afflicts them for his own personal gain. But if a teacher punishes them to teach them Torah or a trade or to guide them along the proper path, then it is permissible. But even so, he should not treat them as he would any other person. Rather, he should make a distinction in their case, leading them gently and with great compassion and honor, as it is stated: "For their Redeemer is mighty, He shall plead their cause" [Prov. 23:11]. This applies whether the orphan is fatherless or motherless. And until when is someone regarded as an orphan in respect to this matter? Until he no longer requires an adult to lean upon who will train him and care for him, and he is able to take care of all his personal needs like any other grown person.

---

58. Avi Shemuel used to keep orphans' money in trust. He stored their funds with his own in such a manner that if any of the money in the storage place rotted away or was stolen, it was the part belonging to himself that would be affected, and the orphans' money would be spared (Berakhot 18b).

59. Or prohibitive commandment, i.e., "thou shalt not."

**Chapter Seven**

1. He who bears tales against his fellow transgresses a negative commandment, as it is stated: "Thou shalt not go up and down as a talebearer among thy people" [Lev. 19:16]. And even though the penalty of flogging is not incurred for this offense, it is a grave sin and leads to the death of many souls in Israel.[60] That is why [in the Torah] it is placed close to the injunction: "Neither shalt thou stand idly by the blood of thy neighbor" [ibid.]. Go and learn what happened to Doeg the Edomite.[61]

2. Who is a talebearer? A person who carries reports and goes from this one to that one [cf. Yerushalmi, Peah 1:1] and says: "So-and-so said this"; "Such-and-such have I heard concerning so-and-so." Even though what he says is true, he destroys the world. An even greater sin is included in this negative commandment, and it is the evil tongue. That is, he who speaks degradingly about his fellow, even if what he says is the truth. However, he who speaks falsehoods is called a slanderer. But in regard to a person with an evil tongue, i.e., someone who sits in company and says: "So-and-so did such-and-such," and "Such-and-such were his ancestors," and "Such-and-such did I hear about him," and then relates scandalous things-concerning him, does Scripture state: "May the Lord cut off all smooth lips, the tongue that speaketh proud things" [Ps. 12:4].

3. Our sages stated [cf. Jer. Peah 1:1]: "There are three transgressions for which retribution is exacted in this world and for which man receives no portion in the world-to-come: idolatry, incest, and bloodshed; but the evil tongue outweighs them all" [Arakhin 15b]. The sages further stated: "He who speaks with an evil tongue is as if he denies the fundamental principle [i.e., belief in God], as it is said: "Who said, 'Our tongue will we make mighty, our lips are

---

60. Talebearing may lead to bloodshed, and a talebearer may be likened to a murderer (Derekh Eretz, chap. 1).

61. Because he brought about the destruction of the city of Nob and the deaths of eighty-five priests (I Sam. 22:23).

with us; who is lord over us?'" [Ps. 12:5]. And further did the sages say: "The evil tongue kills three people: he who utters it, he who receives it, and the one of whom it is spoken; and he who receives it is harmed more than he who utters it" [Shabbat 56b].[62]

4. There are words which are called a semblance of the evil tongue [lit. dust of the evil tongue]. For example: "Who will tell so-and-so to remain as he is now?" Or "Be silent about so-and-so. I do not wish to make known what happened and what went on," and similar phrases. And he who speaks well of his fellow in front of his enemies is also guilty of a semblance of the evil tongue, for this causes them to speak degradingly of him [cf. Bava Batra 164b]. And concerning this matter did Solomon say: "He that blesseth his friend with a loud voice, rising early in the morning, it shall be counted a curse unto him" [Prov. 27:14]. For because of the good-ness said of him, it brings about evil to him. Similarly, he who speaks with an evil tongue in a joking manner or in a light-headed manner, i.e., he does not speak out of hatred—of him too did Solomon in his wisdom state: "As a madman who casteth fire-brands, arrows and death . . . and saith, am I not jesting?" [Prov. 26:18–19]. Similarly reprehensible is he who speaks with an evil tongue in a deceitful manner, that is to say, he speaks innocently as if he did not know that the tale he spoke represents evil speech, and when there is a protest against him he says, "I did not know that this tale represented evil speech or that such was really the conduct of so-and-so" [Shabbat 33a, Jer. Peah 1:1].

5. Regardless of whether you speak with an evil tongue in the presence of your fellow or in his absence, or if you speak words which, if heard from man to man, would cause him to be hurt either physically or financially, or even just to distress him or to frighten him—this is all evil speech. And if such words are uttered

---

62. "Had not David lent an ear to Ziba concerning Mephiboshet, his kingdom would have remained undivided, Israel would not have served foreign gods and suffered disper-sion for it" (Shabbat 56b); i.e., the blame rests with David, the listener, rather than with Ziba, the speaker.

before three people [Arakhin 16a], the matter is considered to have been heard and publicized. If one of the three repeats the matter once more, there is no sin of evil speech, provided he did not intend to spread the rumor and disseminate it further.

6. All the aforementioned are people with evil tongues in whose neighborhood it is prohibited to reside; and certainly to sit in their company and listen to their tales is also prohibited. And the sentence passed against our ancestors in the wilderness was sealed only because they were guilty of the evil tongue [Arakhin 15a].

7. He who takes vengeance of his fellow violates a negative commandment, as it is said: "Thou shalt not take vengeance" [Lev. 19:18]. And even though flogging is not incurred for this, it is still an extremely bad characteristic. More properly, one should be forbearing in all matters of the world, for to those who understand, these are all vain, empty things and not worth taking vengeance for. What is meant by taking vengeance? For example, your fellow says to you, "Lend me your ax," and you answer, "I will not lend it to you." On the morrow, you need to borrow an ax yourself. You say to your fellow, "Lend me your ax." He answers, "I will not lend it to you just as you did not lend it to me when I asked for it." This is called taking vengeance [Yoma 23a]. Rather, when he comes to borrow, you should give with a full heart and not treat him as he treated you. Similarly in all related matters. And so, too, did David state in expressing his good temperaments [Ps. 7:5]: "If I have requited him that did evil unto me, or spoiled mine adversary unto emptiness" [Rosh Hashanah 17a].

8. And, similarly, anyone who bears a grudge against a fellow Israelite transgresses a negative commandment, as it is said: "Nor bear a grudge against the children of thy people" [Lev. 18:18]. What is meant by bearing a grudge? Reuben said to Simeon, "Lease this house to me or lend me this ox," and Simeon refused. After an interval, Simeon came to Reuben to borrow from him or to lease from him. And Reuben said to him, "Here it is for you. Behold, I am lending it to you because I am not like you. I will not pay you back according to your deeds." He who does this transgresses "thou shalt bear no grudge." Rather, he should delete the

matter from his heart and not bear a grudge. For as long as he begrudges the matter and remembers it, he may come to take revenge. Therefore, the Torah admonished against resentment to the point that one should obliterate the sin from his heart and not remember it at all. And this is the proper temperament that makes it possible for society to exist and for people to conduct their business affairs one with the other.

# ⅋ 19 ⅋

# Therapeutic Efficacy
# of Chicken Soup

The therapeutic efficacy of chicken, chicken soup, and other fowl
is extensively described in the medical writings of Moses Maimonides. In his *On the Causes of Symptoms*, also known as *Medical
Responsa*, he recommends the meat of hens or roosters (or chickens
or pullets) and their broth because this type of fowl has the property of rectifying corrupted humors, especially the black humor
(i.e., black bile, an excess of which was thought to cause melancholy), so much so that physicians mention that chicken broth is
beneficial in leprosy.[1] The type of chicken to be used is described as
follows:

> One should not use the too large, i.e., of more than two years of age; nor
> the too small, i.e., those in whom the mucus still prevails; neither the too
> lean nor those who through feeding become obese; but those that are fat by
> nature, without being stuffed.[2]

The chicken or pullet can be boiled, stewed, steamed, or boiled
with fresh coriander or some green fennel added to the soup. This
dish is especially suitable in winter. The soup, however, where

---

1. See J. O. Leibowitz and S. Marcus, *Moses Maimonides on the Causes of Symptoms*, pp.
113–14.
2. F. Rosner and S. Muntner, *The Medical Writings of Moses Maimonides*, vol. 3, pp. 60–62.

lemon juice or citron juice or lemon slices are added to the broth, is better suited for summertime. The method of breeding and feeding the chickens is also discussed in some detail. Maimonides concludes that "these procedures have been verified and their usefulness is clear."[3] He does not state, however, whether or not he conducted a double-blind randomized study.

In the chapter on diet in the *Medical Aphorisms of Moses*, Maimonides states that boiled chicken soup neutralizes bodily constitution. Chicken soup is both an excellent food, as well as a medication for the beginning of leprosy, and fattens the bodily substance of the emaciated and those convalescing from illness. Turtle doves increase memory, improve intellect, and sharpen the senses. The consumption of fowl, continues Maimonides, is beneficial for feebleness, hemiplegia, facial paresis, and the pain of edema. It also increases sexual potency. House pigeons that graze in the streets increase natural body heat. Soup made from the bird called *kanaber* loosens cramps of colic. The quail helps the healthy, as well as those convalescing from illness; its flesh is fine, it dissolves kidney stones and stimulates urine flow. Maimonides further states that chicken testicles provide excellent nourishment. They are especially useful to nourish a weakened or convalescent individual. Testicles of all living creatures are warming and moistening in their action and aid the libido in a strongly perceptible manner. Pigeon eggs are good aphrodisiacs. Similarly, all eggs help the libido, especially if they are cooked with onion or turnip. Finally, baby chicks that have been separated from their mother alleviate the heat that occurs in the stomach. Soup made from an old chicken is of benefit against the chronic fevers that develop from white bile and also aids the cough which is called asthma.[4]

In his *Treatise on Asthma*, Maimonides advises the consumption of chicken meat that is not fatty for sufferers of asthma. Other small fowl, such as the turtle dove, are also useful. The soup of chickens

---

3. Ibid.
4. F. Rosner and S. Muntner, *The Medical Aphorisms of Moses Maimonides*, vol. 2, pp. 77–81.

or fat hens is said to be an effective remedy for asthma. The ingredients of the chicken soup and the method of preparing it are also described. An enema with sap of linseed and fenugreek or both, with oil and chicken fat, and an admixture of beet juice, is strongly endorsed for the treatment of asthma.[5]

The various reported therapeutic efficacies of chicken, chicken soup, and other fowl are summarized in Table 1. With the recent demonstration that chicken soup mobilizes nasal mucus better than other hot liquids,[6] scientific respectability has now been obtained to prove what the proverbial Jewish mother has always known—that chicken soup can help cure an upper respiratory infection.

As with all medicinal agents, however, the consumption of fowl is not without occasional side effects (see Table 2). The physician is thus cautioned against the indiscriminate application of chicken and chicken soup for the therapy of all ailments, abiding by the dictum *primum non nocere*. However, the judicious use of chicken soup as an important element of the therapeutic approach to upper and lower respiratory tract infections seems to be fully justified.

*Table 1—Therapeutic Efficacy of Chicken and Other Fowl*

| Condition | Beneficial Effects | Type of Fowl |
|---|---|---|
| Corrupted humors[a,b] | rectifies | chicken soup |
| Leprosy[a,b] | beneficial | chicken soup |
| Spiritual faculties[a,b] | kindles | turtle dove |
| Body constitution[c] | excellent food | chicken soup |
| Body constitution[c] | medication | chicken soup |
| Body constitution[c] | neutralizes | chicken soup |
| Emaciation[c] | fattens the body | chicken soup |
| Convalescence from illness[c] | strengthens | quail and chicken soup |
| Memory[c] | increases | turtle doves |
| Intellect[c] | improves | turtle doves |
| Senses[c] | sharpens | turtle doves |
| Constipation[c] | loosens the stool | partridge |
| Colic (or convulsions)[c] | loosens the cramps | *kanaber* soup |
| Feebleness[c] | beneficial | fowl |

5. S. Muntner, *The Medical Writings of Moses Maimonides: Treatise on Asthma*, pp. 18–20, 42, 68.

6. K. Saketkhoo, A. Januszkiewicz, and M. A. Sackner, "Effects of Drinking Hot Water, Cold Water, and Chicken Soup on Nasal Mucus Veolocity."

| | | |
|---|---|---|
| Hemiplegia[c] | beneficial | fowl |
| Facial paresis[c] | beneficial | fowl |
| Pain of edema[c] | beneficial | fowl |
| Sexual potential[c] | increases | pigeon eggs |
| Natural body heat[c] | increases | house pigeons |
| Kidney stone[c] | dissolves | quail |
| Urine flow[c] | stimulates | quail |
| Weakness of convalescence from illness[c] | excellent nourishment | chicken testicles |
| Heat in the stomach[c] | alleviates | chicken sucklings |
| Chronic fevers from white bile[c] | beneficial | soup from an old chicken |
| Cough called asthma[c] | aids | soup from an old chicken |
| Asthma[d] | useful | chicken soup and roasted small fowl |
| Nasal mucus[e] | increases velocity | chicken soup |
| Asthma[d] | effective remedy | soup of fat of hens and enema containing duck or chicken fat |
| Pneumonia[f] | efficacious | chicken soup |
| *In vitro* pneumococci[g] | inhibits growth | chicken soup |
| Male impotence[h] | cures | chicken fat |
| Frustration and anxiety[i] | relieves | chicken fat |
| Aircraft fuel shortage[j] | potentially useful | chicken soup |
| Snakebite[k] | antidote | chicken |

[a]Leibowitz & Marcus, *Moses Maimonides on the Causes of Symptoms*, pp. 113–114.

[b]Rosner & Muntner, *Medical Writings of Moses Maimonides*, vol. 3, pp. 60–62.

[c]Rosner & Muntner, *Medical Aphorisms of Moses Maimonides,* vol. 2, pp. 77–81.

[d]Muntner, *Maimonides' Treatise on Asthma*, pp. 18–20, 42, 68.

[e]K. Saketkhoo et al., "Effects of Drinking Hot Water, Cold Water, and Chicken Soup."

[f]N. L. Caroline & H. Schwartz, "Chicken Soup Rebound and Relapse of Pneumonia."

[g]R. J. Duma, S. M. Markowitz, & M. A. Tipple, letter in *Chest* 68 (1975):604.

[h]L. F. Greene, letter in *Chest* 68 (1975): 605.

[i]J. G. Chutkow, letter in Chest 68 (1975): 605.

[j]D. S. Lawrence, letter in *Chest* 68 (1975): 606.

[k]Preuss, *Biblical and Talmudic Medicine*, p. 198.

*Table 2—Harmful Effects of Chicken and Other Fowl*

| Harmful Effect | Type of Fowl |
|---|---|
| Produce migraine headaches | pigeon sucklings[a, c] |
| Causes constipation | partridge[a, c] |
| Obstructs the bowels | quail[a,b] |
| Powerful stool loosener | hen and rooster[c] |
| Contain harmful thick juices and are hard on digestion | goose and duck[d] |
| Produce many juices | hens' egg yolks[d] |

[a]J. O. Leibowitz & S. Marcus, *Moses Maimonides on the Causes of Symptoms*, pp. 113–14.

[b]F. Rosner & S. Muntner, *Maimonides' Treatise on Hemorrhoids and Medical Answers*, pp. 60–62.

[c]F. Rosner & S. Muntner, *Medical Aphorisms of Moses Maimonides*, vol. 2, pp. 77–81.

[d]S. Muntner, *Maimonides' Treatise on Asthma*, pp. 18–20, 42, 58.

# ⁓ 20 ⁓

# The Responsum on Longevity

Among the rich legacy of writings left by Moses Maimonides are several hundred letters and responsa edited and published by Jehoshua Blau.[1] Maimonides' responsum dealing with the duration of life is not included in Blau's work, however, nor is it found in previously published collections of Maimonides' letters and responsa.[2] This responsum, although mentioned by Steinschneider in 1879,[3] did not appear in print until 1953, when Gotthold Weil of Jerusalem edited and published it in the original Arabic accompanied by a German translation and lengthy critical comments.[4] Maimonides' responsum on lifespan was commented upon by Kaufmann, Steinschneider, and Weil.[5] Further bibliographical, grammatical, and orthographic detail concerning it is available in Weil's Arabic and German edition. Weil's work was reviewed by Leibowitz and Muntner.[6] With kind permission from the publisher,

---

1. J. R. Blau, *Moses ben Maimon Responsa.*

2. H. Freiman, *Moses ben Maimon Responsa.*

3. M. Steinschneider, "Blätter für neuere und altere Literatur des Judenthums," p. 131.

4. G. Weil, *Maimonides: Uber die Lebensdauer.*

5. D. Kaufmann, "Ein Responsum des Gaons R. Haja über Gottes Vorherwissen und die Dauer des menschlichen Lebens (Agal)"; M. Steinschneider, *Die Arabische Literatur der Juden*, p. 212; G. Weil, "Ein Unediertes Responsum des Maimonides."

6. J. O. Leibowitz, "Moses ben Maimon. *Uber die Lebensdauer*" ; S. Muntner, "Rabbi Moshe ben Maimon. *Uber die Lebesdauer.*"

S. Karger, Basel and New York, it is upon Weil's version that the present English translation is based.

The laws dealing with the fundamental principles of the Torah (Hilkhot Yesodei ha-Torah) comprise one of the sections of the first volume of Maimonides' *Mishneh Torah*. Toward the end of the tenth chapter, we find the following:

> As to calamities predicted by a prophet, if, for example, he foretells the death of a certain individual or declares that in a particular year there will be famine or war, and so forth, the non-fulfillment of his forecast does not disprove his prophetic character. We are not to say, "See, he spoke, and his prediction has not come to pass." For God is long-suffering and abounding in kindness, and repents of the evil [He threatened]. It may also be that those who were threatened repented and were forgiven, as happened to the men of Nineveh. Possibly, too, the execution of the sentence is only deferred, as in the case of Hezekiah.

The full story of Hezekiah's serious illness, his supplication to the Lord, the divine promise of a prolongation of his life, and his thanksgiving psalm are recorded in detail in the Hebrew Bible (Isa. 38:1–20). Other discussions of Hezekiah's transgressions are recorded in the Talmud (Berakhot 10a). In Oxford Hebrew manuscript No. 2497 of Maimonides' *Mishneh Torah*, adjacent to the words "deferred, as in the case of Hezekiah," an anonymous commentator added the following explanation in Arabic:

> The suspension of punishment results either from the fact that people repent or because a righteous person is born in their midst or because they receive their full recompense if in the meantime they can demonstrate [that they have done] good deeds. The suspension [in the aforementioned case] consists in God's having added fifteen years to Hezekiah's life.[7]

Based on this passage, there follows the responsum of Maimonides concerning longevity. The fundamental question to which Maimonides addresses himself in it is whether our lifespans are predetermined or not. This problem had already been discussed earlier by two famous Jewish savants, Rav Hai Gaon and Rav Sa'adia Gaon, one and a half and two and a half centuries, respectively,

---

7. A. Neubauer, *Catalogue of the Hebrew Manuscripts in the Bodleian Library*, p. 887. MS no. 2497 is entitled "Arabic Commentaries, or Rather Notes, on Maimonides' Mishneh Torah."

before Maimonides.[8] In addition, lengthy discussions on this subject are found in Islamic literature.[9] Maimonides' approach in giving a negative answer to this question is twofold; he cites evidence from both religious and medical sources.

Medical proof that the human lifespan is not predetermined, he argues, is expressed by Galen's concept that "the reason for death is the deterioration of the equilibrium of innate heat." By this is meant the disruption of normal equilibrium between the four bodily humors, blood, phlegm or white bile, choler or yellow bile, and melancholy or black bile. These humors represent various combinations of the four basic elements that comprise the human organism: fire, air, earth, and water. Each of the latter has two qualities: fire warms and dries, air warms and moistens, earth cools and dries, and water cools and moistens. In blood, these elements are equally distributed; in phlegm or white bile, water predominates; in choler or yellow bile, fire predominates; and in black bile, earth predominates. Every human being is born with a particular combination or mixture of these elements, humors, and qualities. Any change or disruption in this equilibrium results in ill health. This important concept in ancient medicine may be a parallel to modern oxygenization of blood.

Perhaps based upon this theory, Maimonides states that causes detrimental to innate heat can be external and produce deterioration of the organs of warmth, or can cause qualitative or quantitative deterioration of the warmth itself. Each of these three possibilities is exemplified separately. Maimonides further states that external causes which disrupt normal bodily heat arise from one of six reasons: (1) through the expulsion of the innate heat from the body, (2) through its reversal internally, (3) overfilling of the body with other substances, (4) cessation of respiration, (5) deterioration of the substance of body heat, and (6) deterioration of the quality of innate heat. The final part of the medical section of the responsum deals with sudden accidental death.

---

8. On Hai Gaon, see Kaufmann, op. cit.; on Sa'adia Gaon, see Weil, op. cit.
9. Weil, op. cit.

Maimonides concludes from all the physiologic information he presents that "if a person is careful concerning these causes [of premature accidental death or the causes leading to disequilibrium of innate body heat] that we have presented . . . he will more readily attain his natural life's end." Thus, Maimonides feels that lifespan is not predetermined.

The next large body of evidence that Maimonides presents to support his contention that the human lifespan is not predetermined is gleaned from biblical and rabbinic writings. First he cites several verses from the Pentateuch (Deut. 22:8, Num. 35:11–12, Deut. 19:5–6, 20:7) dealing with commandments affecting human life. These verses prove that the termination of life is not fixed and that precautionary measures can prevent premature death. Next follows indirect evidence from five additional scriptural verses, only one of which is from the Pentateuch. These latter verses do not contain clearly prescribed commandments but are teachings, accounts of historical facts, and the like. All these religious writings, according to Maimonides, prove that a person's lifespan can be altered by certain occurrences and is not fixed and predetermined.

There are other biblical and talmudic passages which reflect the opposite viewpoint. For example, in the Pentateuch we find "Behold, thy days approach that thou must die" (Deut. 31:14) and in the prophets we find, "when thy days are fulfilled" (II Sam. 7:12). Also, in the Talmud it is written, "Though a plague last seven years, no one dies before his time" (Sanhedrin 29a).

An English translation of Maimonides' *Responsum on Longevity* follows. Words in brackets are not present in the original and were inserted to help clarify the meaning.

૱ ૱ ૱

*Question.* I consider it appropriate to mention here a problem concerning which the Moses of our time [Maimonides] was once asked. His pupil Joseph ben Yehuda asked him and indeed inquired with the following words: Is the termination of man's life in this world established at a specified time at which he inevitably arrives, so that even accidental occurrences will not prematurely discontinue his life or snatch him away; or do accidental happenings, if they should occur, snatch a person away and rob him of his life, if he is not on guard against them? [In other words: Does the following alternative exist?] If man is not careful and does not prepare himself by taking countermeasures to cast off these occurrences, he will not remain alive. However, if he takes preventive measures and prepares himself to offer resistance thereto, then he will remain alive and his life will last longer than it would have had he not been careful or taken any countermeasures.

*Answer.* For us Jews, there is no predetermined end point of life. The living being exists as long as replenishment is provided for [that amount of] its substantive moisture [i.e., bodily humors] that dissolves. Also, this moisture must remain unspoiled in its natural state, as Galen has mentioned: "The reason for death is the deterioration of the equilibrium of innate heat" [i.e., disruption of normal homeostasis between the four bodily humors]. Its deterioration occurs secondary to causes that affect bodily heat from the inside as well as causes that exert their influence externally.

Regarding the causes that affect [bodily] warmth from the inside, these occur either following the deterioration of the organs of warmth, as befalls the brain or the heart or the liver[10] following a faulty mixing, either too warm or too cold; or they occur following an obstruction which happens in the brain so that the power of motion cannot make its way to the chest and thus breathing ceases. Similarly, an obstruction can occur in the lung; then the pneuma therein cannot reach the heart, so that the innate warmth is extinguished. Likewise an obstruction can occur in the arteries of the liver; then the warmth cannot reach it and the liver becomes cool as a result.[11] These things happen to [the body's] heat following the deterioration of its organs.

Concerning the deterioration that occurs to the innate heat in regard to its quality, this happens [in one of three ways: it can

---

10. Each of these organs is the seat of some bodily function or power.

11. This passage seems to indicate that the humors themselves are not responsible for the extinction of natural heat; rather, Maimonides is describing "solid" pathology of an obstructive nature.

occur] either as a result of excessive warmth, such as the warmth of a burning fever; then the innate heat and that which dissolves therefrom forces itself [externally]. Or that which occurs to someone who ingests a warming medication [a drug that warms the body], such as *afarbiyun* [euphorbium].[12] Or following cold, as occurs in cold illnesses like freezing [from exposure to cold], hemiplegia, or other cold illnesses or following inbibition of a cooling medication such as *ufiyun* [opium][13] or *bang* or *sawkaran* [hemlock],[14] [all of which] produce cooling of innate [bodily] heat.

Concerning the case in which the quantity [of bodily heat] is spoiled, this occurs because of an excessive decrease or an overabundant increase in its quantity. Excessive decrease, for example, occurs to him in whom an excessive amount of one of the four basic secretions is eliminated, so that the innate heat is extinguished. Excessive increase in quantity is that which leads to death in illnesses which arise because of overfilling. The reason for this is as follows: If the body becomes abnormal because of overfilling with basic secretions or with food or beverages, whichever of these it might be, and no room remains for inhaled air to find itself a path, then strangulation of innate heat occurs as a result. This extinguishing of innate heat is what occurs, for example, with excessive overfilling of the arteries[15] and ventricles of the brain. Then the innate heat only flows very slowly and is extinguished, and as a result, sudden death ensues.

These are the causes which affect innate heat from the inside. The causes which affect it externally arise from [one of] six reasons: (1) through the expulsion [from the body] of innate heat, (2) through its reversion internally, (3) as a result of overfilling, (4) as a result of the absence of respiration, (5) as a result of the deterioration of its substance, (6) as a result of the deterioration of its quality.

---

12. Drug no. 25 in Maimonides' *Sar Asma Al-Uqqar* ("Book of Drugs"); see Max Mayerhof, *Un Glossaire de matière medicale composé par Maïmonide.*

13. Drug no. 35 in Maimonides' *Book of Drugs.* See ibid., also M. Meyerhof, "The Medical Work of Maimonides."

14. Drug no. 58; see ibid. and Meyerhof, *Glossaire de matière medicale.*

15. Again a nonhumoral etiology.

Expulsion [of body heat] can arise following the sudden experiencing of extreme happiness. Then the innate warmth passes to the outside of the body and streams out and dissolves itself. Thereby the outside and the inside of the body cool, and as a result death ensues. In this case, that which happens to the innate heat is somewhat analogous to the flame in a lamp when a strong wind blows thereon and extinguishes it.[16] We have, for example, heard of people who succeeded in attaining an exceptionally strong, joyous emotion and thereby suddenly died.[17] Further, [body heat can be dissipated] through that which assails the brain, reaches into its ventricles, and thereby expels the substance of the [body] heat. Finally, [loss of body heat can occur] through an expulsion of its mass [i.e., of the blood that carries the natural heat], as happens in the case of someone who develops a wound, or who severs one of his veins or an artery so that his blood flows out completely and the natural heat is extinguished. Then something happens analogous to a lamp when the oil flows out therefrom.

Concerning the deterioration of the natural heat by virtue of its reversion internally, this occurs in someone struck by sudden fright or fear. Then the natural heat penetrates the insides of the body all at once. Thereby, however, it [i.e., the body heat] is suppressed so that it becomes extinguished, and as a result, sudden death occurs.

---

16. The analogy of a lamp's flame with innate warmth and substantive moisture was used by Galen and Avicenna. Maimonides uses a similar analogy in the *Mishneh Torah*, Hilkhot Avel 4:5, where he states as follows: "One who is in a dying condition is regarded as a living person in all respects. . . . He is not to be rubbed or washed . . . until he expires. He who touches him is guilty of shedding blood. To what may he be compared? To a flickering flame, which is extinguished as soon as one touches it."

The prohibition against doing anything that might hasten death (i.e., active euthanasia) had already been enunciated before Maimonides, in the second century C.E. in the Mishnah (Semaḥot 1), and in the fifth century C.E. in the Babylonian Talmud (Shabbat 151b). Both the Mishnah and the Talmud use the lamp analogy.

17. See also the *Regimen of Health*, p. 25, where Maimonides states that "passions of the psyche produce changes in the body that are great, evident, and manifest to all. . . . his color dims, the brightness of his face departs, he loses stature, his voice becomes hoarse . . . his eyes sink, his eyelids become too heavy to move, the surface of his body cools, and his appetite subsides. The cause of all these signs is the recall of the natural heat and the blood into the interior of the body."

Maimonides further discusses the effects of the emotions on the body in his *Medical Aphorisms* and his *Treatise on Cohabitation*.

Concerning the deterioration of heat following overfilling, this is what occurs in someone who drowns, in that the cavities of his body are overfilled with water. Because of this, breathing becomes impossible for him, and as a result, natural heat asphyxiates and death ensues. In this case, what happens to the [body] heat is somewhat analogous to what occurs to the flame of a lamp when the oiliness in it is too great due to an excess of oil and this thereby extinguishes the flame.

Concerning the deterioration of natural heat because of the absence of respiration, this refers to the death that befalls one who is asphyxiating because the air is prevented from entering the lung. Then the vaporous waste products accumulate in the heart so that natural heat is extinguished. In this case there occurs something analogous to what happens to the light of a lamp when a thick occlusive container is inverted over it. Then vapors accumulate and the light is extinguished.

Concerning what happens to natural heat following the deterioration of its substance, this occurs [in two ways]. Firstly, following the inspiration of cold air which is mixed with harmful, malodorous gases, as is the case with gases which emanate from cadavers as well as emitted gases that rise from sewers and cesspools in which black fetid mud is to be found.[18] Through this, the substance of the natural heat deteriorates. Thus, many people have died suddenly therefrom in that these [gases] arose from sewers and wells in which the brick dust [i.e., mud, dirt] had putrefied. In this case there occurs something analogous to that which happens to the light of a lamp in that it is extinguished when it is placed among strong fumes or at a site where many gases arise. [Deterioration of the

18. Maimonides also speaks of the quality of inspired air in chapter 13 of his *Treatise on Asthma* (see above, chap. 2). He gives similar advice on clean air in his *Regimen of Health*, as follows: " . . . the finer the pneuma is, the more it is altered by changes in the air. . . . In the city, because of the height of its buildings, the narrowness of its streets, and all that pours from its inhabitants and their superfluities, their dead, the carcasses of their animals and the corruption of their decaying food, the air becomes stagnant, turbid, thick, misty, and foggy. The pneumas change accordingly . . . also endeavor to rectify the air and dry it with good aromatics, vapors, and fumigation."

substance of natural body warmth can also occur] following the sting or bite of a poisonous animal. Then the poison flows through the person's body, disseminating therein and thereby deteriorating the substance of the natural warmth so that the person dies as a result.[19]

Concerning that which deteriorates natural heat by deteriorating its quality, this occurs [in two ways]. Firstly, if it [bodily warmth] becomes extremely hot—the same occurs if it dissolves or is excessively cooled—as in someone who remains too long in a very hot bath or in the sun in an unusually warm summer. In this case, there occurs to the natural heat something analogous to what happens to the flame of a lamp when it is placed next to a strong fire or in an unusually hot sun, namely, that it is extinguished.[20] Secondly, when it [bodily warmth] is excessively cooled, as occurs to many people who travel during cold [weather] and when snow falls on them, they freeze, then death ensues following the extinguishing of natural heat. In this case, what happens to natural heat is somewhat similar to what occurs to the fire in the lamp when it is placed in extreme cold, namely, it goes out.

Moreover, death sometimes afflicts a person by the latter's contact with a hard object through cutting, as is the case of a sword or a sharp iron instrument, so that the tightly joined structures of the body are separated.[21] Or [sudden death also occurs] through a blow, as in the case of stones or other hard objects when they hit the body of a living being, whether they strike with force or fall on the [person] from a high place.

If the circumstances of the case are as we have described, then [the following is certain]: If a person is careful concerning the

---

19. See also S. Muntner, *Maimonides' Treatise on Poisons and Their Antidotes.*

20. The analogy here is unclear. Maimonides does not explain why a lamp should be extinguished if placed next to a hot fire.

21. In medieval medicine, the term "separation of the connection" includes all illnesses and occurrences in which the tightly bound structures of the skin, muscle, or bone are separated (e.g., gaping wounds, bites, fractures). Avicenna speaks of these illnesses and their remedy in the *Canon* I, 75 and 217.

causes [of premature accidental death or those leading to disequilibrium of innate heat] that we have presented, then such accidents will not snatch him away [from life], and he will more readily attain his natural life's end.

We will prove what we have said by two types of evidence, of which the first [concerns] proofs from religious laws and the second [pertains to] proofs taken from nature.[22] We will first cite the proofs from religious commandments because of their prominence and importance, and because they represent the goal at which a person arrives through logic after studying the introductory sciences, i.e., mathematics, physics, and metaphysics. These [religious laws] also lead to [eternal] happiness in the world-to-come.

It is written: "When you build a new house, you should make a parapet for your roof so that you bring not bloodshed upon your house should any man fall therefrom" [Deut. 22:8]. This phrase proves that preparing oneself, and adopting precautionary measures—in that one is careful before undertaking dangerous enterprises—can prevent their occurrence.[23] If, indeed, preparation were not efficacious in guarding against mishaps, then this commandment would be meaningless because it would not prevent any damage from occurring. If, on the one hand, it has already been determined that the person in question will fall from this roof, then the parapet serves absolutely no purpose; and if, on the other hand, it is only there for frivolous play, then it provides no advantage. Since we see, however, that God specifically requires the parapet, it is clear that preparing oneself and taking precautionary measures do prevent [mishaps]. This then represents a refutation of those who

---

22. The actual sequence of evidence presentation is just the opposite; proofs from the laws of nature precede the discussion of the religious laws. For further comment on this point, see G. Weil, *Maimonides. Uber die Lebensdauer*, pp. 23–28. As was mentioned at the beginning of the chapter, the entire responsum is based on the following words in the *Mishneh Torah*: "or [the execution of the sentence] is deferred, as in the case of Hezekiah." Therefore, according to Weil, the scribe or copyist reversed the order of the evidence presented by Maimonides, placing the medical before the religious proofs in order to begin and end the responsum with the above key words. An alternative explanation is that the scribe was writing from memory and erroneously or accidentally reversed the sequence.

23. Although the grammatical construction of the text is incorrect, the meaning of the sentence is clear.

state that life in this world [continues] up to a fixed, predetermined time.

Further, concerning the establishment of the six cities of refuge as an asylum [for the accidental manslayer] from the avenger of blood, it is stated both in Numbers 35:11–12: "And you shall appoint yourself cities to be cities of refuge for you. And the manslayer who kills any person through error shall flee there. And the cities shall be unto you for refuge from the avenger, that the manslayer not die, until he stand before the congregation for judgment"; as well as in Deuteronomy 19:5–6: ". . . he shall flee unto one of these cities and live, lest the avenger of blood pursue the manslayer . . . and slay him." These cities have thus been ordained as sites of refuge to which the manslayer can flee so that the avenger of blood will not kill him. Had he [the accidental manslayer] a predetermined moment for his life's end, namely, to die at the hands of the avenger of blood, then what purpose would the establishment of cities of refuge serve, since the avenger of blood would be predestined to slay him [the accidental manslayer]? Since we have received the commandment to establish these confined areas, however, we know that it is sensible to prepare oneself, in order to protect against harm.

Similarly, where the war leader addresses the people in Deuteronomy 20:7, it is written: "And what man is there that has betrothed a wife, and has not taken her? let him go and return into his house, lest he die in the war and another man take her. . . . What man is there that is fearful and soft-hearted? let him go and return unto his house, lest his brethren's heart melt as his heart." This proves that his remaining at home is for him a precautionary measure against the awaited occurrence of death. Thus we see that the adoption of safety measures is of value to protect against harm.

Another precise proof is our belief in the proclamation [in Jonah 3:4, where because of the faults of the city's inhabitants, it is decreed]: "Forty days more and Nineveh shall be overthrown." After the inhabitants repented, however, God forgave them, as is stated in Jonah 3:5: "And the inhabitants of Nineveh believed in God, and they proclaimed a fast and put on sackcloth"; as well as

Jonah 3:10: "And God saw their works, that they turned from their evil path, and God repented of the evil which He said He would do unto them, and He did it not." If their life's end had been firmly predetermined at the conclusion of forty days, then penitence would not have saved them and they would have perished. If, on the other hand, their life's end was firmly predetermined for the time which they [actually] reached after they repented, then their disobedience [to God's commandments] did not harm them and they would not have been coerced or required to do penitence. This too is evidence that the end of life in this world is not firmly established in advance, so that accidental occurrences do not prematurely sever it.[24]

That which we expound [above] we have also found in the verse: "Fear of the Lord prolongeth days, but the years of the wicked are shortened" [Prov. 10:27]. Let no doubt arise on this account that in this world the life of the wicked can also be prolonged and that of the righteous shortened. As the sages have already stated: "The righteous man who prospers is a completely righteous man; the righteous man who is in adversity is not a completely righteous man. The wicked man who is in adversity is a completely wicked man; the wicked man who prospers is not a completely wicked man" [Berakhot 7a].[25] This means that the righteous man's bad deeds are the cause of his misfortune, and if all his deeds had been perfectly [proper], they would have protected him from the adversity. The same applies to the wicked person. Had he no good deeds to point to, misfortune would not have been kept from him.

It also states: "He that resides in this city shall perish by the sword and by the famine and by the pestilence; but he that goes out and falls to the Chaldeans that besiege you, he shall live" [Jer. 21:9]. Thus, one sees that their deaths are dependent upon their remaining in this city and their remaining alive is dependent upon their going out therefrom. This demonstrates, however, that there is no

---

24. The last phrase is unclear.
25. The actual text in the Talmud has "the wicked man who prospers" before "the wicked man who is in adversity."

firmly determined time for death. Moreover, the elimination of harmful things is efficacious in prolonging life, whereas the undertaking of dangerous things is the basis for shortening life.

For this reason it also states regarding certain laws: "That your days may be prolonged and the days of your children" [Deut. 11:21]. This proves that [one's] occupation with commandments [of the Bible] can retard the expiration of life.

So too can we explain His [God's] statement to Hezekiah: "I have heard your prayer, I have seen your tears: behold, I will add fifteen years unto your days" [Isa. 38:5]. After he [Hezekiah] repented—he had transgressed the law pertaining to procreation [by not fulfilling it], because he had seen by the Holy Spirit that, in the future, unworthy offspring would issue from him; he then repented, however, and for this reason [the decree against him] "thou shalt die and not live" [Isa. 38:1] was withdrawn—God added to his life.

We will now return to our subject matter to keep this digression from becoming too lengthy. This is because the analysis by the highly respected teacher is complete; we have nevertheless extracted more than amply therefrom regarding the explanation of the words "or [the execution of the sentence] is deferred, as in the case of Hezekiah."

# Miscellaneous

# ♦ 21 ♦

# Medicine in Maimonides'
# Mishnah Commentary

## Introduction

The present essay is a compilation of the statements or discussions pertaining to medicine in Maimonides' *Commentary on the Mishnah*, including his famous assertion that the biblical phrase "And thou shalt restore it to him" (Deut. 22:2) refers to the physician's divine mandate to heal the sick, as discussed in the Talmud (Bava Kamma 81b, Sanhedrin 73a).

## Veterinary Medicine

The Talmud (Ḥullin 3:1) enumerates eighteen anatomical defects which render an animal unfit for consumption (*terefah*). Maimonides comments on some of them as follows:

> The esophagus has two membranes ... the brain has two membranes, one of which is attached to bone. The heart has two chambers, one larger than the second; the larger one is on the left side. The spinal cord, which comes out from the brain, has a membrane surrounding it. There are two very thin membranes on the lung. There are three lobes in the right lung and two in the left lung. A large vessel exists from the liver from which veins branch out throughout the body. Bronchi [Heb. *samponot*] are the tubes of the lung, and these are the round cartilagenous structures which spread out in the body of the lung.

Maimonides also states that animals have eleven ribs on each side (ibid.). The large ones contain marrow. An animal can survive if some of its ribs are broken, but a ruptured spleen is incompatible with life. He further asserts that the presence of three kidneys or only one kidney instead of the normal two is compatible with life, but shrunken kidneys or even one shrunken kidney results in a fatal outcome (ibid. 3:2). He also describes pus in the kidney (renal abscess?) and clear water on the kidneys (renal cysts?). He suggests that the lungs of an animal can dry up by an act of God, such as fright from thunder and/or lightning. He describes how to examine dried-up lungs by inflating them and then placing them in water for twenty-four hours to see whether they return to normal. If they do, the animal is fit for consumption (*kasher*). He also discusses the various colors of lungs: black like ink, red like fresh meat, yellow like egg yolk, green like cassia.

Elsewhere, Maimonides speak about the cricoid cartilage and the esophagus and windpipe which are attached to it (Ḥullin 1: 3). Within the body of the cricoid cartilage are "two structures resembling berries which the sages call grains." He also describes the "two tense, pulsating vessels in the neck on the two sides of the wind-pipe [carotid arteries?]" (ibid. 2:1). According to Maimonides, the leg of an animal is composed of sections which are readily visible (ibid. 4:6). The uppermost section, which is attached to the body, is short in relation to the more distal sections and is clearly seen in a camel. The other end of this section is attached to the knee. A fracture in this section (i.e., the thigh bone) is very serious, whereas a fracture below the knee is not. The danger is also greater if there is a compound fracture.

Tendons, muscles, and blood vessels are also discussed. The Achilles tendon is described, the cutting of which cripples an animal so that it cannot walk. The term "sinews" (Heb. *gidim*) is stated to be a general name which refers to pulsating and non-pulsating vessels, cords, membranes, tendons, and nerves (Ḥullin 9:1, Zevaḥim 3:5, Tohorot 1:4).

The anatomy of birds, including water fowl (Ḥullin 3:3), also comes into Maimonides' purview. He states that the crop in a bird is like the stomach in a human being and is attached to the esophagus (ibid. 3:4). Each of a bird's legs is composed of three sections except for the foot upon which the bird stands, which is composed of many sections. Simple and compound fractures of birds' legs and broken wings are discusssed. The prohibition of eating the sciatic nerve of cattle, Maimonides explains, is not applicable to birds because they do not have a spoon- or club-shaped hip. They do not have a spoon-shaped hip like that of man, which is round (ibid. 7:1). The convex prominence of the thigh where the hip muscles attach is flat in birds.

Maimonides also describes a variety of physical abnormalities that render animals unfit to be sacrificed in the Temple (Bekhorot 6:1–12, 7:1–7). Among the physical blemishes that do not render animals unfit are defects involving the white of the eye, a blood spot or "worm" on the eye, and the like (Zevaḥim 9:3). Temporary blemishes in an animal include eczema, dislocation of a limb, and a fracture that heals. Permanent blemishes include torn or severed limbs (Bekhorot 2:2). Plethora in an animal is defined as meaning that an animal is overcome by its blood, which chokes it (Ḥullin 3:5). In some animals, he says, black bile or white bile (phlegma) predominates.[1] He further affirms that a predominance of yellow bile "rarely occurs in animals, as is explained in veterinary medical books." He also cites animal poisons "which are well known to physicians" (ibid.) and describes an animal footsoreness called *aichaja* in Arabic (Makhshirin 3:8).

**Human Anatomy**

Maimonides enumerates the two hundred and forty-eight members of the human body (Oholot 1:8). The chest, he says, is called "the key of the heart" because chest movement inflates the lungs against the heart and, therefore, serves as a key in that it opens a passageway through which air can enter and exit. A Canaanite slave obtains his freedom if his master causes the loss of one of twenty-

---

1. See the discussion of the four bodily humors (black bile, yellow bile, white bile, i.e., phlegm, and blood) in Maimonides' *Medical Aphorisms*. Melchanoly was thought to be caused by an excess of black bile.

four specified limbs or organs (Kiddushin 1: 3), which Maimonides lists as the fingers of the hands and the feet, the earlobes, the tip of the nose, the tip of the breast in a woman, and the tip of the membrum in a man.

Sexual development in both male and female is described by Maimonides several times. An adolescent girl (*bogeret*) is one who is six months past the time when she developed signs of puberty (Yevamot 6:4). And the tokens of puberty are that she have two pubic hairs after she is a full twelve years of age, because if two hairs are present during the twelve years, they do not represent a token but are only a mole (ibid., Niddah 5:7–8, Ketubbot 3:7). Similarly, as long as she does not develop the two hairs after twelve years of age she is considered a minor until she is twenty full years old. A barren woman cannot give birth because of the characteristics of her body. The tokens are that she does not have breasts like other women's breasts, she has no hair growing on her body like other women, her voice is deep so that one cannot distinguish between it and the voices of men, and the female pudenda do not project from her body as they do in other women. It is for this reason that the sages use the expression "she has no abdominal curvature like other women . . . and she has difficulty during sexual intercourse and has no desire for it" (Yevamot 1:1).

A sterile man can be naturally sterile (lit. "eunuch of the sun") like a barren woman, or secondary to an acquired illness or disorder (ibid. 8:5). Elsewhere Maimonides describes minors, pubertal girls, adolescents, and the signs of barrenness and eunuchism (Ketubbot 1:2, 3:7; Niddah 5:9; Yevamot 1:1, 10:11). He cites the Talmud passage that states that if intercourse takes place in a girl under three years of age, her physical signs of virginity return (Ketubbot 1: 2, Yevamot 7:7, 10:7–8). He also describes the anatomy of the female internal genitalia, including the uterus, cervix, ovaries, and fallopian tubes (Niddah 2:5). A *tumtum* is an individual of indeterminate sex who cannot be definitively recognized as either male or female (Bikkurim 1:5). An *androginos* (i.e., hermaphrodite) is one who has both male and female genital organs (ibid., Yevamot 8:6).

## Human Physiology and Physiopathology

Sexual physiology is discussed in some detail by Maimonides in his *Treatise on Cohabitation* as well as in his *Commentary on the Mishnah.* Menstruation and other genital emissions (gonorrhea?) are pre- cisely defined (Arakhin 2:1), as are the physical signs of the immi- nent onset of menstruation (Niddah 9:8). Maimonides states that flux in a man is an illness of the genitalia in which the retentive and digestive power has weakened, whereas the other powers of the body remain in their normal state. Then the sperm drips and issues forth "incompletely cooked," without pleasure and without erec- tion, and its appearance is a little reddish and thin in consistency (Zavim 2:2). Often, dilute "uncooked" semen issues from the membrum after an issue of semen. People who frequently indulge in sexual intercourse suffer from this the most. They tell their phy- sician that when they indulge excessively in sexual intercourse, their sperm issues from them extremely dilute in consistency and reddish in appearance and they have pain (ibid. 2:3).

Galactorrhea in a male (lit. "the milk of a male") is also described (Makhshirim 6:7). Healthy men ejaculate completely and with force and do not retain sperm in their bodies. Such is not the case with sick or elderly men who do not ejaculate with force (Mikva'ot 8:4). A woman can feel whether a man's sperm "shoots like an arrow," but the man cannot feel after that which separates from his body (Nedarim 11:12). If sperm reaches its place in the woman, "it congeals the essence that it finds there and a fetus is produced, as is known in natural science" (Berakhot 3:6). If a woman discharges semen within three days of cohabitation, she is ritually unclean because sperm can survive for that long (Shabbat 9:3). After three days, sperm putrifies (Mikva'ot 8:3, Berakhot 3:6). Of interest to the hematologist is the fact that Maimonides speaks of menstrual blood, the blood of parturition, and other types of blood in a woman (Eduyyot 5:4, 6). Four types of blood are red, bright crocus, like earthy water, and like wine mixed with water (Niddah 2:5). The blood which flows during phlebotomy first spurts forth and then flows more slowly as the vessels and the body become depleted of blood, with resultant weakness and eventually death (Keritot 5:1). Bloodflow from wounds and from a corpse are also described (Oholot 3:5), as are seven substances which can be used to cleanse a garment to determine whether a stain is blood or dye (Niddah 9:6–7). According to Maimonides, it is well known that most of the blood is not in the head but in the rest of the body, because the main blood is in the liver and the heart and the vessels which emanate from them. And this is what the sages meant when they said that most of the blood is found in the body (Zevaḥim 6:6).

In terms of general physiology, Maimonides quotes Rabbi Eliezer, who states that the navel is the source of life because it is the center of the abdomen, which surrounds all the organs of digestion and within which lies the continuation of life. But Rabbi Akiva states that the most important determinant of life is the respiratory system, as it is written: "all in whose nostrils was the breath of the spirit of life [died]" (Gen. 7:22). The final ruling, concludes Maimonides, is in accord with the opinion of Rabbi Akiva (Sotah 9:4). The constitution of boys is "hotter" than that of girls. Hence, the latter tolerate fasting better than boys and must fast on Yom Kippur beginning at age twelve, whereas boys are not so obligated until thirteen years of age (Yoma 8:2).

The subject of death and dying is covered in some detail in Maimonides' *Mishneh Torah*. However, a few brief statements are found in his *Commentary on the Mishnah*. A person who was decapitated is dead even if the body is still moving. Such movements of limbs after death are called *pirkhus* (lit. "jerking movements," i.e., spasms or convulsions) and are analogous to the severed tail of a lizard, which moves jerkingly for a short time after it is cut off. Postmortem movements of this kind occur in some living beings in whom the motive force is not disseminated through all the organs from a central controlling center but is segmented throughout the body (Oholot 1:7). A body decomposes in three days and the face becomes unrecognizable (Yevamot 16:3). A person in whom death is imminent (Heb. *goses*) is one who is breathing his last breaths (Arakhin 1:3, Oholot 1:7). Most people defined as a *goses* die, but a very rare case may survive (Shevu'ot 4:4).

## Obstetrics

Maimonides states, in accordance with the talmudic sages, that a fetus begins to take form forty days after conception (Niddah 3:7). Prior to forty days, it has no form or shape (Keritot 1:4). Various types of abortuses and monster births are described (Niddah 3:2–6), including those that look like a sandal (i.e., a fish-shaped abortion), an afterbirth (i.e., placenta), or a fully-fashioned fetus (Keritot 1:3). The afterbirth is "the sac which contains the fetus and which is unfurled" (Ḥullin 4:7). One must do everything necessary even on the Sabbath for a parturient woman, including cooking for her and cutting and tying the navel (Shabbat 18:3). Maimonides speaks of a woman in labor giving birth to twins, one dead and one alive (Oholot 7:6). Elsewhere (Eduyyot 4:10) he also speaks of multiple births. He states that a woman pregnant with twins can give birth to one by cesarian section and the second vaginally in the normal manner and then she dies (Bekhorot 8:2). It is very unusual for a woman who has had a cesarian section to become pregnant again and give birth (ibid.). Cesarian section means that one tears open the uterine wall of an animal and extracts the fetus therefrom. The same is done for a woman who is having difficulty in giving birth and whose life is in danger (ibid. 2:9). Maimonides also speaks of postmortem cesarian sections (Ḥullin 4:1) and embryotomies (ibid. 4:2).

## Human Pathology and Diseases

The physical defects in a woman that can nullify a marriage are listed (Ketubbot 7:5). These include a bad body odor, profuse perspiration, a facial mole with or without hair, bad breath, a thick unusual voice (hypothyroidism?), excessively enlarged or widely spaced breasts, and a large scar or keloid secondary to an animal bite; in addition, blindness, an amputated hand, or a broken leg (ibid. 7:6). Defects specific to men are mentioned in the discussion of a priest's fitness to serve in the Temple if he is wounded in his testicles (Heb. *petzu'ah dakah*) or if his membrum is cut off (Heb. *kerut shafkhah*). Maimonides states that:

It is important to note that whether the membrum or the threads of the testicles are wounded, or whether the testicles are cut off, or whether the membrum is punctured or whether the testicles are punctured—the general rule is that any defect that occurs in the reproductive organs results, as is well known in nature, in an inability to procreate. Therefore, such a priest is disqualified [from serving in the Temple and from eating the Heave Offering].

(Yevamot 8:12)

In regard to personal injuries, Maimonides states that someone who cuts off his neighbor's hand or foot is obligated to pay the five forms of restitution (pain, damages, shame, medical bills, compensation for inability to work). But if the victim fails to follow the doctor's instructions, thereby aggravating his illness or causing a new medical condition, the perpetrator is not obligated to pay for the new condition, because the victim brought it upon himself (Bava Kamma 8:1).

Other passages describe the various signs of leprosy (Mo'ed Katan 1:5, Eduyyot 5:6). Elsewhere Maimonides states that a deaf-mute is silent because he developed deafness in his mother's womb and thus is unable to hear (Terumot 1:2). One who is dumb can hear and understand but cannot speak because of an affliction in the organs of the voice (ibid. 1:6).

According to Maimonides, drinking water from Lake Tiberias (the Sea of Galilee) may cause watery diarrhea (Makhshirin 6:7). Another cause of diarrhea is walking barefoot on marble floors, as did the priests in the Temple, who

walked [barefooted] on the floor all day and worked with water and only wore a single [layer of] garments in all seasons because it was prohibited for them to serve [in the Temple] except with the four garments: shirt, pants, turban, and girdle, no more and no less. And they ate meat. And because of this type of activity, their bowels were loosened and the strength of their internal organs weakened. And the son of Aḥiyah was appointed to heal them. This is what the sages meant when they said "over the sickness of the bowels."

(Shekalim 5:1)

Maimonides speaks of pus on the outside of a wound (Mikva'ot 9:2) and infections in the eye (ibid. 9:4). He states that people who are sick with serious illnesses develop confusion (Niddah 2:1). He discusses a disorder called *kordiakos* which he considered to be "'a type of epilepsy" (Gittin 7:1, Yoma 8:4) or "an illness that occurs when the chambers of the brain are filled and the intellect becomes confused as a result, and it is a type of faintness."[2] Others interpret *kordiakos* to be delirium tremens in a chronic alcoholic.[3] Elsewhere Maimonides describes a patient with an evil spirit, referring to "any injury which is not caused by man for any known cause" (Eruvin 4:1). Another type of patient with an evil spirit is one suffering from one of several forms of melancholy (Shabbat 2:5). There is one type of melancholy in which the patient flees and goes out of his mind when he sees light or when he is among people. Such a patient, continues Maimonides, finds peace of mind and tranquility of conscience in darkness and in solitude and in desolate places. This illness is common among people with black bile.

Maimonides asserts that man should pray for good weather because when the weather is not too hot and not too cold but intermediate, sick people are healed and healthy people remain healthy (Yoma 5:1). Maimonides confides the rule that all Jewish laws and commandments (except the cardinal three prohibiting idolatry, incest, and murder) are suspended when there is danger to life. Thus, an abscess may be incised on the Sabbath to drain out the pus because of danger to life (Eduyyot 2:5). A newborn circumcised baby may be washed on the Sabbath in warm water even if the water is heated on the Sabbath because there is danger to life (Shabbat 9:3).

In commenting on the talmudic assertion that a dish may be inverted over a scorpion on the Sabbath to prevent it from biting (Shabbat 16:7), Maimonides states that:

> Among the harmful creatures there are some that invariably produce a fatal outcome if they bite a human being, such as certain types of vipers and snakes and a rabid dog. These may be immediately killed on the Sabbath if one encounters them, and on this point there is no difference of opinion.

---

2. This quotation is translated from Kappach's critical Hebrew edition and new translation of Maimonides' *Commentary on the Mishnah*. The phrase "a type of epilepsy" is found in the standard Hebrew versions of Maimonides' *Commentary*.

3. See F. Rosner, "*Kordiakos* in the Talmud."

Other types of poisonous animals that sting or bite may or may not produce a fatal outcome, or they may produce pain for several days or similar injuries. If these animals pursue a person and come near him, it is permissible to kill them, but if they do not attack but remain in their place, one may place a dish over them to prevent them from moving [i.e., attacking]. And if one desires to step on them and kill them while walking [on the Sabbath], it is permissible to do so. And if one traps a snake or the like on the Sabbath, and one's intent is to prevent it from biting, it is permissible to do so.

An animal bitten by a snake may not be consumed, because the snake's poison may have spread throughout the animal's body and the person who eats it may die (Terumot 8:6). It is prohibited to drink from water, wine, or milk that was left uncovered lest "a snake or viper or similar poisonous animal drank from it and the imbiber die, because such animals spit [poison] into these liquids" (ibid. 8:4).[4] If the quantity of water is very large, however, the poison is diluted out and the water is permitted (ibid. 8:5). An ordinary snake does not usually bite, but a scorpion, rattlesnake, or viper nearly always bites. Maimonides considers it useless for the victim of the bite of a mad dog to consume the liver of that dog even though one sage permits it (Yoma 8:4).

Warriors in a camp, says Maimonides, are exempt from washing their hands before meals but must do so after meals, because the salt they used during the meal may harm their eyes if they touch them with salty hands (Eruvin 1:10). A sick person does not fast on the Day of Atonement but is fed at the word of experts, defined as physicians (Yoma 8:3). A person who is seized by a ravenous hunger (i.e., bulimy) may be given food on the Day of Atonement until his eyes are enlightened (ibid. 8:4). Bulimy is defined by Maimonides as a type of faintness produced by the sensation of hunger in the mouth of the stomach; when the patient eats, the faintness passes and the darkness disappears from his eyes. Water may be warmed on the Day of Atonement for a high priest who is old or whose body is cold (ibid. 3:5). Maimonides explains bodily coldness elsewhere (Berakhot 2:6).

---

4. For a detailed discussion of snakes and serpents in the Bible and Talmud, including the prohibition of drinking from uncovered water, see Rosner, *Medicine in the Bible and Talmud*, pp. 179–94.

**Nutrition**

Maimonides states that vegetables like cabbage and beets can be eaten cooked or raw (Berakhot 6:1). People drink brine to counteract the constipating effect of certain foods and fruits (ibid. 6:7). One knows that food has been digested when one again feels hungry for that food (ibid. 8:7). Food takes three days to be digested in the intestines of dogs (Oholot 11:7, Zavim 2:3). Meat cooked with turnips but not other vegetables imparts its taste to the turnips (Ḥullin 7:4), but nerves cooked with meat do not give any taste to the meat (ibid. 7:5).

According to Maimonides, Jews eat garlic on Fridays because it is an aphrodisiac (Nedarim 3:8, 4:8, 8:6). Fish and milk products and spiced eggs were withheld from the high priest on the eve of the Day of Atonement because these foods increase semen production or may stimulate an erection. The nutritional value of oats, eggs, cucumbers, and other cooked dishes is discussed (Nedarim 6:1 ff., 7:1–2), as is the relationship of the seasons of the year to the ripening of fruits and vegetables (ibid. 9:2–3). Yellow roots of the crocus plant are used by physicians to make compresses (Niddah 2: 5). Asphodel is a plant well known to physicians (Shevi'it 7:1). The Babylonians ate shewbread raw without baking it because they had strong stomachs (Menaḥot 11:7). *Anfakinon* is the oil which physicians squeeze out from unripe olives and has a bitter taste (ibid. 8:3); it is used as an ointment to remove hair and soften the skin.

Detailed discussions of dietetics and nutrition are found in Maimonides' other writings.

**Medical Instruments**

Among the medical instruments mentioned by Maimonides are a physician's drill used by surgeons to incise swollen wounds, i.e., abscesses (Oholot 2:3); a box in which physicians store their medications (Eduyyot 3:9); a large ladle used by physicians to remove solid and liquid medicines from jars (Kelim 17:12); a basket or box used by physicians to store their bandages (ibid. 12:3), the cover of which was used to prepare the bandages; and a bloodletter's lancet (ibid. 12:4).

## Conclusion

Maimonides' medical writings include extracts from Greek medical literature, a series of monographs on health in general and several diseases in particular, and a pharmacopoeia demonstrating extensive knowledge of Arabic medical literature. In addition, there are medical statements and discussions throughout his theological and rabbinic writings. The present chapter has extracted and systematically organized the statements and discussions pertaining to medicine in his *Commentary on the Mishnah*.

# ⸙ 22 ⸙

# The Physician's Prayer Attributed to Moses Maimonides

The Physician's Prayer attributed to Moses Maimonides is a lofty and beautiful prayer which first appeared in print in a German periodical in 1783.[1] The editor of this journal, Heinrich Christian Boie, and his associate, Christian Wilhelm Dohm, provided no notes or commentaries nor any indication as to who the author was. The prayer bears only the title, "Daily Prayer of a Physician Before He Visits His Patients: From the Hebrew Manuscript of a Renowned Jewish Physician in Egypt from the Twelfth Century." A photostatic reproduction of this earliest version of the prayer appeared in 1954 in a Hebrew medical journal.[2] Since the 1783 German edition, numerous versions, abbreviations, or excerpts of the prayer have been presented in English, German, Hebrew, French, Dutch, and Spanish. There are undoubtedly others besides those mentioned in this chapter. Much heated debate exists among the various writers concerning the true authorship of the prayer. This controversy will be presented chronologically, and an attempt

---

1. "Tägliches Gebet eines Arztes bevor er seine Kranken besucht—Aus der hebräischen Handschrift eines berühmten jüdischen Arztes in Egypten aus dem zwölften Jahrhundert," *Deustsches Museum* 1 (1783): 43–45.
2. J. O. Leibowitz, "The Physician's Prayer Ascribed to Maimonides," *Dappim Refu'iyyim* 13 (1954): 77–81.

will be made to arrive at a reasonable conclusion as to whether or not Moses Maimonides actually wrote the "Prayer of Maimonides."

The first Hebrew version of the prayer was published by Isaac Euchel, editor of the Hebrew periodical *Ha-Me'assef*, in 1790.[3] The title indicates that Marcus Herz was its author and that it was translated at his request from German into Hebrew. Half a century later, in 1841, the *Voice of Jacob*, a London newspaper, published the first English rendering from the Hebrew, under the title "Daily Prayer of a Physician."[4] The translator, using the pen name Medicus, states:

> The composition of this prayer has erroneously been attributed to Maimonides, but it is the production of the late Dr. Marcus Herz, a celebrated physician of Berlin. It was published by him in the German language, and the Hebrew version, which is to be found in the [Ha] maasef, owes its existence to the prolific pen of Itzig Eichel.

We next find the prayer, again in German, in a German–Jewish newspaper, the *Allgemeine Zeitung des Judenthums* for 1863.[5] The editor, Ludwig Philippson, makes no mention of authorship at all, but the title reads, "Daily Prayer of a Physician Before the Visits to His Patients: From the Hebrew Manuscript of a Celebrated Jewish Physician from the Twelfth Century." This title is nearly identical with that of the first German version, which appeared eighty years earlier. Philippson again reprinted the German version six years later in his voluminous book, *Weltbewegende Fragen in Politik und Religion aus den letzten dreissig Jahren.*[6] In 1892 yet another German version appeared in the *Allgemeine Zeitung des Judenthums*, this time by Julius Pagel, entitled "The Prayer of the Physician."[7]

In the last year of the nineteenth century, Rev. Madison C.

---

3. I. Euchel, "Prayer for the Physician as He Pours Out His Anxieties Before God Prior to Visiting the Sick: Composed by Sir Hofrat Professor Herz," *Ha-Me'assef* 6 (1790): 242–44.

4. "Daily Prayer of a Physician," *Voice of Jacob* 1, no. 7 (1814): 49–50.

5. L. Philippson, "Tägliches Gebet eines Arztes vor dem Besuch seiner Kranken (Aus der hebr. Handschrift eines berühmtem jüdischen Arztes aus dem zwölften Jahrhundert)," *Allgemeine Zeitung des Judenthums* 27, no. 4 (1863): 49–50.

6. L. Philippson, *Weltbewegende Fragen in Politik und Religion aus den letzten dreissig Jahren*, Zweiter Theil: Religion (Leipzig: Baumgärtner, 1869), pp. 159–60.

7. J. Pagel, "Das Gebet des Arztes," *Allgemeine Zeitung des Judenthums* 56, no. 25 (1892): 294–95.

Peters, pastor of the Bloomingdale Church in New York City, published a short English version of the prayer in his *Justice to the Jew.*[8] This English version, in which authorship is not mentioned at all, later initiated heated debates among Jewish scholars.

In the same year, Moïse Schwab, the celebrated bibliographer, published his *Répertoire*, in which he states that Marcus Herz authored the prayer published over a century earlier in *Ha-Me'assef.*[9] At the turn of the century, Golden published excerpts of the prayer in English in an American medical journal.[10] His article, entitled "Maimonides' Prayer for Physicians," states that Maimonides composed the prayer. A later letter addressed to the *American Israelite* is evidence that he extracted the prayer from Peters's book.

In 1902 the prayer appeared again in German under the title "Prayer of a Jewish Physician in the Twelfth Century."[11] The writer, Dr. Theodor Distel, specifically states that the prayer was published originally in 1783 in the *Deutsches Museum* and that its importance had prompted him to reprint it verbatim. Another quarter-century was to pass before the 1783 version was again mentioned in spite of the rather widespread interest in the prayer and its authorship, manifested by numerous articles on the subject during this period.

In 1902, the same year that Distel reprinted the original German version of the prayer, it was again copied in German in a Swiss newspaper, using Distel's title, "Prayer of a Jewish Physician in the Twelfth Century."[12] No commentary or discussion of authorship is to be found in this Swiss version. Rabbi Jules Wolff of La Chaux-de-Fonds, reading the prayer in the Swiss newspaper, was so

8. M. C. Peters, *Justice to the Jew: The Story of What He Has Done for the World* (London & New York: Neely, 1899), pp. 173–75.

9. M. Schwab, *Répertoire des articles relatifs à l'histoire et à la littérature juives parus dans les périodiques de 1783 à 1898* (Paris: Durlacher, 1899), p. 167.

10. W. W. Golden, "Maimonides' Prayer for Physicians," *Transactions of the Medical Society of West Virginia* 33 (1900): 414–15.

11. Th. Distel, "Gebet eines jüdischen Arztes im 12. Jahrhundert," *Deutsche medizinische Wochenschrift* 28, no. 32 (1902): 580.

12. "Gebet eines jüdischen Arztes im 12. Jahrhundert," *Cor.-Bl. f. Schweiz Aerzte* 32, no. 19 (1902): 611–13.

impressed that he promptly translated it into French. In a letter, dated February 26, 1903, to the editor of the periodical *L'Univers Israélite*, which was published the following day, Wolff provided the first, and excellent, French version of the prayer.[13] He states that it was a "prayer composed by a famous Jewish physician from Egypt in the twelfth century (Maimonides?)." Thus Wolff seemed to assume, perhaps with a little doubt, that Maimonides was the true author of the prayer; Moïse Schwab, however, was quick to reply three weeks later, in another letter to the editor of the same periodical, that the prayer could have been written by any Parisian physician.[14] He further stated that the prayer was definitely the work of Marcus Herz, friend and physician of Moses Mendelssohn, that Herz wrote it in German in Berlin, and that a Hebrew translation was published by Isaac Euchel in *Ha-Me'assef* in 1790.

Although later authors state that German versions of the prayer appeared in the February 4 and August 21, 1904 issues of the *Israelitisches Familienblatt*, this writer has been unable to locate copies of these journals in numerous libraries in the United States. I cannot, therefore, verify this for myself and must leave it in doubt, since numerous errors in bibliography have crept into various subsequent papers published on this subject.

In 1908 Dr. Gotthard Deutsch, professor of Jewish history and literature at the Hebrew Union College in Cincinnati, wrote a letter to the editor of the *American Israelite*, vehemently denouncing those who believed that Maimonides actually wrote the famous prayer.[15] The first part of his letter, tracing the prayer from 1790 to 1903, was reproduced in the miscellany section of the *Journal of the American Medical Association* in 1929.[16] The letter continues as follows:

13. J. Wolff, "Prière d'un médecin juif à l'usage de ses confrères," *Univers israélite* 58 (1903): 753–55.

14. M. Schwab, "La prière d'un médecin juif," *L'Univers Israélite* 58 (1903): 818–19.

15. G. Deutsch, "Maimonides' Prayer," *American Israelite*, March 19, 1908, p. 5, cols. 5–6.

16. "The 'Prayer of Maimonides' and Its True Author," *Journal of the American Medical Association* 92 (1929): 836.

God only knows into how many medical journals, textbooks of medicine, etc., this prayer found its way. The first source of the error is evidently Philippson. How he could commit this blunder is inconceivable to me. He could not have quoted from memory, for he gives a fairly accurate translation and he could not have translated from the original without seeing in his text that the prayer was written by Marcus Herz in German and translated into Hebrew by Euchel. Philippson, however, does not give Maimonides as the author, and I would like to know who was the author of this additional piece of historic information which I notice is stated by Wolff with a question mark. To me, this wandering hoax was a valuable piece of illustration of historic criticism.

Six years later, William W. Golden, superintendent of the Davis Memorial Hospital in Elkins, West Virginia, wrote a letter to the editor of the *American Israelite*. It was published in the June 25, 1914, issue as follows:

Sir: Reverend Madison C. Peters in one of the editions of his book "Justice to the Jew" quotes a prayer for physicians by Maimonides. Can you tell me where the original can be found, or at least in what authoritative work on history, literature or medicine can it be found, and oblige?

Yours very truly . . .

Golden, who in 1900 had published excerpts of the prayer, and in no uncertain terms had attributed authorship to Maimonides, as described earlier in this paper, now seems to have had second thoughts on the matter. The reply to his letter came from Dr. Gotthard Deutsch in the same June 25, 1914, issue of the *American Israelite* and was subsequently reprinted in chapter 6 ("The Maimonides Prayer Myth") of Deutsch's *Scrolls*.[17]

Deutsch's reply begins as follows: "This so-called prayer of Maimonides is an old hoax. It was actually written by Marcus Herz, a prominent physician of Berlin (1747–1803) who attended Moses Mendelssohn in his last illness." Deutsch thus reiterated all the arguments expounded in his earlier letter of 1908. He further stated that

Haeser embodied it in his "Geschichte der Medizin" 1, p. 837, Jena 1875. Having thus been recognized by a standard publication, it was accepted by Julius Pagel, professor of the history of medicine at the Berlin University

---

17. G. Deutsch, *Scrolls*, vol. 3, *Jew and Gentile: Essays on Jewish Apologetics and Kindred Historical Subjects* (Boston: Stratford Co., 1920), pp. 93–95.

(1851–1912), also a Jew, in his essay on Maimonides as physician, which forms part of the memorial volume "Moses Ben Maimon," edited by the Gesellschaft zur Foerderung der Wissenschaft des Judentums, I, p. 244, Leipzic, 1908. Following all this, its authenticity could no more be doubted than the authenticity of the gospel of St. John. The Israelite (March 12, 1908) gave it its seal of approval, although I contested it in the subsequent issue, but repeatedly since it has been proclaimed as being written in distinctly Maimonidean spirit. Recently I wrote a letter to the editor of "Ost und West," who had published it as Maimonidean. He thanked me, but preferred not to publish it. As the very popular "Medizinische Wochenschrift" of Berlin published it in 1902, and any number of medical journals reprinted it, no amount of argument will rob Maimonides of the credit for having written this typically sweet-lemonade prayer, characteristic of the rationalistic tendencies of the era of "Aufklaerung," and I still have hopes that one hundred years hence, somebody will credit Herodotus or at least Rabbi Jose Ben Halafta, the genuine author of Seder Olam, with my "Foreign Notes."

It seems quite evident that Deutsch was unaware of the 1783 edition of the prayer, and thus attributed the authorship of the prayer to Marcus Herz, whose version did not appear until 1790. This ignorance of the 1783 edition of the prayer must have been shared by Schwab and numerous later writers who also ascribed the prayer to Marcus Herz in spite of the specific mention by Distel in 1902 of the existence of the 1783 edition antedating Herz by seven years.

Thus, Deutsch's criticism of Philippson seems unfounded. Philippson was probably aware of the *Deutsches Museum* edition of 1783, and in his own 1863 and 1869 versions of the prayer, he used the same title as in the 1783 original, namely "Daily Prayer of a Physician Before He Visits His Patients: From a Hebrew Manuscript of a Renowned Jewish Physician of the Twelfth Century." Deutsch further perpetuated the misconception, later quoted by Friedenwald,[18] that the prayer was embodied in Haeser's textbook on the history of medicine.[19] In actuality, there is only a brief footnote in Haeser's text, which, translated from the German, states: "Compare the beautiful morning prayer of a Jewish physician from

---

18. H. Friedenwald, *The Jews and Medicine* (Baltimore: Johns Hopkins Press, 1944), vol. 1, pp. 28–30.

19. H. Haeser, *Lehrbuch der Geschichte der Medicin und der epidemischen Krankheiten*, 3rd ed. (Jena: Dufft, 1875), vol. 1, p. 837.

the twelfth century in L. Philippson's Weltbewegende Fragen." No mention is made of the prayer in Haeser's discussion of Maimonides in the same work.[20] Nor is there any mention of the prayer in the two earlier editions of Haeser's textbook in 1845 and 1859 respectively. This indicates that Haeser, too, was unaware of the 1783 edition and first saw the prayer printed in Philippson's paper in 1863.

Seeligmann in Holland wrote in 1928, in response to an inquiry regarding a Hebrew version of Maimonides' prayer, that he remembered that it was probably not composed by Maimonides.[21] He then states that Marcus Herz wrote it and traces its history from *Ha-Me'assef* in 1790 through Philippson and Haeser. Seeligmann further writes that the first Dutch version was by Hektor Treub and was published by Dr. M. J. Premsela.[22]

Emil Bogen, in response to the reprinting of part of one of Gotthard Deutsch's letters in the *Journal of the American Medical Association*, correctly pointed out the existence of the 1783 version, which was not known to Deutsch.[23] Bogen agreed with Kroner, who showed the harmony between the other writings of Maimonides and the so-called Prayer of Maimonides in both form and spirit.[24]

Bennigson and his colleagues reprinted the German version in Leipzig in 1931;[25] they briefly trace the history of the prayer from its origin in the *Deutsches Museum*, erroneously stating that it was reprinted in German by Distel in the *Deutsche Medizinische Wochenschrift* in August 1904, when they probably mean 1902. This error was perpetuated by Kagan and Muntner, probably neither of

---

20. Ibid., pp. 595–97.

21. S. Seeligmann, "Morgengebed van den arts naar Maimonides," *Vrijdagavond* 5, no. 1 (1928): 404–6.

22. M. J. Premsela, *Medische Fastoensleer* (Amsterdam, 1903), pp. 52–53.

23. E. Bogen, "The Daily Prayer of a Physician," *Journal of the American Medical Association* 92 (1929): 2128.

24. H. Kroner, "Arzt und Patient in der Medizin des Maimonides," *Ost und West* 12 (1912): 745–50.

25. W. Bennigson et al., *Des Moses Maimonides Morgengebet bevor er seine Kranken besuchte* (Leipzig, 1931), p. 6.

whom had access to the periodical in question.[26] Another, probably typographical, error in Bennigson's paper is the June 1893 date given for Pagel's version of the prayer, an error again perpetuated by Kagan. The correct date is June 1892.

Keller, in 1931, in an essay entitled "The Ideal Practice of Medicine from the Rabbinical Point of View," compared the Prayer of Maimonides to the Hippocratic Oath and quoted excerpts from both.[27] Maimonides, he said, considered the patient important because he is the creation of the Almighty, so that the responsibility for the outcome of our treatment rests partly with us as an instrument of the Almighty. Hippocrates, on the other hand, considered the preciousness of a human being from the sociological viewpoint.

To commemorate the eight-hundredth anniversary of the birth of Maimonides, in 1935, numerous publications on all aspects of Maimonides appeared in various periodicals, newspapers, journals, and books around the world. Among these were several references to the prayer. Gershenfeld provided excerpts of the English version.[28] Illevitz and Meyerhof emphatically stated that Maimonides did not write the prayer.[29] A Spanish version of the prayer appeared in 1935.[30] The author, E. Singer, stated that it had previously been published in the *Allgemeine Zeitung des Judenthums* in 1863, in *Sulamit* in 1842, in *Abend Zeitung* in 1840, and in the *Medizinischer Almanach*.

---

26. S. R. Kagan, "Maimonides' Prayer," *Annals of Medical History* 10 (1938): 329–32; S. Muntner, *The Deutero Prayer of Moses: With an Introduction About the History of the Prayer, Attributed to the Physician Maimonides and a Contemplation on the State of the Praying and on the Valour of the Prayer in General* (Jerusalem: Geniza, 1946), p. 57.

27. H. Keller, "Comparison Between Hippocratic Oath and Maimonides' Prayer in the Ideal Practice of Medicine from the Rabbinical Point of View," in *Modern Hebrew Orthopedic Terminology and Jewish Medical Essays* (Boston: Stratford Co., 1931), pp. 142–46.

28. L. Gershenfeld, "The Medical Works of Maimonides and His Treatise on Personal Hygiene and Dietetics," *American Journal of Pharmacology* 107 (1935): 14–28. Two other English versions, one published two years before Gershenfeld's, and the other two years later, are: D. Roman, "Maimonides' Prayer," *Hanhneman. Monthly* 67 (1932): 244–50; [anon.] "Physician's Prayer by Maimonides," *Medical Leaves* 1 (1937): 9.

29. A. B. Illevitz, "Maimonides the Physician," *Canadian Medical Association Journal* 32 (1935): 440–42; M. Meyerhof, "The Medical Work of Maimonides," in *Essays on Maimonides: An Octocentennial Volume*, ed. S. W. Baron (New York: Columbia University Press, 1941), pp. 265–99.

30. E. Singer, "Maimonides, Medico," *Semana méd.* 2 (1930): 1960–65.

An interesting inquiry by Sir William Osler concerning the authorship of the prayer was answered by the Chief Rabbi of the British Empire, Dr. Joseph H. Hertz, in a letter dated May 23, 1917, but published in the *Canadian Jewish Chronicle* in 1935.[31] The letter reads as follows:

Dear Sir William:

Some 2 years ago you inquired of me as to the "Physician's Prayer" attributed to Maimonides. I can now give you the following information on the subject:

This prayer is the production of Dr. Markus Herz (1747–1802), a friend and pupil of Immanuel Kant and of Moses Mendelssohn. He was a physician to the Jewish Hospital in Berlin. The prayer was composed by him in the German language and was published in a Hebrew translation in the Periodical Ha-Meassef. The current English version seems to be from this Hebrew translation and first appeared in the London paper "Voice of Jacob" on the 24th December, 1841.

Sincerely yours,
J. H. Hertz.

Also published in 1935, the English translation of Münz's book on Maimonides ascribed the prayer to the great medieval physician, although he had questioned the authorship in the earlier German edition of his book.[32]

In 1938, as mentioned earlier, Kagan reprinted excerpts of the English version of the prayer and traced its history. He based his article mainly on two previous papers, those of Bogen and Bennigson et al., as evidenced by his incorporation of the bibliographical errors in Bennigson's article into his own paper. Kagan concluded with six arguments favoring Maimonides as the true author of the prayer. These arguments can be summarized as follows:

1. The medieval form and style of the prayer conform with Maimonides' other writings.

2. If Marcus Herz was the author, he would have laid claim to its authorship.

---

31. J. H. Hertz, letter to Sir William Osler, *Canadian Jewish Chronicle* 22 (April 12, 1935): 7.

32. I. Münz, *Maimonides (the Rambam): The Story of His Life and Genius*, trans. and ed. H. T. Schnittkind (Boston: Winchell-Thomas, 1935), p. 191; idem, *Moses ben Maimon (Maimonides): Sein Leben und seine Werke* (Frankfurt a.M.: Kauffmann, 1912), pp. 267–68.

3. Dr. Herz, a master of the German language, would have published the original prayer in German and would only later have arranged for a Hebrew translation.

4. If the later German version omitted Herz's name at his request, he would not have requested Euchel, editor of *Ha-Me'assef*, to mention his name in the Hebrew translation.

5. Herz probably knew of the 1783 German version and sent the document for Hebrew translation to Euchel, who erroneously ascribed the German text to Herz. Herz did not know Hebrew, since he did not translate it himself and probably was unaware of the Hebrew editor's note making him the author.

6. All the professional ethics expressed in the prayer are also expressed in some of Maimonides' letters and books.

In 1939 Levinson reprinted the prayer in English as part of a larger review of Maimonides' medical contributions.[33] In 1944, in his two-volume classic, *The Jews and Medicine*, Friedenwald also reprinted the prayer in English.[34]

In 1946, in his *Deutero Prayer of Moses*, mentioned earlier, Muntner published a most interesting discussion comparing the Prayer of Maimonides to the Oath of Asaph[35] and the physician's prayer of Jacob Zahalon.[36] In addition to publishing both Hebrew and German versions, Muntner provided a brief bibliographical sketch tracing the background of the prayer, a sketch which he had found in a 1928 Berlin version of the prayer by Professor Heinrich Levy. Muntner notes that the August 1904 date quoted for Distel's version in the *Deutsche Medizinische Wochenschrift* is incorrect and should properly be August 1902. He also calls attention to the existence of a Hebrew manuscript in the Bibliothèque Nationale de Paris which is entitled "The Prayer of Moses Maimonides." It is Hebrew manuscript no. 873, pt. 7, fol. 98V°, described in the cata-

---

33. A. Levinson, "Maimonides, the Physician," *Medical Leaves* 2 (1939): 96–105.

34. Friedenwald, *Jews and Medicine*, vol. 1, pp. 28–30.

35. F. Rosner and S. Muntner, "The Oath of Asaph," *Annals of Internal Medicine* 63 (1965): 317–20.

36. H. Savitz, "Jacob Zahalon and His Book, *The Treasure of Life*," *New England Journal of Medicine* 213 (1935): 167–76; I. Simon, "La prière des médecins, 'Tephilat Harofim,' de Jacob Zahalon, médecin et rabbin en Italie (1630–1693)," *Revue d'histoire de la médecine hébraïque*, no. 8 (1955): 38–51; Friedenwald, *Jews and Medicine*, pp. 268–79.

logue as follows: "Prayer of Rabbi Moses Maimonides, beginning with *Tefila Lisegulas Eeshim* and terminating by the piece of verse *Galgal Soveiv*."[37] The great bibliographer Moritz Steinschneider described an identical Hebrew work as manuscript Warner no. 41, pt. 11, fol. 150, and referred to the Paris Hebrew manuscript as no. 285 (perhaps an error or perhaps an earlier, different numbering system).[38] In addition, this medieval Hebrew manuscript version of the Prayer of Maimonides was published in 1867 in the weekly Hebrew newspaper *Ha-Karmel*.[39]

Muntner correctly points out that this manuscript version of the prayer was a forgery and could not possibly have been written by Maimonides, since the numerous references to astrology are not in keeping with Maimonides' vehement opposition to the "pseudo-science" of astrology.[40]

Muntner further claimed that the versions of the prayer, beginning with the 1783 German edition, although written in the spirit and form of Maimonides, and omitting any reference to astrology, were also forgeries and can all be traced back to Marcus Herz.

Probably the most comprehensive review of the subject to date is the one published in Hebrew by Leibowitz in 1954.[41] A photocopy of the 1783 original German version is presented, as well as the first page of the 1790 Hebrew version. Leibowitz must have consulted the original sources, since the bibliographical errors described above, first made by Bennigson et al. and later perpetuated by Kagan and others, are absent from his paper. A new Hebrew translation, made directly from the 1783 German version, is also provided in this article.

---

37. *Catalogues des manuscripts hébreux et samaritains de la Bibliothèque impériale* (Paris, 1866), p. 142.

38. M. Steinschneider, *Catalogus codicum hebraeorum Bibliothecae academiae Lugduno Batavae* ([Leiden:] E. J. Brill, 1858), p. 188.

39. R. Meshash, "The Prayer of Rabbi Moses Attributed to Rabbi Moses ben Maimon (Maimonides)," *Ha-Karmel* 6 (1867): 350.

40. Muntner, *Deutero Prayer of Moses*, p. 57; see also A. Marx, "The Correspondence Between the Rabbis of Southern France and Maimonides About Astrology," *Hebrew Union College Annual* 3 (1926): 311–58.

41. See above, n. 2.

A second French edition of the prayer appeared in 1956,[42] and a short English version was reprinted in 1957.[43] A brief version of "The Oath and Prayer of Maimonides" was published in the *Journal of the American Medical Association* in 1955, in which Maimonides was falsely called an Islamic philosopher, an error that was corrected by Lanzkron and Berner in two separate letters to the editor.[44]

The most recent version of the prayer that I have been able to find is a 1962 French one.[45] According to the author, Dr. J. Pines, only parts of the prayer were translated into French from the Paris Hebrew manuscript no. 837 described above.

I have been fortunate in being able to obtain copies of every reference enumerated in the notes to this chapter. There are undoubtedly other versions, editions, and printings of the prayer in numerous languages in various newspapers, periodicals, and books throughout the world. The popularity of the prayer is attested to by its frequent quotation and publication. Whether Maimonides actually wrote the prayer or not remains an open question. Certainly most of those who are of the opinion that Maimonides did not write it, including Illevitz, Meyerhof, Simon, Hertz, Seeligmann, and others, base their remarks on the statements of Deutsch and Schwab, although "Medicus" had already attributed authorship of the prayer to Marcus Herz in 1841. As has been pointed out, both Deutsch and Schwab were probably unaware of the 1783 German version of the prayer, which antedated Herz by seven years, and thus they perpetuated the concept that Marcus Herz composed the prayer. This thesis may or may not be valid.

Other writers, such as Bogen, Kagan, and perhaps Wolff, agree

---

42. I. Simon, "L'oeuvre médicale de Maïmonide," *Revue d'histoire de la médicine hébraïque* 31 (1956): 107–20.

43. J. S. Minkin, *The World of Moses Maimonides, with Selections from His Writings* (New York: Yoseloff, 1957), pp. 149–50.

44. "The Oath and Prayer of Maimonides," *Journal of the American Medical Association* 157 (1955): 1158; J. Lanzkron and H. Berner, "Maimonides: Physician, Astronomer, Philosopher, Talmudist," ibid., p. 1637.

45. J. Pines, "La contribution juive à la médecine arabe au moyen âge," *Scalpel* (Brussels) 115 (1962): 207–18.

with Kroner that the prayer was probably truly composed by Maimonides, since it conforms completely with the ideals, medical ethics, and spirit of Maimonides; they believe that the original will yet be found. Pagel also supports this viewpoint.[46] Certainly, at this point in history, this suggestion is no more than wishful thinking. However, it is conceivable that Marcus Herz saw an original manuscript in Hebrew; he may have based his version, in which he does not claim authorship, on such an original. This proposal seems unlikely. Alternatively, Herz may have seen the 1783 German version and asked his friend Isaac Euchel to translate it into Hebrew. The latter may have erroneously ascribed the German to Herz, as Kagan postulates. This theory, too, seems unlikely. It is also possible that neither Maimonides nor Herz wrote the prayer, but that a twelfth-century astrologer wrote it in what became the Paris Hebrew manuscript, from which was extracted an abbreviated German version. A further possibility is that Maimonides did indeed write the prayer, but that an astrologer amended it and only the amended versions are extant today. These two latter possibilities are extremely remote.

It seems clear that the manuscript version of the prayer in Paris and Oxford, mentioned above, is a forgery and was not written by Maimonides. This was proved by Muntner, who states that the numerous references to astrology in this work make it impossible to ascribe authorship to Maimonides, who was vehemently opposed to this "pseudoscience."

The question remains whether the 1783 *Deutsches Museum* edition of the prayer, upon which many versions in numerous languages are based, was truly written by Maimonides or not. As already mentioned, Kroner, Pagel, Wolff, Bogen, and Kagan support the former view, whereas Leibowitz, Muntner, Schwab, Deutsch, Illevitz, Meyerhof, Seeligmann, "Medicus," and Hertz believe the prayer to be spurious.

The most potent arguments favoring the rejection of Mai-

---

46. J. Pagel, *Maimuni als medizinischer Schriftsteller* (Frankfurt a.M.: Kauffmann, 1908), p. 17.

monides as author come from Professor Leibowitz, who states that no prominent medical historian supports the view of Maimonides' authorship. Furthermore, in Euchel's Hebrew version of 1790, it is specifically stated that the prayer was composed by Marcus Herz and translated from German into Hebrew at his request. The confusion arose from the discovery of an earlier German edition bearing the unfortunate title ". . . From the Hebrew Manuscript of a Renowned Jewish Physician in Egypt from the Twelfth Century." This title leads logically to the supposition that Maimonides was the renowned physician referred to. However, if one carefully reads the text of 1783, one notes that, contrary to what Kagan states, style, phrasing, and concepts are not compatible with a medieval dating. A phrase such as "art is great, but the mind of man is ever expanding" is typical and characteristic of eighteenth-century Europe and is at variance with Maimonidean medieval thought. Here, according to Leibowitz, is the idea of progress, which became even more popular in the nineteenth century.[47]

Further evidence for an eighteenth-century author lies in the phrase "that act unceasingly and harmoniously to preserve the whole in all its beauty." This concept of "beauty," or *das Schöne*, is characteristic of German literature of the Enlightenment. Moreover, a phrase such as "ten thousand times ten thousand organs hast Thou combined" presupposes knowledge of the newer sciences of anatomy, biology, and microscopy. The tensions between colleagues discussed in the prayer are also products of a more modern period and dictated by the new academic hierarchy.

Leibowitz further writes:

> Markus Herz probably wrote the Prayer as a contribution to medical ethics and as a comment on prevailing low standards of the practice. It was usual to insert in almanachs anonymous short contributions. Markus Herz was a warm Jew, proud of the history of his people; he clad his literary piece into the colorful frame indicated in the caption, probably indeed meaning Maimonides, but not based on a manuscript, which did not exist, but as belonging to the belles-lettres. Editions of Hebrew medical manuscripts began only in 1867 (Steinschneider's Donnolo).[48]

---

47. J. O. Leibowitz, personal communication.
48. Ibid.

One of the greatest authorities on the medical writings of Maimonides was Suessman Muntner. His book on the subject of Maimonides' prayer has already been mentioned in this chapter. Muntner also strongly believed that Marcus Herz composed this prayer in beautiful German and that a very poor translation into Hebrew was produced by Euchel.[49] Furthermore, an anonymous or unknown writer added the confusing caption to this earliest (1790) Hebrew version. Muntner further states that Herz based his version of the prayer on the earlier Prayer of Jacob Zahalon, written in the seventeenth century, and was greatly influenced and stimulated by it.

From all the foregoing discussion, the evidence overwhelmingly favors the concept that the physician's prayer attributed to Maimonides is a spurious work, not written by Maimonides but composed by an eighteenth-century writer, probably Marcus Herz. Absolute proof that this is so, however, is lacking and may never be discovered.

In a comparative and historical study of the Jewish religious attitude to medicine and its practice published in 1959, Dr. Immanuel Jakobovits, Chief Rabbi of the British Commonwealth, emphasized the ethical and moral responsibilities of the physician as a divine agent in the alleviation of human suffering.[50] Deeply pious and moving prayers of gratitude for divine help, such as those of Asaph, Judah Halevi,[51] Jacob Zahalon, and Abraham Zacutus,[52] as well as the Physician's Prayer attributed to Maimonides, says Jakobovits, all recognize God as the ultimate healer of disease, while also asserting "the indispensable part played by the physician, his art and his medicines" in the preservation of health.

The Physician's Prayer attributed to Maimonides contains moral and ethical standards by which physicians should conduct their professional lives. The daily recitation of this prayer serves to remind physicians of the standards that have been set up for them and that they should attempt to live up to. Physicians should constantly be

---

49. S. Muntner, personal communication.
50. I. Jakobovits, *Jewish Medical Ethics* (New York: Bloch, 1959), pp. 15–18.
51. Friedenwald, *Jews and Medicine*, vol. 1, p. 27.
52. Friedenwald, *Jews and Medicine*, vol. 2, pp. 295–321.

motivated by the highest code of medical philanthropy and professional ethics. The medical profession's noble philosophy and high aspirations are embodied in the Physician's Prayer.

There follows below Dr. Harry Friedenwald's English version of the Prayer, reprinted from his "Daily Prayer of a Physician," *Bulletin of the Johns Hopkins Hospital* 28 (1917): 256–61, with kind permission from the editors and publishers.

## Daily Prayer of a Physician

Almighty God, Thou hast created the human body with infinite wisdom. Ten thousand times ten thousand organs hast Thou combined in it that act unceasingly and harmoniously to preserve the whole in all its beauty—the body which is the envelope of the immortal soul. They are ever acting in perfect order, agreement and accord. Yet, when the frailty of matter or the unbridling of passions deranges this order or interrupts this accord, then forces clash and the body crumbles into the primal dust from which it came. Thou sendest to man diseases as beneficent messengers to foretell approaching danger and to urge him to avert it.

Thou hast blest Thine earth, Thy rivers and Thy mountains with healing substances; they enable Thy creatures to alleviate their sufferings and to heal their illnesses. Thou hast endowed man with the wisdom to relieve the suffering of his brother, to recognize his disorders, to extract the healing substances, to discover their powers and to prepare and to apply them to suit every ill. In Thine Eternal Providence Thou hast chosen me to watch over the life and health of Thy creatures. I am now about to apply myself to the duties of my profession. Support me, Almighty God, in these great labors that they may benefit mankind, for without Thy help not even the least thing will succeed.

Inspire me with love for my art and for Thy creatures. Do not allow thirst for profit, ambition for renown and admiration, to interfere with my profession, for these are the enemies of truth and of love for mankind and they can lead astray in the great task of attending to the welfare of Thy creatures. Preserve the strength of my body and of my soul that they ever be ready to cheerfully help and support rich and poor, good and bad, enemy as well as friend. In the sufferer let me see only the human being. Illumine my mind that it recognize what presents itself and that it may comprehend what is absent or hidden. Let it not fail to see what is visible, but do not permit it to arrogate to itself the power to see what cannot be seen, for delicate and indefinite are the bounds of the great art of caring for the lives and health of Thy creatures. Let me never be absent-minded. May no strange thoughts divert my attention at the bedside of the sick, or disturb my mind in its silent labors, for great and sacred are the thoughtful deliberations required to preserve the lives and health of Thy creatures.

Grant that my patients have confidence in me and my art and follow my directions and my counsel. Remove from their midst all charlatans and the whole host of officious relatives and know-all nurses, cruel people who arrogantly frustrate the wisest purposes of our art and often lead Thy creatures to their death.

Should those who are wiser than I wish to improve and instruct me, let my soul gratefully follow their guidance; for vast is the extent of our art. Should conceited fools, however, censure me, then let love for my profession steer me against them, so that I remain steadfast without regard for age, for reputation, or for honor, because surrender would bring to Thy creatures sickness and death.

Imbue my soul with gentleness and calmness when older colleagues, proud of their age, wish to displace me or to scorn me or disdainfully to teach me. May even this be of advantage to me, for they know many things of which I am ignorant, but let not their arrogance give me pain. For they are old and old age is not master of the passions. I also hope to attain old age upon this earth, before Thee, Almighty God!

Let me be contented in everything except in the great science of my profession. Never allow the thought to arise in me that I have attained to sufficient knowledge, but vouchsafe to me the strength, the leisure and the ambition ever to extend my knowledge. For art is great, but the mind of man is ever expanding.

Almighty God! Thou hast chosen me in Thy mercy to watch over the life and death of Thy creatures. I now apply myself to my profession. Support me in this great task so that it may benefit mankind, for without Thy help not even the least thing will succeed.

# Bibliography

Aharoni, J. "Maimonides the Zoologist." *Harefuah* 10 (1936): 105.

Asbell, M. B. "A Review of Hebraic Dentistry from Earliest Times Through the Middle Ages." *Medical Leaves* 5 (1943): 31–42.

———. "Vignettes in Dental History: Moses Maimonides (1135–1204)." *Alpha Omegan* 40 (1946): 4–8.

Bar Sela, A., and H. E. Hoff. "Maimonides' Interpretation of the First Aphorism of Hippocrates." *Bulletin of the History of Medicine* 37 (1968): 347–54.

Bar Sela, A., H. E. Hoff, and E. Faris. *Moses Maimonides' Two Treatises on the Regimen of Health.* Philadelphia: American Philosophical Society (*Transactions*, n.s. vol. 54), 1964.

Barzel, U. "The Art of Cure: A Non-Published Medical Book by Maimonides." *Harofe Haivri* 2 (1955) 82–83 (Heb.) and 165–77 (Eng.).

———. *Moses Maimonides' The Art of Cure: Extracts from Galen.* Haifa: Maimonides Research Institute, 1992.

Blau, J. R. *Moses ben Maimon Responsa.* 3 vols. Jerusalem: Mekizei Nirdamin, 1958–61.

Bloch, S. "Mikhtav ha-Rav Rabbenu Moshe ben Maimon be'ad ha-Sultan." *Kerem Ḥemed* 3 (1838): 31–39.

Bragman, L. J. "Maimonides on Physical Hygiene." *Annals of Medical History* 7 (1925): 140–43.

————. "Maimonides' Treatise on Hemorrhoids." *New York State Medical Journal* 27 (1927): 598–601.

————. "Maimonides' Treatise on Poisons." *Medical Journal and Record* 124 (1926): 103–7.

Brockelman, C. *Geschichte der Arabischen Literatur*. Leiden: E. J. Brill, 1943.

Butterworth, C. E. "On the Management of Health." In *Ethical Writings of Maimonides*, ed. R. L. Weiss and C. E. Butterworth, pp. 105–111. New York: New York University Press, 1975.

Caroline, N. L., and H. Schwartz. "Chicken Soup Rebound and Relapse of Pneumonia: Report of a Case." *Chest* 67 (1975): 215–16.

Castiglioni, A. *A History of Medicine*. New York: Knopf, 1941.

Chavel, C. B. *The Book of Divine Commandments (The Sefer Ha-Mitzvoth of Moses Maimonides)*. London: Soncino Press, 1940.

Chelminski, E. "La preservación de la juventud de Maimonides, versión Castellana." *Anales de ars medici* (Mexico) 5 (1961): 303–44.

————. "Notas introductorias al *Guia sobre el contacto sexual* de Maimonides." *Anales de ars medici* (Mexico) 5(4) (1961): 240–48.

Dienstag, J. I. Review of S. Muntner, *Moshe ben Maimon: Sefer ha-Katzeret*. *Jewish Social Studies* 28 (1966): 38–39.

————. "Translators and Editors of Maimonides' Medical Works: A Bio-Bibliographical Survey." In *Memorial Volume in Honor of S. Muntner*, ed. J. O. Leibowitz, pp. 95–135. Jerusalem: Israel Institute for the History of Medicine, 1983.

DeMartini, U. *Maimonides, Segreto dei segreti*. Rome: Istituto di storia della Medicina dell'Università de Roma, 1960.

DiCyan, E. "Treatise on Poisons and Their Antidotes by Moses Maimonides." *Archives of Internal Medicine* 119 (1967): 431.

Ebstein, W. *Die Medizin im Neuen Testament und im Talmud*. Munich: Werner Fritzch, 1965.

Efros, I. *Maimonides' Treatise on Logic (Makalah Fi-Sin at Al-Mantik)*. New York: American Academy of Jewish Research, 1938.

Ehrlich, D. "Neonatal Purpura in the Talmud." *Harefuah* 76 (1969): 1 ff.

Etziony, M. "Apropos of Maimonides' Aphorisms." *Bulletin of the History of Medicine* 35 (1961): 1163–68.

Feldman, D. M. *Marital Relations, Birth Control and Abortion in Jewish Law.* New York: Schocken, 1974.

Finkel, J. *Maimonides' Treatise on Resurrection (Maqala Fi Tehiyyat ha-Metim).* New York: American Academy of Jewish Research, 1939.

Freiman, H. *Moses ben Maimon Responsa.* Jerusalem: Mekize Nir-damin, 1934.

Friedenwald, H. *Jewish Luminaries in Medical History and a Catalogue of Works Bearing on the Subject of the Jews and Medicine from the Private Library of Harry Friedenwald.* Baltimore: Johns Hopkins Press, 1946.

Gordon, H. L. *Moses ben Maimon: The Preservation of Youth; Essays on Health (Fi Tadbir as-Sihha).* New York: Philosophical Library, 1958.

Gorlin, M. *Maimonides' On Sexual Intercourse (Fi'l-Jima).* Brooklyn: Rambash, 1961.

Hasida (Bocian), M. Z. "Perush le-Pirkei Abukrat shel ha-Rambam." *Ha-Segullah* (Jerusalem), nos. 1–30 (1934–35).

Heilperin, L. "Perush Pirkei Abukrat le-Rabbi Moshe ben Maimon." *Harefuah* 9 (1935): 162–68.

Herscovici, H. "Le traitement des morsures venimeuses d'après Maïmonide." *Practicien du Nord de l'Afrique* 11 (1938): 505.

Hyamson, M. *Mishneh Torah: The Book of Knowledge by Maimonides.* Jerusalem: Boys' Town Publishers, 1962.

Jakobovits, I. *Jewish Medical Ethics.* New York: Bloch, 1975.

———. "Jewish Views on Abortion." In *Jewish Bioethics,* ed. F. Rosner and J. D. Bleich, pp. 118–33. New York: Sanhedrin Press, 1979.

Kapach, D. *Mishneh with the Commentary of Rabbi Moses ben Maimon.* 6 vols. Jerusalem: Mosad Harav Kook, 1962–68.

Kahle, P. "Moses Maimonides Aphorismorum Praefatio et Excerpta." In *Galeni in Platonis tinalum commentarii fragmenta,* ed. H. O. Schroeder. Leipzig: Thebner, 1934.

Katzenelson, Il. *Ha-Talmud ve-Ḥokhmat ha-Refuah*. Berlin: Chaim, 1928.

Kaufmann, D. "Ein Responsum des Gaons R. Haja über Gottes Vorherwissen und die Dauer des menschlichen Lebens (Agal)." *Zeitschrift für Deutsche Morgenlandische Gesellschaft* 49 (1895): 73–84.

Khalifah, E. S. "Dentistry in the Twelfth Century as Revealed in the Medical Writings of Maimonides." *British Dental Journal* 67 (1939): 133–39.

Kook, H. "Genitourinary Items in the Writings of Maimonides." *Korot* 6, nos. 3–4 (February 1973): 216–21.

––––––. "Genito-Urological Items in the Scripts of Rambam." *Korot* 4, nos. 5–7 (December 1967): 448–51.

––––––. "Maimonides as Seen by a Modern Urologist." *International Surgery* 61 (August 1976): 390–92.

––––––. "Maimonides the Physician as Seen by a Modern Urologist." *Korot* 6, nos. 7–8 (June 1974): 489–96.

Krauss, S. *Talmudische Archaeologie*. Leipzig, 1910.

Kroner, H. "Der medizinische Schwanengesang des Maimonides." *Janus* 32 (1928): 12–116.

––––––. "Die Haemorrhoiden in der Medizin des XII und XIII Jahrhunderts." *Janus* 16 (1911): 441–565, 644–718.

––––––. *Die Seelenhygiene des Maimonides, Auszug aus der 3 Kapital des diatetischen Sendschreibens des Maimonides an den Sultan al Malik Alafdahl (ca. 1198)*. Frankfurt a.M.: J. Kauffmann, 1914.

––––––. *Ein Beitrag zur Geschichte der Medizin des XII Jahrhunderts an der Hand Zweier Medizinischer Abhandlungen des Maimonides auf Grund von 6 unedierten Handschriften*. Oberdorf-Bopfingen: Itzowski, 1906.

––––––. "Eine Medizinische Maimonides Handschrift aus Granada. Ein Beitrag zur Stilistik des Maimonides und Charakteristik der Hebräischen Ueberzetzungsliteratur." *Janus* 21 (1916): 203–47.

––––––. "*Fi tadbir as sikhat*. Gesundheitsanleitung des Maimonides für den Sultan al-Malik al-Afdhal." *Janus* 27 (1923): 101–16, 286–330; 28 (1924): 61–74, 143–52, 199–217, 408–19, 455–72; 29 (1925): 235–58.

Lanzkowsky, P. "Twin-to-Twin Transfusion." *Pediatrics* 64 (September 1979): 309.

Leibowitz, J. O. "Harveian Items in Hebrew Medicine." *Harofe Haivri* 2 (1957): 74–79 (Heb.), 134–38 (Eng.).

———. *The History of Coronary Heart Disease.* Berkeley: University of California Press, 1970.

———. "The Latin Translations of Maimonides' Aphorisms." *Korot* 6 (1973): 273–81 (Heb.), xciii–xciv (Eng. summary).

———. "Maimonides' Aphorisms." *Korot* 1 (1955): 213–19 (Heb.), i–iii (Eng. summary).

———. "Moses ben Maimon. *Uber die Lebensdauer*, ein unediertes Responsum herausgegeben, übersetzt und erklärt von Gotthold Weil." *Kiryat Sefer* 29 (1954): 67.

——— and S. Marcus. *Moses Maimonides on the Causes of Symptoms.* Berkeley: University of California Press, 1974.

———. "The Physician's Prayer Ascribed to Maimonides." *Dappim Refu'iyyim* 13 (1954): 77–81.

Levy, A. J. "He'arot le-Sefer ha-Katzeret le-ha-Rambam" [Comments on the treatise on asthma by Maimonides]. *Harofe Haivri* 2 (1940): 129–32.

Lieber, E. "A Medieval Hebrew Presage of the Circulation of the Blood, Based on Biblical and Talmudic Concepts." *Korot* 9, nos. 1–2 (1985): 157–63.

Magid, Z., ed. *Pirkei Moshe* [Medical aphorisms of Maimonides]. Lemberg, 1834. Vilna: L. Matz, 1888.

Margalith, D. "The First Anticipations of the Idea of Circulation in Ancient Jewish Sources." *Harofe Haivri* 2 (1957): 79–88 (Heb.), 130–34 (Eng.).

Meyerhof, M. "Sur un glossaire de matière médicale arabe composé par Maïmonide." *Bull. Inst. Egypte* 17 (1935): 223–35.

———. "Sur un ouvrage médicale inconnu de Maïmonide." *Mélanges Maspéro* 3 (1935–40): 1–7.

———. "The Medical Work of Maimonides." In *Essays on Maimonides: Octocentennial Volume*, edited by S. W. Baron, pp. 265–99. New York: Columbia University Press, 1941.

———. *Un Glossaire de matière médicale, composé par Maïmonide (Sarh Asma al'Uqqar).* Cairo: Mém. d'Inst. d'Egypte, 1940.

Mildner, T. "Eine gewissensfrage an Maimonides." *Med. Klin.* 67 (1972): 1091–93.

Morais, S. "A Letter by Maimonides to the Jews of South Arabia Entitled 'The Inspired Hope.'" *Jewish Quarterly Review* 25 (1934–35): 330–69.

Muntner, S. "Maimonides' Book for Al-Fadil." *Isis* 35 (1944): 3.

———. *The Medical Writings of Moses Maimonides: Treatise on Asthma.* Philadelphia: Lippincott, 1963.

———. *Treatise on Poisons and Their Antidotes.* Philadelphia: Lippincott, 1966.

———. *Moshe ben Maimon: Pirkei Moshe be-Refuah* [(Medical) Aphorisms of Moses in twenty-five treatises]. Jerusalem: Mosad Harav Kook, 1959.

———. *Moshe ben Maimon: Bi-Refuot ha-Teḥorim* [On hemorrhoids]. Jerusalem: Mosad Harav Kook, 1965.

———. *Moshe ben Maimon: Biyur Shemot ha-Refuot* [Lexicography of drugs and medical responses]. Jerusalem: Mosad Harav Kook, 1969.

———. *Moshe ben Maimon: Hanhagat ha-Beriut* [*Regimen Sanitatis*; Letters on the hygiene of the body and of the soul]. Jerusalem: Mosad Harav Kook, 1956.

———. *Moshe ben Maimon: Ma'amar al Ḥizzuk Ko'aḥ ha-Gavra* [On the increase of physical vigor]. Jerusalem: Mosad Harav Kook, 1965.

———. *Moshe ben Maimon: Perush le-Pirkei Abukrat* [Commentary on the Aphorisms of Hippocrates]. Jerusalem: Mosad Harav Kook, 1961.

———. *Moshe ben Maimon: Samei ha-Mavet ve-ha-Refuot ke-Negdam.* [Poisons and their antidotes; or, "The Treatise to the Honored One"]. Jerusalem: Rubin Mass, 1942.

———. *Moshe ben Maimon: Sefer ha-Katzeret* [Treatise on asthma]. Jerusalem: Rubin Mass, 1940.

———. *Moshe ben Maimon on Asthma (Sefer ha-Katzeret).* Jerusalem: Mosad Harav Kook, 1965.

————. "Pseudo-Maimonides on Sexual Life." In *Sexual Life: Collection of Medical Treatises (Ma'amar al-Razei ha-Ḥayyim ha-Miniyim)*. Jerusalem: Geniza, 1965.

————. *Rabbi Moses ben Maimon: Sefer ha-Katzeret or Sefer ha-Misadim* [Treatise on asthma]. Jerusalem: Geniza, 1963.

————. "Rabbi Moshe ben Maimon. *Uber die Lebensdauer*, Edited, translated, and with commentary by G. Weil." *Harefuah* 44, no. 4 (1953): 95.

————. "Reexamination of Galen's Books Listed by Maimonides in *Pirkei Moshe*." *Harofe Haivri* 2 (1954): 120–33 (Heb.), 160–61 (Eng.).

————. *Regimen Sanitatis oder Diätetik für die Seele und den Körper mit Anhang der Medizinischen Responsen und Ethik des Maimonides.* Basel: S. Karger, 1966.

————. *Samei ha-Mavet ve-ha-Refuot ke-Negdam* [Poisons and their antidotes]. Jerusalem: Rubin Mass, 1942.

———— and I. Simon. "Le Traité de l'Asthme de Maïmonide (1135–1304) traduit pour la première fois en Français d'après le texte hébreu." *Revue d'histoire de la médicine hébraïque* 16 (1963): 171–86; 17 (1964): 5–13, 83–97, 127–39, 187–96; 18 (1965): 5–15.

Nasse, C. F. "Von Einer Erblichen Neigung zu Todtlichen Blutungen." *Arch. Med. Erfahr.* 1 (1820): 385 ff.

Nebauer, A. *Catalogue of the Hebrew Manuscripts in the Bodleian Library and in the College Libraries of Oxford, including Mss in other languages, which are written with Hebrew characters, or relating to the Hebrew language or literature; and a few Samaritan Mss.* Oxford: Clarendon Press, 1886.

Nemoy, L. "Rabbenu Moshe ben Maimon: Sefer ha-Katzeret" [Maimonides' treatise on asthma]. *Harofe Haivri* 2 (1940): 133–34.

Nobel, G. *Zur Geschichte der Zahnheilkunde in Talmud.* Leipzig: Drugulin, 1909.

Otto, J. C. "An Account of an Hemorrhagic Disposition Existing in Certain Families." *Medical Respository* 6 (1803): 1 ff.

Perel, L. "Sur quelques ideés modernes dans le 'Traité des Poisons' de Maïmonide (1135–1204)." *Paris M.* 96, no. 4 (1935).

Pines, S., ed. and trans. *The Guide of the Perplexed of Moses Maimonides.* Chicago: University of Chicago Press, 1963.

Preuss, J. *Biblical and Talmudic Medicine.* Trans. F. Rosner. New York: Sanhedrin Press, 1978. (Reprinted by Jason Aaronson, Inc., 1993).

Rabbinowicz, I. M. *Maïmonide (Abou-Amram Moussa Ibn-Maimon, 1135–1204): Traité des Poisons.* 1865. 2nd ed. Paris: Librairie Lipschutz, 1935.

Richards, D. W. "The First Aphorism of Hippocrates." *Perspectives in Biol. Med.* 5 (1961): 61–64.

Rosenthal, F. "Life Is Short, the Art Is Long": Arabic Commentaries on the First Hippocratic Aphorism." *Bulletin of the History of Medicine* 40 (1966): 226–45.

Rosner, F. "Bloodletting in Talmudic Times." *Bulletin of the New York Academy of Medicine* 62 (1986): 935–46.

———. "Circumcision: Attempt at Clearer Understanding." *New York State Journal of Medicine* 66 (1966): 2919–22.

———. "Dentistry in the Bible and Talmud." *Bulletin of the History of Dentistry* 23 (1975): 25–30.

———. "Geriatrics in the Medical Aphorisms of Moses Maimonides." *Postgraduate Medicine* 55 (1974): 229–33.

———. "Hemophilia in the Talmud and Rabbinic Writings." *Annals of Internal Medicine* 70 (April 1969): 833–37.

———. "The Hygienic Principles of Moses Maimonides." *Journal of the American Medical Association* 194 (1965): 1352–54.

———. "The Introduction of Maimonides to his *Commentary on the Aphorisms of Hippocrates.*" *Clio Medica* 11 (1976): 59–64.

———. "The Jewish Attitude Toward Abortion." In *Modern Medicine and Jewish Law,* ed., pp. 53–78. New York: Yeshiva University Press, 1972.

———. "*Kordiakos* in the Talmud." In *Medicine in the Bible and Talmud,* pp. 61–65. New York: Ktav, 1977.

———. "Maimonides the Physician: A Bibliography." *Clio Medica* 15 (1980): 75–79.

————. "Maimonides, the Physician: A Bibliography." *Bulletin of the History of Medicine* 43 (1969): 221–35.

————. "Mar Samuel the Physician." In *Medicine in the Bible and Talmud*, pp. 156–70. New York: Ktav, 1977.

————. "The Medical Aphorisms of Moses Maimonides." In *Memorial Volume in Honor of S. Muntner*, ed. J. O. Leibowitz, pp. 6–30. Jerusalem: Israel Institute for the History of Medicine, 1983.

————. "Medical Writings of Moses Maimonides." *New York State Journal of Medicine* 73 (1973): 2185–90.

————. "The Medical Writings of Moses Maimonides." *New York State Journal of Medicine* 87 (1987): 656–61.

————. *Medicine in the Bible and Talmud.* New York: Ktav, 1977. 2nd edition, 1995.

————. *Medicine in the Mishneh Torah of Maimonides.* New York: Ktav, 1984.

————. *Modern Medicine and Jewish Ethics.* 2nd ed. New York: Ktav and Yeshiva University Press, 1991.

————. "Moses Maimonides (1135–1204)." *Annals of Internal Medicine* 62 (1965): 373–75.

————. "Moses Maimonides and Diseases of the Chest." *Chest* 60 (1971): 68–72.

————. *Moses Maimonides' Commentary on the Aphorisms of Hippocrates.* Haifa: Maimonides Research Institute, 1987.

————. *Moses Maimonides' Contribution to Medicine.* Chicago: College of Jewish Studies Press, 1969.

————. *Moses Maimonides' Glossary of Drug Names.* Philadelphia: American Philosophical Society, 1979.

————. "Moses Maimonides' Responsum on Longevity." *Geriatrics* 23 (October 1968): 170–78.

————. *Moses Maimonides' Three Treatises on Health.* Haifa: Maimonides Research Institute, 1990.

————. "Moses Maimonides' Treatise on Asthma." *Medical Times* 94 (1966): 1227–30.

————. "Moses Maimonides' Treatise on Asthma." *Thorax* 36 (1981): 245–51. *J. Asthma* 21 (1984): 118–129

————. *Moses Maimonides' Treatise on Asthma.* Haifa: Maimonides Research Institute, 1994.

————. "Moses Maimonides' Treatise on Poisons." *Journal of the American Medical Association* 205 (1968): 914–16.

————. "Moses Maimonides' Treatise on Poisons." *New York State Journal of Medicine* 80 (1980): 1627–30.

————. *Moses Maimonides' Treatises on Poisons, Hemorrhoids, and Cohabitation.* Haifa: Maimonides Research Institute, 1984.

————. "Ophthalmology in the Medical Aphorisms of Moses Maimonides." *New York State Journal of Medicine* 74 (1974): 699–703.

————. "The Physician's Prayer Attributed to Maimonides." *Bulletin of the History of Medicine* 41 (1967): 440–54.

————. *Sex Ethics in the Writings of Moses Maimonides.* New York: Bloch, 1974.

————. *Six Treatises Attributed to Maimonides.* Northvale, N.J.: Jason Aronson, 1991.

———— and S. Muntner. *The Medical Aphorisms of Moses Maimonides.* 2 vols. New York: Yeshiva University Press, 1970–71. Reprinted. New York: Bloch Publishing Co., 1973.

———— and S. Muntner. *The Medical Writings of Moses Maimonides: Treatise on Hemorrhoids and Maimonides' Answers to Queries.* Philadelphia: Lippincott, 1969.

———— and S. Muntner. "Moses Maimonides' Aphorisms Regarding Analysis of Urine." *Annals of Internal Medicine* 71 (1969): 217–20.

———— and S. Muntner. "The Surgical Aphorisms of Moses Maimonides." *American Journal of Surgery* 119 (1970): 718–25.

Roy, P. S. "Historical Development of Our Knowledge of the Circulation and Its Disorders." *Annals of Medical History* 1 (1917): 141–54.

Saketkhoo, K., A. Jansuzkiewicz, and M. A. Sackner. "Effects of Drinking Hot Water, Cold Water, and Chicken Soup on Nasal Mucus Velocity and Nasal Airflow Resistance." *Chest* 74 (1978): 408–10.

Savitz, H. "Maimonides' Hygiene of the Soul." *Annals of Medical History* 4 (1932): 80–86.

Schacht, J., and M. Meyerhof. "Maimonides Against Galen on Philosophy and Cosmology." *Bulletin of the Faculty of Arts* (Cairo), 5, pt. I (1939).

Schlueter, R. E. "The First Aphorism of Hippocrates as Explained by Paracelsus." *Annals of Science* 1 (1936): 453–61.

Shmukler, I. K. *Pismo Moiseh Maimonida k Egipetskomu Sultanu.* Gugienicheskie Sovetia Perevod s Drevneevreiskogo Doctora I. K. Shmuklera (Kiev). Otdelnii Ottisk Iz, "Vrach Dela" # 14–15 and 16. Kharkov: Nauchnaja Misl. Uchr. NKZ., 1930.

Skoss, S. K. "The Treatises of Maimonides on Health Care." In *Portraits of a Jewish Scholar: Essays and Addresses*, pp. 99–116. New York: Bloch, 1957.

Steinberg, W., and S. Muntner. "Maimonides' Views on Gynecology and Obstetrics." *American Journal of Obstetrics and Gynecology* 91 (1965): 443–48.

Steinschneider, M. *Die Arabische Literatur der Juden: Ein Beitrag zur Literaturgeschichte der Araber. Grossenteils aus Handschriftlichen Quellen.* Frankfurt: Kauffmann, 1902.

———. *Die Hebraeischen Uebersetzungen des Mittelalters und die Juden als Dolmetscher: Ein Beitrag zur Literaturgeschichte des Mittelalters Meist nach handschriftlichen Quellen.* Berlin, 1893.

———. "Die Vorrede des Maimonides zu Seinem Commentar über die Aphorismen des Hippokrates." *Zeitschrift für Deutschen Morgenländischen Gesellschaft* 48 (1894): 213–34.

——— "Gifte und ihre Heilung: Eine Abhandlung des Moses Maimonides, auf Befehl des Aegyptischen Wezirs (1198) Verfasst, nach Einer Unedierten Hebraischen Ubersetzung bearbeit." *Virchows Archiv für pathologische Anatomie* 57 (1873): 62–120.

———, ed. *Hamazkir, Hebraeische Bibliographie. Blätter für neuere und altere Literatur des Judenthums, nebst einer literarischen Beilage.* Berlin: Julius Benzian, 1879. vol. 19, p. 131.

Theodorides, J. "Les sciences naturelles et particulièrement la zoologie dans le Traité des Poisons de Maïmonide." *Revue d'histoire de la médecine hébraïque* 9 (1956): 87.

Weil, G. "Ein Unediertes Responsum des Maimonides." *Deutsche literaturzeitung für Kritik der Internationalen Wissenschaft* [o.s. 47] 3, no. 39 (1926): 1933–38.

———. *Maimonides. Uber die Lebensdauer.* Basel and New York: S. Karger, 1953.

Wallerstein, E. *Circumcision: An American Health Fallacy.* New York: Springer, 1980.

Winternitz, D. *Das Diatetische Sendschreiben des Maimonides an den Sultan Saladin.* Vienna: Braumueller & Seidel, 1843.

Zimmels, H. J. *Magicians, Theologians, and Doctors.* London: Goldston, 1952.

# Index